Emergency Nursing Examination

R·E·V·I·E·W

Second Edition

Emergency Nursing Examination

R·E·V·I·E·W

Second Edition

Laura Gasparis Vonfrolio, RN, MA, CCRN, CEN

Assistant Professor of Nursing
College of Staten Island
Staten Island, New York

Joanne Noone, RN, MSN, CCRN, CEN

Medical-Surgical Nursing Instructor
Kauai Community College
Lihue, Hawaii

Springhouse Corporation
Springhouse, Pennsylvania

Staff

Executive Director, Editorial
Stanley Loeb

Director of Trade and Textbooks
Minnie B. Rose, RN, BSN, MEd

Art Director
John Hubbard

Senior Acquisitions Editor
Susan L. Mease

Clinical Editor
Maryann Foley, RN, BSN

Editor
Diane Labus

Copy Editor
Mary Hohenhaus Hardy

Designers
Stephanie Peters (associate art director), Hillary Shnycer

Art Production
Robert Perry (manager), Anna Brindisi, Donald Knauss, Tom Robbins, Robert Wieder

Typography
David Kosten (director), Diane Paluba (manager), Elizabeth Bergman, Joyce Rossi Biletz, Phyllis Marron, Robin Rantz, Valerie Rosenberger

Manufacturing
Deborah Meiris (manager), T.A. Landis, Jennifer Suter

Production Coordination
Colleen M. Hayman, Laurie J. Sander

Library of Congress Cataloging-in-Publication Data
Vonfrolio, Laura Gasparis, 1952-
    Emergency nursing examination review/ Laura Gasparis Vonfrolio, Joanne Noone. — 2nd ed.
        p. cm.
    Includes bibliographical references and index.
        1. Emergency nursing — Examinations, questions, etc. I. Noone, Joanne, 1956- II. Title.
        [DNLM: 1. Critical Care — examination questions.   2. Emergencies — examination questions.   3. Emergency Service, Hospital — examination questions.   4. Nursing — examination questions. WY 18 V944e]
    RT120.E4V66 1991
    610.73'61 — dc20
    DNLM/DLC
    ISBN 0-87434-359-3   90-10402

Contents

Contributors

Alice Belcher, RN, BSN, CCRN
Former Critical Care Educator;
Director of Nursing, Critical Care
Dover General Hospital
Dover, N.J.

Mary Blum, RN, MSN
Former Instructor of Nursing
Rutgers—The State University
Newark, N.J.

Carol A. Bottin, RN
Lecturer-Consultant and
Procurement Coordinator
Organ Retrieval Program
Department of Surgery
University of Florida
Jacksonville

Patrice Case, RN, MA
Adjunct Faculty
College of Staten Island
Staten Island, N.Y.

Elizabeth Connelly, RN, MS, CCRN
Staff Development Instructor
Staten Island University Hospital
Staten Island, N.Y.

Kathy Daly, RN, CCRN, CEN
Former Staff Nurse II, Emergency Department
Beth Israel Medical Center
New York

Marcia Downs, RN, CEN
Educational Coordinator, Life Flight
Baptist Medical Center
Jacksonville, Fla.

Vincent J. Ferragano, MD
Attending Physician, Obstetrics & Gynecology
Staten Island University Hospital;
Assistant Clinical Professor
State University of New York Health Sciences Center
New York

Deborah S. Gough, RN, MSN, CCRN, CEN
Clinical Education Coordinator
Bayley Seton Hospital
Staten Island, N.Y.

Stephanie Higie, RN, BSN, CEN
Trauma Nurse Coordinator
University Medical Center
Tucson, Ariz.

Catherine T. Kelly, RN, MSN, EMT-P, CCRN, CEN
Clinical Nurse Specialist-Chief Flight Nurse
Emergency Department
St. Francis Hospital
Poughkeepsie, N.Y.

Linda Anne Laner, RN, MSN, CS, CCRN, CEN
Staff Nurse, Emergency Department
Staten Island University Hospital
Staten Island, N.Y.

Joanne Lapidus-Graham, RN, MA
Instructor, Maternal-Child Nursing
Rockville Center, N.Y.

Lisa Mayercik, RN, BSN
Former Assistant Head Nurse, Maternity
Staten Island University Hospital
Staten Island, N.Y.

Marilyn McDonald, RN, MA
Assistant Professor of Nursing
College of Staten Island
Staten Island, N.Y.

Kathleen McMahon, RN, MSN, CEN
Assistant Director of Nurses
Treat and Release Center
Brooklyn, N.Y.

Patricia Murphy, MD
Attending Physician, EENT
Long Island College Hospital
New York

Theresa Nauta, RN, MSN
Obstetrical Inservice Clinician
Maimonides Medical Center
Brooklyn, N.Y.

Janet A. Neff, RN, MN, CCRN, CEN
Editorial Board, Journal of Emergency Nursing;
Instructor of Nursing
University of Arizona
Tucson

Neil Nepola, MD
Family Physician and
Attending Physician, Emergency Department
Bayley Seton Hospital
Staten Island, N.Y.

Joanne Noone, RN, MSN, CCRN, CEN
Medical-Surgical Nursing Instructor
Kauai Community College
Lihue, Hawaii

June L. Olsen, RN, MS
Former Deputy Chairperson and
Associate Professor of Nursing
College of Staten Island
Staten Island, N.Y.

Catherine Paradiso, RN, MSN, CCRN, CEN
Former Clinical Nurse Specialist for Critical Care
Veterans Administration Hospital;
Instructor of Nursing
Kingsborough Community College
Brooklyn, N.Y.

Linda Reese, RN, MA
Assistant Professor of Nursing
College of Staten Island
Staten Island, N.Y.

Deborah Reilly, RN, MSN, CEN
Former Nurse Care Coordinator, Emergency Department
Staten Island University Hospital
Staten Island, N.Y.

John P. Reilly, MD
Fellow, Orthopedic Traumatology
Maryland Institute for Emergency Medical Services
Baltimore

Patricia Robertazza, RN, MSN, CCRN
Critical Care Educator
Kimball Medical Center
Lakewood, N.J.

Susan Schulmerich, RN, MS, MA, CNA, CEN
Administrator, Emergency Department
North Central Bronx Hospital
New York

Joanne Scotto, RN, BSN
Clinical Nurse, Ambulatory Care
Staten Island University Hospital;
President, Health Awareness, Inc.
Staten Island, N.Y.

Eva Scripps, RN, BVSN, CCRN, CEN
Nurse Care Coordinator,
Emergency Department
Staten Island University Hospital
Staten Island, N.Y.

Nancy C. Seddio, RN, CS, PhD
Clinical Nurse Specialist in Psychiatry
Interfaith Medical Center
Brooklyn, N.Y.;
Psychotherapist, Private Practice
New York

Maureen Sheehy, RN, CCRN, CEN
Staff Nurse, Emergency Department
Bayley Seton Hospital
Staten Island, N.Y.

Patricia Tooker, RN, MSN, CCRN
Supervisor, Critical Care
Bayley Seton Hospital
Staten Island, N.Y.

Debra Toth, RN, BSN
Transplant Coordinator
New York University Hospital
New York

David Unkle, RN, CCRN, CEN
Clinical Research Coordinator,
Division of Trauma and Emergency Services
Cooper Hospital-University Medical Center
Camden, N.J.

Charles T. Vonfrolio, MD
Former Chief of Anesthesia,
Anesthesia Department
Staten Island University Hospital
Staten Island, N.Y.

Laura Gasparis Vonfrolio, RN, MA, CCRN, CEN
Assistant Professor of Nursing
College of Staten Island
Staten Island, N.Y.

David Weaver, Esq.
Trapasso, Dolan & Hollander
Newton, N.J.

Acknowledgments

We would like to express our heartfelt gratitude to many people. First, we owe our deepest thanks to our contributing authors for their inspiring commitment to the creation of this book.

Secondly, we want to thank Fay Gasparis, who demonstrated a nearly psychic ability to decipher reams of handwritten material accompanied by complicated format directions. From these piles of scribbled sheets, she consistently produced beautiful manuscript pages in time for every deadline, all the while enthusiastically responding to the material she was typing.

L.G.V. and J.N.

To my mom, Fay Gasparis, whose continuous encouragement and endless assistance brighten my life.

L.G.V.

To my son, Jesse Noone.

J.N.

Introduction

We applaud the professionalism of members of the emergency health care team who have decided to update and validate their knowledge and skills through certification by the Emergency Nurses Association. To them we dedicate this second edition of *Emergency Nursing Examination Review* as a support tool for passing the certification examination.

Nurses preparing to take the Certification Examination for Emergency Nurses (the CEN examination) will find this an especially useful study guide. This book focuses on various aspects of nursing practice and professional issues (the two main areas of concentration in the CEN examination) and offers an integrated approach to the entire nursing process. Each nursing practice chapter contains specific questions on assessment, nursing diagnoses, interventions, and evaluation—key areas representative of the CEN exam and real-life clinical settings. Nurses who are already certified but wish to build on their current knowledge will find this book beneficial, since each chapter also contains advanced clinical information.

Emergency Nursing Examination Review, Second Edition, reviews topics relevant to emergency nursing as defined in the *Emergency Nursing Core Curriculum* and includes questions on abdominal, environmental, facial, cardiovascular, orthopedic, EENT, neurologic, respiratory, obstetric, and psychiatric emergencies, as well as shock, surface trauma, substance abuse, and organ donation. Questions are arranged in a multiple-choice format, as on the CEN exam. An answer sheet follows the questions section of each chapter, so you can complete each group of questions before reviewing the answers. Answers include the rationale for the correct choice and, where appropriate, explain why the other choices are incorrect.

About the CEN Examination
The Certification Examination for Emergency Nurses, first offered in July 1980, was developed to help measure the knowledge of nurses working in emergency care settings. Each nurse who passes the examination is recognized as a Certified Emergency Nurse (CEN); recertification is required every 4 years.

The examination consists of a maximum of 250 multiple-choice, objective questions to be completed within 4 hours. Content is roughly divided into the following areas:

I. Nursing Practice
Assessment 30.5%
Analysis and Nursing Diagnosis 15.0%
Planning and Intervention 30.0%
Evaluation 14.5%
II. Professional Issues 10.0%
————
100.0%

Although the examination begins at 9:00 a.m., you should arrive at the test center by 8:00 a.m. Test takers are seated alphabetically in various rooms, with two proctors usually in each room. Be sure to bring a form of identification to the examination, such as any photo I.D. (a valid driver's license or passport) and your examination admission ticket. You'll also need at least two #2 pencils. Since a few rhythm strips typically appear on the examination, you may want to bring calipers if you need them to decipher rhythms. A nonprinting, battery-operated calculator also is allowed.

Immediately before the test, you'll have time to review the instructions for filling out the answer sheet. Note that your test results may be delayed if you don't follow these instructions precisely. The test comes in a sealed booklet. Do not break the seal before you are told to do so. After the test begins, the proctors periodically will write the time remaining on a chalkboard.

Test-Taking Tips
● Take a vacation from studying a few days before the test. Too much studying may tire you so much that you may not do well on the test. If possible, take the day before the test off and relax.
● Get a good night's sleep the night before the test. Being rested will give you an advantage that you won't have if you're exhausted.
● When you see the test for the first time, scan the first page for a question you can easily answer. This will give you the confidence you need to approach the test without panic.
● Check the answer sheet frequently during the test to make sure you aren't making small but serious errors, such as answering Question 2 in Question 3's box. Such an error will affect your overall test score.

• Stick to the first answer you choose. It is probably correct. The more you fret over which answer to select, the more indecisive you may become. If you don't know an answer, come back to that question later. Try to narrow your choices to the point where your guess has fair odds of being correct. For example, if you can narrow your choices to two answers and then guess, you have a 50% chance of being correct.

• Try to relax. Remember, overwhelming anxiety will hamper you. Don't let this test intimidate you, even though passing it is important for you. Also, remember you've prepared well for this test if you have studied this book. And if you have taken the test before, you've already had a valuable test-taking experience.

Good luck! We hope our efforts increase your knowledge and help you to pass the examination.

Laura Gasparis Vonfrolio
Joanne Noone

CHAPTER 1

Abdominal Emergencies

1 A patient arrives in the emergency department (ED) with an ice pick protruding from his left lower abdominal quadrant. An appropriate nursing action would be to:

A. Immediately remove the object and apply firm pressure to the wound
B. Leave the object in place until the patient is taken to the operating room
C. Establish two large-bore I.V. lines, then remove the object
D. Obtain an abdominal X-ray, then remove the object

2 Which type of penetrating injury would the nurse document in the assessment findings for a patient with a gunshot wound at the sixth intercostal space?

A. Chest
B. Abdominal
C. Thoracoabdominal
D. Pelvic

3 A patient with a gunshot wound to the left lower abdominal quadrant arrives at the ED with the following vital signs: blood pressure (BP), 110/70 mm Hg; pulse rate, 96 beats/minute; and respirations, 24 breaths/minute. What would be the highest priority at this time?

A. Emergency exploratory laparotomy
B. Abdominal computed tomography (CT) scan
C. Diagnostic peritoneal lavage
D. Close observation in the ED over the next several hours

4 A patient arrives at the ED with a penetrating gunshot wound to the abdomen and hematuria. Which diagnostic test would the nurse expect the physician to order before surgery?

A. Diagnostic peritoneal lavage
B. Abdominal X-ray
C. Intravenous pyelography (IVP)
D. Abdominal CT scan

5 When assessing a patient for potential complications from a gunshot wound to the right upper abdominal quadrant, the nurse should observe the patient closely for injury to the:

A. Liver
B. Transverse colon
C. Stomach
D. All of the above

6 Which nursing action would the nurse expect to perform preoperatively for a patient with a penetrating abdominal wound?

A. Establishment of two large-bore I.V. lines
B. Insertion of a nasogastric (NG) tube
C. Insertion of an indwelling urinary catheter
D. All of the above

7 The nurse would expect to note early signs of shock in a young male patient who has sustained a penetrating abdominal wound after the patient has suffered a blood volume loss of:

A. 15%
B. 25%
C. 30%
D. 50%

8 All of the following injuries are considered penetrating *except:*

A. A stab wound to the right upper abdominal quadrant
B. A severe abdominal laceration caused by a fall
C. A gunshot wound to the left lower abdominal quadrant
D. A BB pellet to the lower abdomen

9 All of the following assessment findings would lead the nurse to suspect a perforated gastric ulcer *except:*

A. Absent bowel sounds
B. Hypotension and tachycardia
C. Anxiety and respiratory difficulty
D. Severe upper abdominal pain radiating to the jaw

10 Which of the following can cause chemical peritonitis in a patient with a perforated gastric ulcer?

A. Overuse of antacids
B. Salicylate ingestion
C. Gastric and intestinal content spillage
D. Sodium and calcium imbalance

11 Perforated ulcers occur most commonly in the:

A. Stomach
B. Jejunum
C. Duodenum
D. Ileum

12 The nurse knows that such abdominal emergencies as obstruction, perforation, and acute intractable hemorrhage are typically treated by:

A. Surgery
B. Fluid and blood replacement
C. Antacids, anticholinergics, and sedatives
D. Stress reduction and dietary changes

13 The most common causes of upper GI bleeding include:

A. Neoplasms, gastritis, and duodenal ulcers
B. Peptic ulcers, acute mucosal lesions, and esophageal varices
C. Esophagitis, gastric ulcers, and hematologic disorders
D. Mallory-Weiss tears, peptic ulcers, and vascular anomalies

14 Esophageal varices are:

A. Always caused by abnormal circulation within the splenic artery
B. Nearly always caused by portal hypertension
C. The result of frequent intake of alcohol, tobacco, or spicy foods
D. Almost always the result of an existing esophageal carcinoma

15 Nursing care of the patient with a three-lumen, double-balloon esophageal tube includes all of the following *except:*

A. Maintaining constant observation during balloon inflation
B. Ensuring that the balloon pressures are kept at the levels required to control bleeding
C. Remaining alert for any complaints of chest pain
D. Placing the patient in a supine position to prevent shock

SITUATION

A 38-year-old man is admitted to the ED with complaints of severe epigastric pain. His vital signs upon admission are within normal limits. His diagnosis is acute pancreatitis.

Questions 16 to 24 relate to the above situation.

16 Of the following history findings, the most likely cause of pancreatitis is:

A. Excessive alcohol intake
B. Excessive fat intake
C. Heredity
D. Stress

17 The nurse knows that pancreatitis also may occur as a complication of a perforated duodenal ulcer when:

A. Serum amylase is elevated to dangerous levels
B. The perforation erodes into the pancreas
C. The patient's alcohol intake is high
D. The pancreatic duct is obstructed

18 Which nursing diagnosis is most appropriate for a patient at risk for complications from pancreatitis?

A. Potential for injury related to seizures
B. Potential for injury related to hyperkalemia
C. Altered thought processes related to hypoglycemia
D. Impaired gas exchange related to pulmonary edema

19 The nurse normally assesses a patient with acute pancreatitis for elevated levels of serum:

A. Cholesterol
B. Amylase
C. Potassium
D. Calcium

20 The nurse knows that meperidine hydrochloride (Demerol) is typically used to treat acute pancreatitis because it:

A. Does not cause respiratory depression
B. Suppresses hydrochloric acid secretion
C. Does not cause spasm of the sphincter of Oddi
D. Does not decrease GI motility

21 The nurse should assess the patient for all of the following symptoms of hemorrhagic pancreatitis *except:*

A. Jaundice
B. Extreme epigastric or umbilical pain extending to the back or flank
C. Shock
D. Hypertension

22 Nursing interventions for a patient with acute hemorrhagic pancreatitis include all of the following *except:*

A. Administration of large volumes of colloid and electrolyte solutions
B. Administration of calcium gluconate
C. Monitoring of central venous pressure and urine output
D. Administering a clear liquid diet

6

Abdominal Emergencies
Questions

23 Over the course of several months of caring for various patients with pancreatitis, the nurse would expect the physician to order broad-spectrum antibiotics:

A. Frequently
B. Only when surgery is required
C. Rarely
D. Never

24 The patient is being admitted to the medical-surgical unit for further treatment and observation. Which dietary regimen would the nurse expect the physician to order for this patient?

A. Low-fat, no-alcohol, no-caffeine
B. Low-fat, low-cholesterol
C. Low-salt, low-sugar, no-alcohol
D. No-alcohol, no-caffeine, no-sugar

SITUATION

A 21-year-old man arrives at the ED with abdominal pain of sudden onset. The physician diagnoses the patient as having acute appendicitis.

Questions 25 to 27 relate to the above situation.

25 Which assessment finding is characteristic of acute appendicitis?

A. Rovsing's sign
B. Leukopenia
C. Abdominal distention
D. Audible borborygmi

26 Which practice is considered unsafe when caring for a patient with sudden abdominal pain?

A. Infusing the patient with lactated Ringer's solution
B. Inserting an NG tube attached to a suction device
C. Promptly administering analgesics to decrease discomfort
D. Monitoring the patient's rectal temperature

27 When compared with older children and adults, young children have a higher incidence of perforation of the appendix with ensuing peritonitis because they typically have:

A. Difficulty describing symptoms
B. A greater pain tolerance
C. A weaker appendiceal wall
D. Less resistance to infection

SITUATION

A 26-year-old man arrives at the ED in an ambulance after an automobile accident. The physician notes that the patient has no obvious fractures or injuries and diagnoses him as having a possible blunt abdominal trauma.

Questions 28 to 32 relate to the above situation.

28 Which internal organ is typically injured in a patient with a blunt abdominal trauma?

A. Pancreas
B. Spleen
C. Small intestine
D. Gallbladder

29 Which type of solution would the nurse expect to infuse to restore circulatory dynamics in a patient with this type of injury?

A. Hypertonic
B. Hypotonic
C. Isotonic
D. Hypo-osmolar

30 The physician may order paracentesis or peritoneal lavage to detect any intra-abdominal injuries. The nurse knows that peritoneal lavage is contraindicated in a patient who:

A. Has a colostomy
B. Is unconscious
C. Has multiple abdominal surgical scars
D. All of the above

31 Which statement regarding the spleen is *false?*

A. The normal spleen is palpable below the lower left costal margin
B. The spleen is injured more frequently than any other abdominal organ
C. The high incidence of splenic complications is directly related to the organ's high vascularity
D. Approximately 50% of patients with splenic bleeding exhibit a positive Kehr's sign

32 The nurse would suspect splenic injury in the patient with an injury to the:

A. Bladder
B. Sternum
C. 11th or 12th rib on the right side
D. 8th, 9th, or 10th rib on the left side

SITUATION

A 74-year-old man is brought to the hospital by his nephew after complaining of severe abdominal cramping and swelling. He claims to have had a stomach virus for the past few days. His symptoms include nausea, anorexia, mild discomfort, and constipation. Within the last 12 hours, his pain has increased in intensity, and he has vomited small amounts of greenish liquid several times. The physician diagnoses his condition as a possible bowel obstruction.

Questions 33 to 37 relate to the above situation.

33 The nurse understands that bowel obstruction occurs most commonly in extremely young and old patients and that its hallmark signs and symptoms include:

A. Pain, distention, vomiting, and prolonged constipation
B. Absence of pain, nausea and vomiting, and prolonged constipation
C. Loss of bowel sounds, distention, constipation, and nausea
D. Hyperactive bowel sounds, diarrhea, vomiting, and cramping

34 An appropriate nursing diagnosis for this patient would be:

A. Fluid volume deficit related to fluid shifting and vomiting
B. Decreased cardiac output related to impaired myocardial contractility
C. Fluid volume excess related to decreased renal perfusion
D. Fluid volume excess related to increased water absorption from stool

35 Which condition is the primary cause of large-bowel obstruction in an adult?

A. Adhesions
B. Volvulus
C. Carcinoma
D. Diverticulitis

36 While the nurse is completing the initial physical assessment and history, the patient becomes increasingly restless and confused. The nurse obtains a second set of vital signs and notifies the physician. The vital signs—BP, 90/58 mm Hg; pulse rate, 134 beats/minute and weak; temperature, 96.6° F (35.9° C) with a cool skin surface; and respirations, 16 breaths/minute and shallow—indicate development of:

A. Cerebrovascular accident
B. Congestive heart failure
C. Shock
D. Anxiety

37 Which is the correct sequence for assessing and evaluating a patient's abdomen?

A. Auscultation, percussion, inspection, and palpation
B. Auscultation, inspection, percussion, and palpation
C. Inspection, auscultation, percussion, and palpation
D. Inspection, auscultation, palpation, and percussion

SITUATION

A 38-year-old stockbroker is brought to the ED by a coworker after experiencing an episode of severe weakness after a business luncheon. Although the patient claims to have no medical or surgical history, he admits to taking large amounts of liquid antacids to calm his stomach. He has had several episodes of bloody vomitus within the past 3 to 4 days. The physician diagnoses the patient as having upper GI bleeding.

Questions 38 to 40 relate to the above situation.

38 Which nursing intervention would be most helpful in determining the cause of the patient's bleeding?

A. Inserting an NG tube to measure the pH of gastric fluids
B. Collecting blood specimens for a complete blood count, type and screen, and coagulation profiles
C. Prompt scheduling of an endoscopy
D. Determining the patient's shock status, then obtaining a thorough history and performing a physical examination

39 In assessing the patient's health status, the nurse should know that hematemesis is most commonly caused by:

A. Malignant tumors
B. Peptic ulcers
C. Blood dyscrasias
D. Esophageal varices

40 Anticholinergic drugs, commonly used to treat peptic ulcer disease, typically produce which pharmacologic action?

A. Decreased patient responsiveness
B. Increased gastric emptying
C. Inhibited histamine formation
D. Blockage of the effects of vagal nerve impulses on smooth muscles

SITUATION

A 72-year-old man is brought to the ED by his daughter after an episode of rectal bleeding. He has been previously treated for hemorrhoidal discomfort and bleeding.

Questions 41 to 46 relate to the above situation.

41 Which diagnostic test would the nurse expect the physician to order first if clinical findings suggest that the lower bowel is the source of the patient's bleeding?

A. Angiography
B. Abdominal CT scan
C. Esophagogastroduodenoscopy
D. Proctoscopy

42 After initial treatment in the ED, the patient will probably be:

A. Prepared for emergency surgery
B. Admitted to the intensive care unit
C. Admitted to a medical unit
D. Sent home and referred to an outpatient clinic

43 In a patient with prolonged bleeding, anemia is a potential complication. The nurse assesses for anemia by noting signs of pallor in the patient's:

A. Lips
B. Gums
C. Sclera
D. Nail beds

44 Which condition is the most common cause of lower GI bleeding?

A. Diverticulitis
B. Hemorrhoids
C. Ischemic bowel disease
D. Neoplasm

45 When a patient is undergoing emergency endoscopy, the nurse should assess for all of the following potential complications *except:*

A. Cardiac arrhythmias
B. Perforation
C. Aspiration
D. Paralytic ileus

46 Lower GI bleeding is characterized by bleeding from:

A. The colon
B. Any source below the ligament of Treitz
C. Any source below the appendix
D. Diverticuli

SITUATION

A 28-year-old man is admitted to the ED after a high-speed, head-on automobile accident. He is conscious and alert; his skin is cool and dry. Vital signs are BP, 110/70 mm Hg; pulse rate, 100 beats/minute; and respirations, 24 breaths/minute. The emergency medical technicians report severe front-end damage to the car and a broken steering wheel.

Questions 47 to 53 relate to the above situation.

47 After assessing the patient's airway, breathing, and circulation, the nurse's primary concern would be to:

A. Ask the patient when he ate his last meal
B. Establish two large-bore I.V. lines
C. Insert an indwelling urinary catheter
D. Insert an NG tube

48 Which assessment finding is the earliest indication of impending shock?

A. Tachycardia
B. Hypotension
C. Narrowing pulse pressure
D. Cool and clammy skin

49 The patient's BP suddenly drops to 88/60 mm Hg and his pulse increases to 130 beats/minute. After administration of 500 ml of lactated Ringer's solution, the patient's BP increases to 100/70 mm Hg and his pulse rate decreases to 100 beats/minute. The nurse's priority at this time would be to:

A. Prepare the patient for an IVP
B. Prepare the patient for a diagnostic peritoneal lavage
C. Prepare the patient for surgery
D. Immediately transfuse the patient with O-positive or O-negative blood, depending on availability

50 Results of a diagnostic peritoneal lavage may be falsely negative in a patient with a:

A. Splenic hemorrhage
B. Diaphragmatic rupture
C. Bladder tear
D. Retroperitoneal hematoma

51 Which sign is not an indication for IVP?

A. Blood at the urinary meatus
B. A high-riding prostate on rectal examination
C. Hematuria
D. Lower abdominal crepitus

52 During the assessment, the nurse notes a large mass in the left upper abdominal qudrant, displacement of the stomach, and associated rib fractures in the left lower thorax. These signs are consistent with injury to the:

A. Liver
B. Small intestine
C. Spleen
D. Colon

53 Based on the above assessment findings, the nurse identifies the patient's primary nursing diagnosis as:

A. Potential for infection related to abdominal contamination
B. Impaired gas exchange related to respiratory trauma
C. Fluid volume deficit related to blood loss
D. Decreased cardiac output related to cardiac trauma

SITUATION

A 60-year-old man is transferred to the ED by ambulance from his physician's office with a diagnosis of a possible abdominal aortic aneurysm.

Questions 54 to 57 refer to the above situation.

54 When eliciting the patient's history, the nurse keeps in mind that one of the most common factors predisposing a patient to abdominal aortic aneurysm is:

A. Diabetes
B. Congestive heart failure
C. Renal disease
D. Abdominal carcinoma

55 Which assessment finding would be typical for a patient with an abdominal aortic aneurysm?

A. Hoarseness
B. Abdominal distention
C. Difficulty swallowing
D. Midscapular back pain

56 The patient's abdominal X-ray reveals a fusiform infrarenal nondissecting aortic aneurysm. Which nursing diagnosis would be the highest priority for this patient?

A. Altered renal tissue perfusion related to decreased blood flow to the kidneys
B. Impaired gas exchange related to blood loss
C. Decreased cardiac output related to decreased preload
D. Altered peripheral tissue perfusion related to decreased arterial blood flow

57 While in the ED, which is the best parameter for evaluating expected patient outcomes for the above nursing diagnosis?

A. Urine output studies
B. Respiratory rate measurements
C. Arterial blood gas studies
D. Femoral pulse assessments

Answer Sheet

	A	B	C	D			A	B	C	D
1	○	○	○	○		31	○	○	○	○
2	○	○	○	○		32	○	○	○	○
3	○	○	○	○		33	○	○	○	○
4	○	○	○	○		34	○	○	○	○
5	○	○	○	○		35	○	○	○	○
6	○	○	○	○		36	○	○	○	○
7	○	○	○	○		37	○	○	○	○
8	○	○	○	○		38	○	○	○	○
9	○	○	○	○		39	○	○	○	○
10	○	○	○	○		40	○	○	○	○
11	○	○	○	○		41	○	○	○	○
12	○	○	○	○		42	○	○	○	○
13	○	○	○	○		43	○	○	○	○
14	○	○	○	○		44	○	○	○	○
15	○	○	○	○		45	○	○	○	○
16	○	○	○	○		46	○	○	○	○
17	○	○	○	○		47	○	○	○	○
18	○	○	○	○		48	○	○	○	○
19	○	○	○	○		49	○	○	○	○
20	○	○	○	○		50	○	○	○	○
21	○	○	○	○		51	○	○	○	○
22	○	○	○	○		52	○	○	○	○
23	○	○	○	○		53	○	○	○	○
24	○	○	○	○		54	○	○	○	○
25	○	○	○	○		55	○	○	○	○
26	○	○	○	○		56	○	○	○	○
27	○	○	○	○		57	○	○	○	○
28	○	○	○	○						
29	○	○	○	○						
30	○	○	○	○						

1 Correct answer – **B**

The appropriate nursing action in this situation would be to leave the object in place until the patient is taken to the operating room, where hemorrhage can be surgically controlled once the object is removed. Removing the object may cause further exsanguination and the development of shock.

2 Correct answer – **C**

The diaphragm, which separates the chest (thoracic cavity) from the abdomen, rises to the level of the sixth intercostal space on respiratory exhalation. Therefore, a gunshot wound at the sixth intercostal space is considered a thoracoabdominal injury because a bullet may enter both the abdomen and the chest.

3 Correct answer – **A**

Emergency exploratory laparotomy is the highest priority for a patient with a gunshot wound to the left lower abdominal quadrant. This procedure is necessary to determine which structures have been penetrated by the bullet so that hemorrhage can be controlled. Abdominal computed tomography (CT) scan and peritoneal lavage cannot help to identify the extent of injury to vessels. Also, these procedures take considerable time, thereby predisposing the patient to hemorrhage, as would observing the patient in the ED over the next several hours.

4 Correct answer – **C**

The nurse should expect the physician to order intravenous pyelography (IVP) to ensure that at least one kidney is functioning in case the patient must undergo nephrectomy. The existence of hematuria signifies that renal trauma may have resulted from the gunshot wound. Diagnostic peritoneal lavage, abdominal X-ray, and abdominal CT scan do not provide information on renal function.

5 Correct answer – **D**

Predicting the direction a bullet takes once it enters the abdomen is impossible; therefore, the nurse must closely observe the liver, transverse colon, and stomach for signs of penetration.

6 Correct answer – **D**

The nurse would expect to perform all of the nursing actions preoperatively. Establishing two large-bore I.V. lines provides access for administration of fluids and blood products. Inserting a nasogastric

(NG) tube empties the stomach, thereby preventing aspiration and relieving distention. Inserting an indwelling urinary catheter empties the bladder and provides a means by which to measure hourly urine output; output of less than 30 ml/hour indicates shock.

7 Correct answer—A

The nurse would expect to note the early signs of hypovolemic shock, especially tachycardia and orthostatic hypotension, after a patient sustains a blood loss of 15%. Significant hypotension (below 90/60 mm Hg or a 30-mm Hg drop from the patient's baseline) typically occurs after a blood loss of 25%. Irreversible shock, which does not respond to treatment and leads to cardiac arrest, is common after a blood loss of 40% to 50%.

8 Correct answer—B

All injuries that penetrate the surface of the skin, except abrasions or lacerations, and that are not caused by blunt trauma are classified as penetrating.

9 Correct answer—D

A patient with a perforated gastric ulcer does not typically complain of severe upper abdominal pain radiating to the jaw; however, he may complain of severe upper abdominal pain radiating to the neck, which is caused by irritation of the diaphragm and phrenic nerves. Other signs of perforated gastric ulcer include absent bowel sounds, hypotension, tachycardia, anxiety, and respiratory difficulty.

10 Correct answer—C

Chemical peritonitis, the inflammation of a portion or all of the parietal and visceral surfaces of the abdominal cavity, results from the rapid escape or spillage of gastric and intestinal contents after perforation. The peritoneum's primary response to injury includes edema in the subperitoneal tissues, bowel hypermotility, and an outpouring of plasmalike fluid from the extracellular, vascular, and interstitial compartments into the peritoneal space. Neither overuse of antacids nor sodium and calcium imbalance is associated with perforated ulcer. Salicylate ingestion may initiate ulcer formation but does not cause the resulting chemical peritonitis that occurs after perforation.

11 Correct answer—C

The most common site of perforated ulcers is the duodenum, constituting approximately 80% of all ulcers; the remaining 20% are considered gastric and occur in the stomach. Duodenal ulcers typically manifest in those between ages 30 and 50; gastric ulcers are more common in those over age 50. The jejunum and the ileum are not sites of ulcer formation.

12 Correct answer—A

Surgery usually is indicated in life-threatening abdominal emergencies involving perforation, acute obstruction, and acute intractable hemorrhage. Other forms of treatment—including fluid and blood replacement; antacids, anticholinergics, and sedatives; and stress reduction and dietary changes—may be indicated for less serious abdominal illnesses.

13 Correct answer—B

The most common causes of upper GI bleeding are peptic ulcers, acute mucosal lesions (resulting from gastritis, esophagitis, or Mallory-Weiss tears), and esophageal or gastric varices. Neoplasms, hematologic disorders, and vascular anomalies rarely cause upper GI bleeding.

14 Correct answer—B

Esophageal varices—dilated, tortuous veins found in the submucosa of the lower esophagus that may extend throughout the esophagus and into the stomach—are nearly always caused by portal hypertension, resulting from obstruction of the portal venous circulation or cirrhosis of the liver (from excessive alcohol intake). Abnormal circulation within the splenic artery or superior vena cava may also cause esophageal varices; however, such abnormalities are not the most common cause. Frequent intake of alcohol, tobacco, or spicy foods may lead to esophageal carcinoma; however, this is not directly related to the development of esophageal varices.

15 Correct answer—D

Placing the patient in a supine position is not a part of the normal nursing care of a patient with a three lumen, double-balloon esophageal tube. The tube helps to control esophageal bleeding through the inflation of gastric and esophageal balloons. During inflation, the nurse must maintain the head of the bed in a slightly elevated position, unless the patient is in shock, in which case a supine position may be necessary. Such elevation helps prevent gastric regurgitation and diminishes nausea and gagging. The nurse must observe the patient closely for signs of airway obstruction from migration of the esophageal balloon into the trachea. The nurse should also ensure that balloon pressures are kept at levels required to control bleeding and should remain alert for any signs of chest pain, which may indicate that the balloon pressures are excessive and causing tissue ischemia.

16 Correct answer — A

The most common cause of pancreatitis is excessive alcohol intake, which typically causes toxic effects on the pancreas or backup of pancreatic juices into the pancreas. Biliary tract disease, another common cause of pancreatitis, typically causes pancreatic duct obstruction, a backup of pancreatic juices, and cholecystitis (which is caused by reflux of bile components into the pancreatic duct). Although decreasing fat intake and reducing stress can help to reduce symptoms of pancreatitis, fat intake and stress are not necessarily precipitating causes. Heredity is also not a causal factor.

17 Correct answer — B

Pancreatitis may result as a complication of a perforated duodenal ulcer when the perforation erodes through the pancreatic wall and into the pancreas. An elevated serum amylase level is a sign, not a cause, of pancreatitis. Alcohol levels and pancreatic duct obstruction are not associated with ulcer perforation.

18 Correct answer — D

The most appropriate nursing diagnosis for a patient at risk for complications from pancreatitis is *Impaired gas exchange related to pulmonary edema,* as adult respiratory distress syndrome (ARDS) is an associated pulmonary complication of pancreatitis. ARDS may result from the pancreatitis itself or from ensuing sepsis or hypovolemia. Researchers theorize that pancreatic exudate destroys surfactant, which leads to the development of ARDS. The other diagnoses would be inappropriate because seizures are not associated with pancreatitis and because hyperkalemia and hypoglycemia are not common complications of pancreatitis, whereas hypokalemia and hyperglycemia are.

19 Correct answer — B

Within a few hours after onset of acute pancreatitis, serum amylase levels rise and remain elevated for about 3 days. After 24 hours, serum lipase levels also rise and remain elevated for up to 10 days. Serum levels of cholesterol, potassium, and calcium reveal nothing about acute pancreatitis.

20 Correct answer — C

Meperidine hydrochloride (Demerol) is typically used to treat acute pancreatitis because, unlike other opiates, it does not cause spasms of the sphincter of Oddi, which can increase the severity of pancreatic pain. Meperidine, like morphine, can cause respiratory depression and decreased GI motility; it does not affect hydrochloric acid secretion.

21 Correct answer — D

Hypertension is not a symptom of hemorrhagic pancreatitis. Jaundice is caused by common bile duct obstruction that occurs as a result of pancreatic edema. Shock develops when trypsin, a chemical found in the inflammatory fluid that spills into the peritoneum and causes pancreatitis, activates kinin, a vasodilator. Hemorrhage occurs when activated elastase dissolves the fibers of surrounding blood vessels. The pooling of blood caused by vasodilation compounded by blood loss leads to the development of signs of shock, such as hypotension. Pain results from distention of the pancreatic capsule, ductal spasm, or increased secretion of enzymes after eating.

22 Correct answer — D

Administering a clear liquid diet would be inappropriate in this situation. A patient with acute hemorrhagic pancreatitis should receive nothing by mouth (NPO) but should have a nasogastric tube inserted and attached to low suction, to drain gastric secretions and prevent further pancreatic stimulation. The nurse normally administers large quantities of volume expanders, such as colloid and electrolyte solutions, to combat shock and also administers calcium gluconate to correct the hypocalcemia that commonly occurs in acute pancreatitis. Central venous pressure and urine output should be monitored hourly to assess for impending shock and its treatment.

23 Correct answer — C

Antibiotics are rarely used to treat pancreatitis, except when infection has been established. In cases of infection, broad-spectrum antibiotics, such as ampicillin (Amcill) and gentamicin sulfate (Garamycin), may be ordered to help combat bacteria, which readily multiply in necrotic tissue.

24 Correct answer — A

The nurse would expect the physician to order a low-fat, no-alcohol, no-caffeine diet for a patient with acute pancreatitis. Limiting fat intake and avoiding alcohol helps prevent pancreatic stimulation. Avoiding caffeine prevents stimulation of gastric acid secretion, which activates pancreatic activity. Although a low-cholesterol, low-sodium, and low-sugar diet is beneficial, it does not stimulate the pancreas or gastric acid secretion.

25 Correct answer—A

Rovsing's sign, which is pain in the right lower abdominal quadrant that intensifies when pressure is applied to the left lower abdominal quadrant, is characteristic of acute appendicitis. Other classic signs include a slightly elevated temperature (99° to 101° F, or 37.2° to 38.3° C) and moderate leukocytosis (an elevated white blood cell count). The patient may also have anorexia, nausea, and vomiting. Abdominal distention and audible borborygmi are commonly associated with bowel obstruction.

26 Correct answer—C

The prompt administration of analgesics to decrease discomfort is considered an unsafe practice when caring for a patient with sudden abdominal pain. Because such drugs can mask important signs and symptoms, they usually are not given until the physician determines the cause of pain and decides whether the patient requires surgery. Appropriate nursing interventions include infusing the patient with lactated Ringer's or normal saline solution, inserting a nasogastric tube for suctioning, monitoring the patient's rectal temperature, obtaining blood cultures, and administering antipyretics and antibiotics, as ordered.

27 Correct answer—A

Young children have a higher incidence of perforated appendixes with ensuing peritonitis because they typically have difficulty describing symptoms. Also, the abdominal omentum (the peritoneal fold extending from the stomach to adjacent organs) is not well developed in children, allowing for rapid development of peritonitis because infection cannot be easily contained. Such children invariably have pain, although they may be unable to articulate the location or degree of pain. Appendicitis should be suspected in any child over age 2 who demonstrates symptoms of persistent abdominal pain, as early recognition can prevent rupture and other serious complications. Although young children are more prone to infection, they do not have a higher incidence of perforation. Also, young children do not have a weaker appendiceal wall.

28 Correct answer—B

Some abdominal organs are more susceptible to injury than others. The frequency of which internal organ is involved depends largely on how the injury is produced and on its location. The spleen, liver, and kidneys are the three most commonly injured organs in blunt abdominal trauma.

29 Correct answer — C

The nurse should expect to administer an infusion of an isotonic solution, such as lactated Ringer's or normal saline solution, to restore circulatory dynamics in a patient with a blunt abdominal injury and suspected injury to internal organs. This type of solution maintains the same osmotic pressure as blood serum and ensures that cellular constituents remain unchanged until surgery can be performed. Hypertonic solutions are better suited for treating electrolyte imbalances, such as dilutional hyponatremia in which the patient has an excess of free water. Hypotonic solutions, which are hypo-osmolar, are indicated in such electrolyte imbalances as hypernatremia to dilute the excess sodium load.

30 Correct answer — C

Peritoneal lavage is contraindicated in any patient who has a history of several abdominal surgeries, which suggests multiple abdominal surgical scars. Adhesions increase the likelihood that lavage fluid will penetrate the bowel and become trapped, making its return difficult. Peritoneal lavage is also contraindicated in pregnant patients because of possible fetal damage. This procedure is not contraindicated in colostomy patients or in those who are unconscious.

31 Correct answer — A

The spleen, which is located in the left upper abdominal quadrant under the diaphragm and near the abdominal wall, is partially protected by the lower left ribs and cannot be palpated until triple its normal size. This organ is injured more frequently than any other abdominal organ. The high incidence of splenic complications is directly related to the fact that the spleen is the most vascular organ in the body. Splenic lacerations and ruptured hematomas are notorious sources of peristent bleeding into the peritoneal cavity. Kehr's sign, which is referred pain to the left shoulder from blood irritating the diaphragm, is evident in about 50% of patients with splenic bleeding.

32 Correct answer — D

Because the spleen is located in the left upper abdominal quadrant, the nurse should suspect splenic injury in fractures involving the 8th, 9th, or 10th rib on the left side.

33 Correct answer — A

The hallmark signs and symptoms of intestinal obstruction include abdominal pain, distention, vomiting, and prolonged constipation (obstipation). All four signs and symptoms are not necessarily present in every case, and the severity varies with the level and type of obstruction. When an obstruction is high in the small intestine, the patient may have copious vomiting early with minimal abdominal distention. When obstruction is low in the colon, the patient may have marked distention with no vomiting. Constipation may be overlooked because the patient may have two or three bowel movements early in its initial stages, until the bowel, distal to the point of obstruction, is evacuated. On physical examination, bowel sounds typically are high-pitched and occur in rushes. The abdomen usually is distended but not tender unless the bowel is ischemic.

34 Correct answer — A

An appropriate nursing diagnosis for a patient with bowel obstruction is *Fluid volume deficit related to fluid shifting and vomiting* because of the loss of fluid through shifting in the intestinal lumen and vomiting. Myocardial contractility usually is not impaired in bowel obstruction. Although decreased renal perfusion may result from hypovolemia, acute renal failure is not a common complication. Although excess water is reabsorbed from impacted stool, it is not enough to cause a fluid volume excess.

35 Correct answer — C

The primary cause of large-bowel obstruction in an adult is carcinoma. Diverticulitis is the second leading cause; volvulus, the third. Adhesions are a less common cause of bowel obstruction. Cancer of the colon and rectum accounts for more than 50,000 deaths annually — the second highest death rate in the United States for any type of cancer. Men are affected more commonly than women. The highest incidence occurs in people about age 50. The 5-year survival rate is 40% to 50%, the best of the visceral cancers.

36 Correct answer — C

Shock, a condition in which effective circulating blood volume decreases, causes inadequate organ and tissue perfusion and can lead to derangements of cellular function. Clinical manifestations include decreasing arterial pressure (systolic pressure falls more rapidly than diastolic), tachycardia, cold and clammy skin, circumoral pallor, altered mental status, and suppressed kidney function.

37 Correct answer — C

The correct sequence for assessing and evaluating a patient's abdomen is inspection, auscultation, percussion, and palpation. Auscultation precedes percussion and palpation to prevent distortion of auscultatory findings related to pressure on the abdominal wall. Percussion precedes palpation to screen for an enlarged spleen before deep palpation.

38 Correct answer — D

Because acute upper GI bleeding is a potentially life-threatening condition, the patient requires immediate assessment to determine the extent and cause of bleeding. Therefore, the most helpful nursing action would be to determine the patient's shock status, then obtain a detailed health history and perform a thorough physical examination. The history and subsequent physical examination help to identify the sequence of events that prompted the patient to seek aid and reveals specific information about the nature of current or previous bleeding episodes, associated symptoms or diseases, and drug use. Inserting a nasogastric tube, collecting blood specimens to evaluate the patient's hematologic status, and scheduling an endoscopy as necessary are all important subsequent interventions.

39 Correct answer — B

In approximately 80% of all patients, hematemesis (the vomiting of blood) is caused by peptic ulcers. Other common causes, in decreasing order of frequency, include gastric and duodenal ulcers, bleeding esophageal varices, and gastric carcinoma.

40 Correct answer — D

Anticholinergic drugs, such as atropine sulfate, methantheline bromide (Banthine), and propantheline bromide (Pro-Banthine), are administered to suppress gastric secretions and to delay gastric emptying by blocking the effects of vagal nerve impulses on smooth muscle. Sedatives are usually administered with anticholinergics to decrease the patient's level of responsiveness. H_2-receptor antagonists, such as cimetidine (Tagamet) and ranitidine (Zantac), inhibit the action of histamine, which causes gastric acid secretion.

41 Correct answer — D

If the clinical findings suggest the lower bowel is the source of bleeding, proctoscopy should be the first diagnostic procedure. Proctoscopy will determine if the bleeding is from the rectosigmoid colon, rectum, or anal canal. Bleeding lesions commonly identified by proctoscopy include diffuse mucosal lesions, such as ulcerative and ischemic colitis; local vascular lesions, such as hemorrhoids; and tumors, such as polyps or cancer. An abdominal CT scan may be necessary as a follow-up to protoscopy. Angiography is not indicated to evaluate GI bleeding. Esophagogastroduodenoscopy is useful in pinpointing the source of upper GI bleeding.

42 Correct answer — D

The treatment for patients in the ED with lower GI bleeding depends on the extent and type of bleeding. If bleeding is caused by hemorrhoids or fissures, emergency admission is rarely necessary, and the patient may be referred to an outpatient clinic. If the bleeding is overt and from polyps, carcinoma, or ulcerative colitis, blood replacement may be necessary. This may be performed in the ED or on a medical unit. A patient with lower GI bleeding would rarely need emergency surgery or admittance to the intensive care unit.

43 Correct answer — D

When the amount of hemoglobin has been significantly reduced, the nail beds or palms will reveal anemia, unless the hand has been held in an awkward position or has been exposed to extreme cold or heat. Skin color, as in lips and gums, is an unreliable index of the degree of anemia because of wide individual variations in the amount of melanin in the skin. Although the sclera is typically pale in anemia, such pallor is not as evident as that of the patient's nail bed or palms.

44 Correct answer — B

Hemorrhoids, the most common cause of lower GI bleeding, typically produce intermittent, minute amounts of bright-red blood on the outside of formed stool or on toilet tissue. Massive bleeding rarely occurs. Bleeding from the colon is much less common than from the stomach or duodenum; however, the blood loss may be abrupt. Perirectal diseases, such as hemorrhoids, fissures, diverticulitis, ischemia, and tumors, usually result in lower GI bleeding.

45 Correct answer — D

Paralytic ileus is not a complication of endoscopy. Emergency endoscopy can be a useful diagnostic tool; however, its use may result in serious complications in certain situations. A patient who is uncooperative or unresponsive or who has esophageal obstruction is at high risk for perforation or aspiration. Also, because the endoscope increases airway resistance, the patient may be at risk for cardiac arrhythmias.

46 Correct answer—B

Lower GI bleeding is characterized by bleeding from any source below the ligament of Treitz, as the ligament of Treitz at the duodenojejunal junction is the dividing point for upper and lower GI bleeding.

47 Correct answer—B

The nurse's primary concern after assessing the patient's airway, breathing, and circulation would be to establish two large-bore I.V. lines in the event that the patient develops hypotension or tachycardia secondary to hemorrhage and requires rapid fluid and blood replacement.

48 Correct answer—A

The earliest indications of shock is tachycardia, a compensatory mechanism initiated by the sympathetic nervous system in an attempt to maintain cardiac output and organ perfusion. Later signs include a narrowing pulse pressure, which indicates a falling cardiac output, followed by hypotension and cool, clammy skin.

49 Correct answer—B

The nurse's priority at this time would be to prepare the patient for a diagnostic peritoneal lavage to determine whether the patient has internal bleeding. A CT scan may be ordered instead of peritoneal lavage, depending on the physician's preference. IVP may be necessary later if renal trauma is suspected. Neither immediate surgery nor blood replacement is warranted at this time.

50 Correct answer—D

Because hemorrhage from retroperitoneal structures does not cause bleeding into the abdominal compartment, the results of a peritoneal lavage in a patient with a retroperitoneal hematoma may be falsely negative. A negative lavage typically yields less than 100,000 red blood cells/mm^3 in the drainage. After injury to the spleen, diaphragm, or bladder, bloody drainage (a positive result) is typically obtained.

51 Correct answer—D

Lower abdominal crepitus may be indicative of a pelvic fracture, not renal trauma. Blood at the urinary meatus, a high-riding prostate on rectal examination, and hematuria all indicate trauma to the genitourinary system. An IVP or abdominal CT scan may be necessary to diagnose the specific site of damage.

52 Correct answer — C

The spleen, located in the left upper abdominal quadrant, is a highly vascular organ that normally cannot be palpated. However, when traumatized, intrasplenic bleeding may occur, resulting in a large mass that may be palpated in the left upper abdominal quadrant and displacement of the stomach. Fractured ribs in the left lower thorax may also signal a possible spleen injury. The liver, located in the right upper abdominal quadrant, cannot be palpated on the left side. Damage to the small intestine or colon usually is associated with lower quadrant injuries.

53 Correct answer — C

Because the assessment findings indicate an injury to the spleen, a highly vascular organ, the patient is at risk for fluid volume deficit related to blood loss. *Potential for infection related to abdominal contamination* would be an appropriate diagnosis for bowel perforation. *Impaired gas exchange related to inspiratory trauma* would be applicable if respiratory trauma were suspected. *Decreased cardiac output related to cardiac trauma* would be appropriate if cardiac trauma were evident.

54 Correct answer — A

One of the most common factors predisposing a patient to abdominal aortic aneurysm in an older adult is a history of diabetes. Other risk factors include hypertension, male sex, advanced age, and smoking. Congestive heart failure, renal disease, and abdominal carcinoma are not considered risk factors for this condition.

55 Correct answer — B

Abdominal distention, a pulsatile abdominal mass, and lower back pain are signs of an abdominal aortic aneurysm. Hoarseness, dysphagia, and midscapular back pain are signs of a thoracic aortic aneurysm.

56 Correct answer — D

The highest priority nursing diagnosis for a patient with a fusiform infrarenal nondissecting aortic aneurysm, the most common type of abdominal aortic aneurysm, would be *Altered peripheral tissue perfusion related to decreased arterial blood flow*. The other diagnoses are inappropriate because blood flow to the kidneys should not be impaired, and the patient's breathing and cardiac output should remain unaffected until late in the dissection, if it occurs.

57 Correct answer — D

Femoral pulse assessments are the best parameter for evaluating tissue perfusion to the lower extremities. The other parameters are indirect measurements of tissue perfusion.

CHAPTER 2

Cardiovascular Emergencies

SITUATION

A 68-year-old man arrives at the emergency department (ED) complaining of frequent episodes of substernal chest pain that have grown increasingly severe throughout the morning. He is alert and denies experiencing nausea, vomiting, or any radiation of the pain. The episodes, which began during the past month, typically occur at rest and last 10 to 15 minutes; they subside when the patient takes nitroglycerin sublingually.

After initiating cardiac monitoring, the nurse begins an infusion of 500 ml of dextrose and water I.V. at a keep-vein-open (KVO) rate and administers oxygen 24% by facemask. The patient's electrocardiogram (ECG) demonstrates ST-segment elevation. After assessing the patient's vital signs, the nurse administers the following medications, as ordered: 1" (2.5 cm) of nitroglycerin paste, 10 mg of propanolol hydrochloride (Inderal), and 10 mg of nifedipine (Procardia). Vital signs are blood pressure, 130/90 mm Hg; pulse rate, 110 beats/minute; and respirations, 24 breaths/minute.

Questions 1 to 6 relate to the above situation.

1 After reviewing the patient's history and ECG, the nurse determines that the findings are consistent with those of:

A. Stable angina
B. Preinfarction angina
C. Prinzmetal's angina
D. Angina decubitus

2 Appropriate nursing diagnoses for a patient with angina include all of the following *except*:

A. Knowledge deficit related to anginal pain
B. Potential for activity intolerance related to pain
C. Noncompliance related to life-style changes
D. Altered cardiopulmonary tissue perfusion related to coronary spasms

3 Which ECG finding is indicative of myocardial ischemia?

A. ST-segment depression
B. ST-segment elevation
C. T-wave elevation
D. U-wave appearance

4 The nurse understands that all of the following precipitating factors can contribute to the development of angina pectoris *except:*

A. Stress
B. Ingestion of heavy meals
C. Bed rest
D. Smoking

5 Which abnormality would the nurse be able to detect during an angina attack?

A. Transient diastolic murmur
B. Transient abnormal point of maximal impulse
C. Pulsus paradoxus
D. Pericardial friction rub

6 The nurse understands that the administration of propranolol to a patient with angina is contraindicated in all of the following circumstances *except:*

A. Heart block
B. Uncompensated congestive heart failure (CHF)
C. Tachycardia
D. Asthma

SITUATION

The triage nurse assesses an anxious and diaphoretic 54-year-old man who arrives at the ED complaining of severe, left-sided, pressurelike chest pain and left arm numbness. The pain began 2 hours ago and is unrelieved by rest. He has no significant medical history.

After initiating cardiac monitoring, the nurse administers oxygen at 2 liters/minute and establishes an I.V. line of dextrose 5% in water (D₅W) at a KVO rate. The patient's vital signs are blood pressure, 120/60 mm Hg; pulse rate, 88 beats/minute and irregular; and respirations, 20 breaths/minute. The cardiac rhythm shows normal sinus rhythm with occasional unifocal premature ventricular contractions (PVCs).

Questions 7 to 11 refer to the above situation.

7 The triage nurse suspects that this patient is exhibiting signs of a myocardial infarction (MI) because the chest pain:

A. Had not occurred previously
B. Is severe and radiating
C. Has lasted for 2 hours
D. Is accompanied by PVCs

8 The 12-lead ECG demonstrates ST elevation in leads V_1 through V_3. The nurse interprets this as an acute MI involving the:

A. Inferior wall
B. Anteroseptal wall
C. Lateral wall
D. Posterior wall

9 The patient's pain is unrelieved by the oxygen and sublingual nitroglycerin ($\frac{1}{150}$ grain every 5 minutes for three doses). The physician orders morphine sulfate I.V. because:

A. It is a powerful analgesic and decreases myocardial work load
B. It dilates coronary arteries when used with nitroglycerin
C. It produces sedation
D. It is an effective sedative and nonaddicting when given in small doses

10 The patient's pain is relieved after 6 mg of morphine. The physician orders a 50-mg bolus of lidocaine hydrochloride (Xylocaine) every 5 minutes for two doses, followed by an infusion at a rate of 2 mg/minute. Lidocaine is indicated because it:

A. Lowers the fibrillation threshold
B. Decreases the heart's need for oxygen
C. Eliminates irritability within necrotic areas of the myocardium
D. Eradicates potentially dangerous PVCs

11 While awaiting transfer to the coronary care unit, the patient becomes tachycardic but his blood pressure remains stable. Which nursing action is most appropriate at this point?

A. Giving additional morphine and reassuring the patient
B. Decreasing the lidocaine to 1 mg/minute and obtaining a lidocaine blood level stat
C. Auscultating the patient's lungs
D. Placing the patient in a low-Fowler's position

12 Which should be the nurse's primary goal when planning the care of a patient with an acute MI?

A. Preventing arrhythmias
B. Minimizing further cardiac damage
C. Decreasing the patient's oxygen needs
D. Alleviating the patient's anxiety

13 When caring for a patient with an MI, the nurse should keep in mind all of the following statements *except:*

A. Most patients with inferior wall MIs develop life-threatening conduction disturbances

B. Arrhythmias associated with atrioventricular (AV) block usually are transient and not dangerous when they occur with an inferior wall MI

C. Severe nausea and vomiting are common with an inferior wall MI

D. Ventricular irritability, demonstrated by PVCs, is dangerous regardless of the type of MI

14 Upon auscultation, the nurse detects a new crescendo-decrescendo systolic murmur, which is indicative of:

A. Aortic insufficiency

B. Papillary muscle dysfunction

C. Ventricular aneurysm

D. Early pericarditis

15 The nurse would suspect the development of a lateral wall MI in a patient who demonstrates:

A. Q waves in leads II, III, and aVF

B. Q waves in leads I, aVL, V_5, and V_6

C. Q waves in leads V_1 through V_3

D. Tall R waves in leads V_1 and V_2

16 Which health history finding would not predispose a patient to developing an MI?

A. Diabetes

B. Hypertension

C. Hyperlipidemia

D. High estrogen levels

SITUATION

A 56-year-old woman is brought to the ED by emergency medical service personnel for evaluation of increasing shortness of breath. Her shortness of breath began 2 days ago and has become increasingly severe. She is pale and diaphoretic, and her skin is warm. Her respirations are 36 breaths/ minute, and she exhibits increasing use of supraclavicular and abdominal muscles. The nurse detects bilateral crackles on auscultation.

The nurse notes that the patient has a history of coronary artery disease and that she had an MI 2 years ago. After assisting the patient into a high Fowler's position, the nurse records the following vital signs: blood pressure, 90/60 mm Hg; and pulse rate, 116 beats/minute and irregular.

Questions 17 to 32 relate to the above situation.

17 Based on the above vital signs, the nurse determines the patient's pulse pressure to be:

A. 30 mm Hg
B. 50 mm Hg
C. 70 mm Hg
D. 75 mm Hg

18 The nurse notes that the patient's presenting symptoms and vital signs are consistent with:

A. Right ventricular failure
B. Left ventricular failure
C. Biventricular failure
D. Backward failure

19 The physical findings of a patient with right ventricular failure would typically include:

A. Gallop rhythm and pulsus alternans
B. Elevated pulmonary artery diastolic pressure and pulmonary capillary wedge pressure
C. Hepatosplenomegaly with or without pain
D. Cough, dyspnea, and crackles

20 Which nursing intervention would be inappropriate for a patient with left ventricular failure?

A. Assessing the patient's fluid intake and output and electrolyte balance
B. Restricting the patient's fluid intake
C. Maintaining an infusion of normal saline solution
D. Maintaining the patient's intake of dietary sodium at 2 g/day

21 The nurse understands that the most common cause of right ventricular failure is:

A. Left ventricular failure
B. MI
C. Pulmonary hypertension
D. Cor pulmonale

22 Which nursing diagnostic category would be appropriate for a patient with CHF?

A. Decreased cardiac output
B. Impaired gas exchange
C. Activity intolerance
D. All of the above

23 The nurse understands that the rationale for administering inotropic and vasodilative drugs to a patient with CHF is to:

A. Decrease preload, increase afterload, and decrease contractility
B. Decrease preload, decrease afterload, and increase contractility
C. Increase preload, decrease afterload, and increase contractility
D. Increase preload, increase afterload, and decrease contractility

24 Which condition would the nurse suspect is a treatment-induced complication of CHF?

A. Hypervolemia
B. Pulmonary hypertension
C. Digitalis toxicity
D. Cor pulmonale

25 The physician orders digoxin (Lanoxin) to treat the patient's congestive heart failure. The nurse understands the pharmacologic effects of digoxin to be:

A. Negative inotropism and positive chronotropism
B. Negative inotropism and negative chronotropism
C. Positive inotropism and negative chronotropism
D. Positive inotropism and positive chronotropism

26 A patient receiving digoxin is at risk for developing toxicity. All of the following ECG changes are indicative of digoxin toxicity *except:*

A. Prolonged PR intervals and shortened QT intervals
B. ST-segment changes and decreased T-wave amplitudes
C. Tachyarrhythmias and ventricular ectopy
D. Prolonged QT intervals and decreased P-wave amplitudes

27 Which nursing action is appropriate when caring for a patient with digoxin toxicity?

A. Monitoring for hyperkalemia
B. Administering quinidine for tachyarrhythmias
C. Administering phenytoin sodium (Dilantin) for ventricular bigeminy
D. Administering calcium to desensitize the heart to the digoxin's effects

28 Which nursing diagnostic category is most appropriate for a patient with digoxin toxicity whose condition has been stabilized?

A. Self-care deficit
B. Activity intolerance
C. Knowledge deficit
D. Sensory-perceptual alteration

29 Which ECG finding would the nurse expect for a patient whose potassium level is 6 mEq/liter?

A. ST-segment depression
B. PVCs
C. Peaked T waves
D. Prominent U waves

30

This ECG tracing is representative of:

A. Ventricular flutter
B. Atrial flutter
C. Atrial fibrillation
D. Paroxysmal atrial tachycardia with block

31

All of the following are consistent with this ECG tracing *except:*

A. Inferior wall MI
B. Digoxin use
C. Hypokalemia
D. Organic heart disease

32

This ECG tracing was taken from a patient on digoxin who, at the time, was experiencing nausea. The pulse indicates perfusion of all beats. This rhythm:

A. May be associated with digoxin toxicity
B. Indicates that the patient should be treated with lidocaine
C. Represents ventricular trigeminy
D. Is caused by multiple ectopic foci in the ventricle

SITUATION

A patient who is experiencing an acute MI suddenly becomes unresponsive and pulseless while speaking with the nurse.

Questions 33 to 38 relate to the above situation.

33

The nurse notes the ECG rhythm above and responds by calling for help and:

A. Administering a 1 mg/kg bolus of lidocaine
B. Defibrillating using 200 joules
C. Performing synchronized cardioversion using 100 joules
D. Administering repeated precordial thumps

34

Which action should the nurse take next if the patient's ECG rhythm takes on the configuration above?

A. Administer a 1 mg/kg bolus of lidocaine
B. Administer a 350- to 500-mg bolus of bretylium (Bretylol) I.V.
C. Defibrillate using 300 joules
D. Perform synchronized cardioversion using 300 joules

35 The nurse observes that the patient's cardiac rhythm converts to sinus bradycardia with a rate of 30 beats/minute and notes that he is exhibiting frequent PVCs. Which of the following is the treatment of choice in this situation?

A. Placement of a temporary pacemaker
B. Administration of a bolus of an appropriate antiarrhythmic agent
C. Administration of a 0.5-mg bolus of atropine sulfate I.V.
D. Infusion of isoproterenol (Isuprel)

36

The nurse interprets the ECG tracing above as indicating:

A. Wandering atrial pacemaker
B. Second-degree AV block, Mobitz type I
C. Second-degree AV block, Mobitz type II
D. Third-degree heart block

37

The nurse notes the rhythm above while monitoring a patient with a temporary pacemaker. Which nursing action would be unsafe in this situation?

A. Turn the patient on his side
B. Increase the pacemaker rate
C. Check the pacemaker connections
D. Turn up the output (milliamperes) dial

38

Which problem is represented by the ECG tracing above?

A. Runaway pacemaker
B. Loss of capture
C. Loss of sensing
D. Inadequate connection between the distal wire of the catheter and the negative terminal of the pulse generator

SITUATION

A 63-year-old man arrives at the ED in an ambulance, complaining of a persistent, dull epigastric pain radiating to the interscapular region; the pain began 2 days ago. The nurse notes that he is alert and has good coloring and that his skin is warm and dry. Vital signs include right-arm blood pressure (BP), 120/60 mm Hg; left-arm BP, 220/100 mm Hg; right radial pulse, 2 +; and left radial pulse, 3 +. The nurse notes bilateral basilar crackles and a systolic cardiac murmur at the second right intercostal space. The patient has a 33-year history of hypertension, for which he is taking 50 mg of chlorthalidone (Hygroton) daily and 250 mg of methyldopa (Aldomet) three times a day.

Questions 39 to 44 relate to the above situation.

39 Aneurysms are classified according to all of the following *except:*

A. Type
B. Shape
C. Consistency
D. Location

40 Which signs would the nurse typically note when assessing a patient with a proximal dissecting aortic aneurysm?

A. Hypotension, tachycardia, and radiating back pain
B. Hypotension, bradycardia, and ECG changes
C. Anterior chest pain, altered consciousness, and paraparesis
D. Hypertension, vomiting, and chest pain

41 The nurse understands that the most helpful studies in diagnosing aortic aneurysms include:

A. Complete blood count (CBC), electrolyte studies, and chest X-ray
B. CBC, lactic dehydrogenase (LDH) level, and chest X-ray
C. LDH level, aspartate aminotransferase (AST) level, and ECG
D. AST level, ECG, and echocardiography

42 The physician prescribes an antihypertensive agent for the patient. The main objective of therapy is to maintain:

A. Systolic blood pressure at 100 to 120 mm Hg
B. Systolic blood pressure at 140 to 160 mm Hg
C. Diastolic blood pressure at 90 to 120 mm Hg
D. Diastolic blood pressure at 130 to 150 mm Hg

43 Most aneurysms occur in the:

A. Cerebral arteries
B. Aorta
C. Iliac artery
D. Popliteal artery

44 Which nursing diagnostic category is most appropriate for a patient with a dissecting aortic aneurysm and a blood pressure of 220/100 mm Hg in the right arm and 140/100 mm Hg in the left arm?

A. Altered tissue perfusion
B. Ineffective breathing pattern
C. Fluid volume deficit
D. Potential for infection

SITUATION

A 20-year-old man is admitted to the ED after being removed from a serious automobile accident. He sustained severe chest injuries as a result of not wearing his seat belt while driving. Chest X-rays reveal fractures to the second, third, and fourth ribs on the left side. The physician diagnoses cardiac tamponade.

Questions 45 to 50 relate to the above situation.

45 The nurse should assess for which sign in a patient with suspected cardiac tamponade?

A. Pulsus alternans
B. Wide pulse pressure
C. Large R waves in V_1 to V_6
D. Restlessness

46 Initially, administering I.V. fluid to a patient with acute cardiac tamponade:

A. Is important to replace lost fluid volume
B. Increases preload, thereby temporarily increasing cardiac output
C. Increases afterload, thereby temporarily increasing blood pressure
D. Usually is contraindicated because of accompanying pulmonary edema

47 Which treatment receives the highest priority in a patient with cardiac tamponade?

A. Thoracotomy
B. Administration of I.V. fluids
C. Pericardiocentesis
D. Application of medical antishock trousers

48 The nurse understands that all of the following are common complications of pericardiocentesis *except:*

A. Ventricular perforation
B. Pneumothorax
C. Complete heart block
D. Ventricular fibrillation

49 Which is the most important nursing intervention during pericardiocentesis?

A. Preparing an infusion of isoproterenol (Isuprel)
B. Monitoring the patient's ECG tracings in V_1 to V_6
C. Positioning the patient flat, if possible
D. Encouraging the patient to perform Valsalva's maneuver, if possible

50 The nurse knows that the most common cause of acute cardiac tamponade is:

A. MI
B. Penetrating chest trauma
C. Blunt chest trauma
D. Cancer

SITUATION

A 50-year-old man arrives at the ED complaining of headache, nausea, vomiting, and blurred vision. His blood pressure is 210/144 mm Hg. When asked about his medication history, the patient states that he usually takes clonidine hydrochloride (Catapres) but that he hasn't taken it for 2 days because he ran out of medication.

Questions 51 to 54 refer to the above situation.

51 Which assessment finding is *least* important in alerting the nurse to the patient's need for prompt medical attention?

A. Systolic blood pressure of 210 mm Hg
B. Diastolic blood pressure of 144 mm Hg
C. Headache and blurred vision
D. Nausea and vomiting

52 The nurse suspects that the patient has hypertensive crisis, which is probably the result of:

A. Retention of sodium and water
B. Renal failure
C. Increased peripheral vascular resistance
D. Increased sympathetic stimulation from the brain

53 Nitroprusside sodium (Nipride) is commonly used in hypertensive emergencies. This medication:

A. Must be administered slowly, through microdrip tubing
B. Has a direct vasodilating effect on the smooth muscles of arteries and veins
C. Has an onset of action of 2 to 3 minutes
D. Stimulates alpha-adrenergic receptors, producing sympathetic inhibition of blood pressure

54 The nurse understands that the most common cause of hypertension is:

A. Renal disease
B. Endocrine system dysfunction
C. Poor dietary habits
D. Idiopathic causes

SITUATION

A patient is brought into the ED by two emergency technicians, who are performing cardiopulmonary resuscitation. The patient is connected to a cardiac monitor and and is receiving 100% oxygen by a hand-held resuscitation (Ambu) bag. He has an endotracheal tube and a subclavian line in place. His ECG tracing shows that he is in ventricular fibrillation. He is defibrillated three times unsuccessfully.

Questions 55 to 65 relate to the above situation.

55 After the patient has been unsuccessfully defibrillated, the nurse should intervene by preparing an administration of:

A. Epinephrine hydrochloride (Adrenalin)
B. Calcium chloride
C. Bretylium tosylate (Bretylol)
D. Lidocaine hydrochloride (Xylocaine)

56 The patient's ventricular fibrillation continues. His arterial blood gas levels are pH, 7.25; PCO_2 35 mm Hg; PO_2, 60 mm Hg; and HCO_3^-, 15 mEq/liter. At this time, the nurse should expect to administer:

A. Sodium bicarbonate
B. Calcium chloride
C. Bretylium
D. Lidocaine

57 Which drug is usually infused after termination of ventricular fibrillation or ventricular tachycardia?

A. Digoxin
B. Lidocaine
C. Verapamil hydrochloride (Isoptin)
D. Dopamine

58 If ventricular fibrillation is refractory to lidocaine, drug therapy would most likely include:

A. Verapamil
B. Calcium chloride
C. Epinephrine
D. Bretylium

59 Treatment of a patient with symptomatic complete heart block that is refractory to atropine typically includes:

A. Dopamine
B. Epinephrine
C. Isoproterenol
D. Propranolol hydrochloride (Inderal)

60 The nurse understands that one of the therapeutic effects of propranolol is:

A. Increased myocardial contractility
B. Decreased cardiac output
C. Decreased myocardial oxygen supply
D. Prolonged AV conduction time

Cardiovascular Emergencies
Questions

61 Which drug is commonly used to treat hypotensive shock in a cardiac patient?

A. Dopamine
B. Dobutamine hydrochloride (Dobutrex)
C. Isoproterenol
D. Epinephrine

62 Which statement about dopamine is *true?*

A. It should be infused thorugh a central line
B. The dose should be regulated through microdrip tubing
C. It is the drug of choice in treating uncontrolled arrhythmias
D. It may increase oxygen demand, when given in low doses

63 Which drug is preferred in treating severe heart failure?

A. Epinephrine
B. Dopamine
C. Dobutamine
D. Digoxin

64 The nurse understands that the most serious adverse effect of I.V. nitroglycerin therapy is:

A. Hypotension
B. Bradycardia
C. Congestive heart failure
D. Ventricular fibrillation

65 Rapid I.V. infusion of nitroprusside can cause:

A. Hypertension and bradycardia
B. Chest pain and muscle twitching
C. Dyspnea and arrhythmias
D. Syncope and vomiting

Cardiovascular Emergencies Questions

SITUATION

A 50-year-old man is brought to the ED complaining of severe chest pain. An ECG tracing demonstrates an acute inferior wall MI. The cardiologist determines that the patient requires tissue plasminogen activator (t-PA) therapy.

Questions 66 to 71 relate to the above situation.

66 The nurse understands that t-PA (Activase) is used to:

A. Dissolve thrombi and reperfuse blood flow to the heart muscle
B. Improve myocardial function
C. Limit the size of an infarction
D. All of the above

67 Which statement about t-PA is *false?*

A. It is contraindicated for anyone with abnormal Q waves
B. Arrhythmias may occur during the infusion process
C. It should be administered within 6 hours of the onset of symptoms
D. It is contraindicated for anyone who has had recent major surgery

68 Which principle is most important to remember when administering
t-PA?

A. It should not be mixed in an I.V. line with any other medications
B. It should be administered via an infusion pump
C. It should be infused along with a heparin drip to prevent
   rethrombosis
D. All of the above

69 Which nursing action is least important during t-PA administration?

A. Monitoring ECG tracings for reperfusion arrhythmias
B. Checking the patient's neurologic status frequently
C. Inspecting the skin for bruising and the urine for blood
D. Measuring QT intervals every ½ hour

70 The nurse knows that lidocaine is administered during t-PA therapy
to:

A. Prevent ventricular arrhythmias caused by reperfusion of blood
   flow
B. Maintain blood pressure
C. Prevent the development of atrial arrhythmias
D. Increase myocardial automaticity

71 Which ECG changes would the nurse expect to see after the
successful administration of t-PA therapy?

A. Elevation of ST segments
B. Presence of Q waves
C. Increased T-wave inversion
D. Return of ST segments to the isoelectric line

SITUATION

A 32-year-old man, the driver of an automobile involved in an accident, is brought to the ED by ambulance. He is complaining of chest pain and shortness of breath. ECG tracings show sinus tachycardia with frequent PVCs.

Questions 72 to 76 relate to the above situation.

72 Based on the presenting signs and symptoms, the nurse suspects that the patient has:

A. An MI
B. Fractured ribs
C. Pericarditis
D. A cardiac contusion

73 The nurse understands that blunt chest trauma commonly results in damage to the:

A. Left ventricle
B. Right ventricle
C. Septum
D. Right atrium

74 Which therapy would be contraindicated for a patient with a myocardial contusion?

A. Nitroglycerin
B. Lidocaine
C. Morphine sulfate
D. Oxygen

75 The nurse should monitor this patient for development of which complication?

A. Adult respiratory distress syndrome
B. Pulmonary embolism
C. CHF
D. Cardiomyopathy

76 Which drug would be contraindicated for a patient with complications from a myocardial contusion?

A. Heparin
B. Digoxin
C. Dopamine
D. Bretylium

SITUATION

A 56-year-old man is being examined in the ED after complaining of chest pain and shortness of breath. His history reveals open-heart surgery, which occurred 1 month ago. He claims that, until today, he has been feeling fine. The physician diagnoses pericarditis.

Questions 77 to 80 relate to the above situation.

77 During the initial assessment, the nurse should check the patient for:

A. Elevated temperature
B. Pericardial friction rub
C. Pulsus paradoxus
D. Kussmaul's sign

78 The nurse would expect a patient with pericarditis to exhibit:

A. Further chest pain when sitting upright
B. Immediate relief of discomfort during deep inspiration
C. Bradycardia with ST-segment depression
D. Dyspnea and tachypnea

79 Administration of which drug may best relieve the patient's symptoms?

A. Indomethacin (Indocin)
B. Penicillin
C. Acetaminophen (Tylenol)
D. Digoxin

80 Which history finding would not predispose a patient to developing pericarditis?

A. Rheumatic fever
B. Postmyocardial infarction
C. Chronic obstructive pulmonary disease
D. Kidney disease

Cardiovascular Emergencies
Questions

SITUATION

A 26-year-old man with a long history of I.V. drug abuse enters the ED complaining of fever, shaking, chills, and severe night sweats. The physician diagnoses his condition as endocarditis.

Questions 81 to 83 relate to the above situation.

81 Which procedure is the nurse's *lowest* priority when assessing a patient with endocarditis?

A. Ausculating for S_3 heart sounds
B. Monitoring ECG tracings for PVCs
C. Monitoring the patient's temperature
D. Auscultating for crackles

82 The nurse would expect the laboratory studies of a patient with endocarditis to reveal:

A. Leukocytopenia
B. Elevated erythrocyte sedimentation rate
C. Polycythemia vera
D. Thrombocytosis

83 Which laboratory study is a prime diagnostic tool for a patient with endocarditis?

A. Blood culture
B. CBC with differential
C. Electrolyte studies
D. Clotting profile

SITUATION

A 42-year-old woman is admitted to the ED with complaints of sudden, severe pain in the right leg. After a thorough assessment, the physician diagnoses her condition as acute arterial occlusion of the right leg.

Questions 84 to 87 relate to the above situation.

84 Which history finding is atypical of a patient with acute arterial occlusion?

A. Atrial fibrillation
B. Postpartum status
C. Prosthetic valve replacement
D. MI

85 Which symptom would the nurse expect in a patient with acute arterial occlusion?

A. A swollen affected extremity with trophic changes
B. Positive Homans' sign with nonpalpable pulses
C. A pale affected extremity that is tender to deep pressure
D. Paresthesias

86 An appropriate action for the ED nurse caring for a patient with an arterial occlusion is to:

A. Apply hot compresses to the extremity
B. Elevate the ischemic extremity
C. Infuse heparin, as ordered
D. Measure the patient's calf width

87 The nurse would anticipate preparing this patient for all of the following procedures *except:*

A. Arteriovenous shunt
B. Embolectomy
C. Thrombolytic infusion
D. Extraction of emboli with a balloon-tipped catheter

Answer Sheet

	A B C D		A B C D		A B C D
1	○ ○ ○ ○	31	○ ○ ○ ○	61	○ ○ ○ ○
2	○ ○ ○ ○	32	○ ○ ○ ○	62	○ ○ ○ ○
3	○ ○ ○ ○	33	○ ○ ○ ○	63	○ ○ ○ ○
4	○ ○ ○ ○	34	○ ○ ○ ○	64	○ ○ ○ ○
5	○ ○ ○ ○	35	○ ○ ○ ○	65	○ ○ ○ ○
6	○ ○ ○ ○	36	○ ○ ○ ○	66	○ ○ ○ ○
7	○ ○ ○ ○	37	○ ○ ○ ○	67	○ ○ ○ ○
8	○ ○ ○ ○	38	○ ○ ○ ○	68	○ ○ ○ ○
9	○ ○ ○ ○	39	○ ○ ○ ○	69	○ ○ ○ ○
10	○ ○ ○ ○	40	○ ○ ○ ○	70	○ ○ ○ ○
11	○ ○ ○ ○	41	○ ○ ○ ○	71	○ ○ ○ ○
12	○ ○ ○ ○	42	○ ○ ○ ○	72	○ ○ ○ ○
13	○ ○ ○ ○	43	○ ○ ○ ○	73	○ ○ ○ ○
14	○ ○ ○ ○	44	○ ○ ○ ○	74	○ ○ ○ ○
15	○ ○ ○ ○	45	○ ○ ○ ○	75	○ ○ ○ ○
16	○ ○ ○ ○	46	○ ○ ○ ○	76	○ ○ ○ ○
17	○ ○ ○ ○	47	○ ○ ○ ○	77	○ ○ ○ ○
18	○ ○ ○ ○	48	○ ○ ○ ○	78	○ ○ ○ ○
19	○ ○ ○ ○	49	○ ○ ○ ○	79	○ ○ ○ ○
20	○ ○ ○ ○	50	○ ○ ○ ○	80	○ ○ ○ ○
21	○ ○ ○ ○	51	○ ○ ○ ○	81	○ ○ ○ ○
22	○ ○ ○ ○	52	○ ○ ○ ○	82	○ ○ ○ ○
23	○ ○ ○ ○	53	○ ○ ○ ○	83	○ ○ ○ ○
24	○ ○ ○ ○	54	○ ○ ○ ○	84	○ ○ ○ ○
25	○ ○ ○ ○	55	○ ○ ○ ○	85	○ ○ ○ ○
26	○ ○ ○ ○	56	○ ○ ○ ○	86	○ ○ ○ ○
27	○ ○ ○ ○	57	○ ○ ○ ○	87	○ ○ ○ ○
28	○ ○ ○ ○	58	○ ○ ○ ○		
29	○ ○ ○ ○	59	○ ○ ○ ○		
30	○ ○ ○ ○	60	○ ○ ○ ○		

Cardiovascular Emergencies
Answer Sheet

1 Correct answer—C

Based on the history and electrocardiogram (ECG), the nurse determines that the patient's findings are consistent with Prinzmetal's angina, a form of severe, non-effort-induced pain that occurs at rest. This type of pain, which occurs cyclically (commonly at the same time each day) and may be of a greater duration than the other types of anginal pain. Prinzmetal's angina, which is most common in women under age 50, is caused by spasms of a large coronary artery. Stable angina is characterized by chronic pain that shows no variance in duration, intensity, or frequency for at least 2 months; it may be debilitating or mild. Preinfarction angina, or unstable angina, is characterized by pain that increases in frequency, duration, and severity and usually develops into a myocardial infarction (MI). Angina decubitus is characterized by pain that occurs upon assuming a recumbent position.

2 Correct answer—C

Noncompliance related to life-style changes would be an inappropriate nursing diagnosis because the ED nurse would not know whether the patient was compliant or not. All of the other diagnoses are appropriate because they identify specific, treatable aspects of the patient's conditions.

3 Correct answer—A

Transient myocardial ischemia, which produces the chest pain or discomfort characteristic of angina pectoris, may be identified by ST-segment depression or T-wave inversion on an ECG tracing. ST-segment elevation on an ECG tracing is typically associated with Prinzmetal's angina. T-wave elevation is common in patients with hyperkalemia. The appearance of U-waves on an ECG is associated with hypokalemia.

4 Correct answer—C

The underlying cause of angina pectoris is a disequilibrium between myocardial oxygen supply and demand, in which too little oxygen is available to meet the demands of the heart. Bed rest decreases myocardial oxygen demand and therefore poses no threat to equilibrium. Stress and ingestion of heavy meals increase oxygen demand; smoking decreases the blood and oxygen supply through vasoconstriction.

5 Correct answer—**B**

During an angina attack, the nurse would be able to detect a transient abnormal point of maximal impulse. Other signs and symptoms of angina include anxiety, diaphoresis, pain or discomfort, cold and clammy skin, dyspnea, increased heart rate, pulsus alternans, atrial gallop (S_4), and a rare transient systolic murmur. Pulsus paradoxus may occur in a patient with cardiac tamponade or hypovolemic shock. Pericardial friction rub may be auscultated in a patient with pericarditis.

6 Correct answer—**C**

Reflex tachycardia, which is induced by the use of nitrates, can be compensated by the bradycardic effects of beta blockade, resulting in a decrease in myocardial contractility, blood pressure, and heart rate. Beta blockers, such as propranolol hydrochloride, usually are administered until the patient obtains relief or experiences adverse reactions. After abrupt cessation of propranolol, the patient may experience exacerbation of angina, which may induce an acute myocardial infarction (MI). Common contraindications to beta-blocker use include heart block, uncompensated congestive heart failure (CHF), and asthma.

7 Correct answer—**C**

Any chest pain lasting longer than 45 minutes is probably caused by an MI. Chest pain associated with angina rarely lasts longer than 30 minutes and may also be severe and radiating, but it is usually relieved by rest. Premature ventricular contractions (PVCs) may result from myocardial ischemia; they may occur during an angina episode.

8 Correct answer—**B**

In this setting, ST-segment elevations are indicative of acute myocardial injury. Because leads V_1, V_2, and V_3 represent the anteroseptal wall of the left ventricle, the nurse would suspect that the patient is experiencing an MI involving the anteroseptal wall. Leads II, III, and aVF represent the inferior wall; leads I, aVL, V_5, and V_6 represent the lateral wall. ST-segment elevations are not characteristic of posterior wall MI; instead, mirror images (represented by ST-segment depression) would be present in leads V_1, V_2, and V_3 along with tall R waves.

9 Correct answer—**A**

Morphine is a powerful analgesic. It reduces preload by causing peripheral vasodilation and reduces sympathetic activity, thereby decreasing myocardial work load. It has no direct effect on coronary arteries. Although morphine may produce sedation and is nonaddictive in small doses, it is not administered for these reasons.

10 Correct answer—D

PVCs, which result from myocardial irritability, are dangerous in a patient with an acute MI because they are precursors to life-threatening ventricular arrhythmias. Lidocaine is an antiarrhythmic that raises the fibrillation threshold and has little effect on myocardial oxygen needs. The ischemic area surrounding the area of infarction, not the necrotic area, is the source of irritability, as necrotic tissue can neither generate nor transmit impulses.

11 Correct answer—C

The most appropriate nursing action at this time would be to auscultate the patient's lungs to identify the cause of the tachycardia. Tachycardia is frequently the first sign of heart failure in the patient with an MI. It is a compensatory mechanism for low stroke volume or cardiac output. Tachycardia may also be caused by anxiety and chest pain, but it is not a symptom of lidocaine toxicity. If heart failure is the cause of the tachycardia, a high Fowler's position would be the most comfortable for the patient. The nurse must assess the patient to determine the cause of tachycardia before administering morphine.

12 Correct answer—C

The primary goal when planning the care of patient with an acute MI is to decrease the patient's oxygen needs. In an MI, the patient has an imbalance between myocardial oxygen supply and demand. Measures that reduce the body's need for oxygen, such as giving supplemental oxygen, promoting rest, and reducing the patient's anxiety, can decrease the occurrence of complications, such as arrhythmias, and prevent further myocardial damage.

13 Correct answer—A

A patient with an anterior wall MI, not an inferior wall MI, is more likely to develop life-threatening conduction disturbances because the left anterior descending coronary artery supplies the His bundle and bundle branches as well as the anterior wall of the left ventricle. Such a patient should be closely monitored because second-degree heart blocks, especially Mobitz type II, are more likely to progress to complete heart block and cardiac arrest. First-degree atrioventricular (AV) blocks and second-degree AV (Mobitz type I, or Wenckebach) blocks are common in patients with an inferior wall MI. Caused by vagus nerve stimulation and AV node ischemia and edema, these blocks are transient and are not considered dangerous to the patient; progression to more dangerous blocks rarely occurs.

14 Correct answer — B

This murmur is characteristic of a papillary muscle dysfunction, namely mitral valve insufficiency. When a papillary muscle becomes infarcted, improper valve closure results in regurgitation of blood from the left ventricle into the left atrium. Aortic insufficiency produces a diastolic murmur, and pericarditis produces a friction rub. Various murmurs can accompany ventricular aneurysm, depending on the aneurysm's location. Alone, none of these is diagnostic.

15 Correct answer — B

Q waves are indicative of myocardial necrosis. Therefore, Q waves in leads I, aVL, V_5, and V_6, which represent the lateral wall of the left ventricle, would lead the nurse to suspect that the patient is experiencing a lateral wall MI. Leads II, III, and aVF represent the inferior wall; leads V_1, V_2, and V_3, the anterior wall. Tall R waves in leads V_1 and V_2, reflecting mirror images of Q waves, are characteristic of a posterior wall infarction.

16 Correct answer — D

Estrogen is thought to decrease lipoprotein levels and help coronary arteries resist atherosclerosis. For this reason, MI rarely occurs in women of childbearing age, as these women typically have high estrogen levels. However, when women reach menopause, estrogen levels decrease and their chance of developing coronary artery disease approaches that of men. Diabetes, hypertension, and hyperlipidemia are considered predisposing factors for the development of an MI.

17 Correct answer — A

Pulse pressure is the difference between the systolic and diastolic blood pressures; therefore, a patient with a blood pressure of 90/60 mm Hg would have a pulse pressure of 30 mm Hg. If arterial pressure falls and sympathetic compensatory vasoconstriction occurs, the pulse pressure is narrowed. The pulse pressure is influenced by stroke volume and peripheral resistance. A narrow pulse pressure indicates a low stroke volume (decreasing systolic pressure) or high peripheral resistance (increasing diastolic pressure).

18 Correct answer — B

A falling blood pressure and narrowing pulse pressure are ominous signs of left ventricular failure, or forward failure. CHF can be described as right-sided or left-sided, although failure of both sides may occur simultaneously (biventricular failure) or one may progress to the other. In left-sided heart failure, fluid accumulates in the pulmonary bed, whereas in right-sided heart failure, fluid accumulates in the systemic circulation. CHF can also be described according to the direction of the main force of blood flow. Cardiac output is decreased in forward failure. Backward failure occurs when blood accumulates in one or both ventricles and the venous system, thus decreasing cardiac output.

19 Correct answer—C

Hepatosplenomegaly, with or without pain, is characteristic of a patient who exhibits signs of right ventricular failure. The signs of right-sided heart failure are a result of venous congestion. With systemic vascular engorgement, the pressure in the capillaries of the abdominal organs will rise, resulting in edema. The edema produces a sense of fullness in the abdomen and may cause anorexia, nausea, and vomiting. Liver congestion causes tenderness over the hepatic area. The liver should be palpated for tenderness and engorgement. (Normally, the liver cannot be palpated.) Gallop rhythm, pulsus alternans, an elevated pulmonary artery diastolic pressure and pulmonary capillary wedge pressure, dyspnea, and crackles are seen in left ventricular failure. Cough is not associated with right or left ventricular failure.

20 Correct answer—C

In this situation, maintaining an infusion of normal saline solution is inappropriate because this would worsen the patient's CHF. Appropriate nursing interventions include monitoring the patient's blood pressure and closely monitoring the patient's fluid and sodium intake. Although the patient's serum sodium concentration level may be low, dilution from excessive fluid retention may be masking the underlying problem of sodium excess. Fluid restriction is necessary to allow the sodium concentration to reach a normal level. Maintaining the patient's intake of dietary sodium at 2 g/day is necessary to control thirst and water intake.

21 Correct answer—A

The most common cause of right ventricular failure is left ventricular failure. This occurs as an increase in pulmonary venous and arterial pressures that is seen in left ventricular failure strains and increases the preload on right ventricular tissue. Other causes of right ventricular failure include intrinsic lung disease, valvular disease, right ventricular infarction, and pulmonary hypertension. Cor

pulmonale is right ventricular failure that occurs from prolonged
pulmonary hypertension.

22 Correct answer—D

All of the diagnostic categories are appropriate because a patient with
CHF has decreased cardiac output, impaired gas exchange, and
activity intolerance—all problems that the nurse can identify and
treat.

23 Correct answer—B

The aim of inotropic and vasodilative drug therapy in a patient with
CHF is to decrease left ventricular demand and increase myocardial
oxygen supply. This is accomplished by decreasing preload, decreasing
afterload, and increasing contractility.

24 Correct answer—C

Digitalis toxicity, a common complication resulting from treatment of
CHF, can result from digoxin overmedication or from hypokalemia or
renal dysfunction, which are commonly seen in patients with CHF.
Other common complications include hypovolemia, hypokalemia,
cardiac arrhythmias, and emboli formation. Hypovolemia and
hypokalemia may occur from excessive use of diuretic therapy,
resulting in sodium, potassium, and water loss. Hypokalemia may lead
to cardiac arrhythmias. Arrhythmias may occur in response to
electrolyte imbalances, sympathomimetic drugs, or digoxin (Lanoxin).
Emboli formation can be caused by bed rest or excessive diuretic
therapy, resulting in an elevated hematocrit hemoconcentration. Cor
pulmonale, the dilation and hypertrophy of the right ventricle
resulting from lung disease, develops as a result of pulmonary
hypertension.

25 Correct answer—C

Digoxin, a widely used drug in the treatment of CHF and
supraventricular arrhythmias (especially atrial fibrillation), exerts a
positive inotropic action, thereby increasing contractility in normal and
failing hearts. In the failing heart, digoxin decreases ventricular size
and reduces wall tension. Antiarrhythmic action of the drug prolongs
conduction time and the refractory features of the AV node. As a
negative chronotropic agent, digoxin produces vagotonia, resulting in a
slow heart rate.

26 Correct answer — D

Prolonged QT intervals and decreased P-wave amplitudes are not indicative of digoxin toxicity. The patient who is receiving digoxin should be closely monitored for changes in the PR interval, QT interval, and QRS complex (especially prolonged PR intervals, shortened QT intervals, ST-segment changes, and decreased T-wave amplitudes) as well as for changes in atrial and ventricular rates. The cardiac rhythm should also be noted, as the enhanced automaticity and facilitation of reentry produced by the drug can result in atrial, junctional, or ventricular tachyarrhythmias. Other manifestations of digoxin toxicity include paroxysmal atrial tachycardia with block, AV blocks, atrial ectopic beats, atrial fibrillation, sinus arrest, and sinoatrial block. However, the hallmark arrhythmia in digoxin toxicity is ventricular bigeminy. In diseased hearts, digoxin toxicity is more likely to result in tachyarrhythmias; in normal hearts, AV blocks.

27 Correct answer — C

The appropriate nursing action in this situation is to administer phenytoin sodium (Dilantin), as phenytoin is the antiarrhythmic drug of choice in digoxin toxicity. The patient should be monitored for hypokalemia because a low potassium level enhances digoxin toxicity. Administering quinidine would potentiate digoxin's effect and may precipitate digoxin toxicity. Administering calcium may sensitize the heart to the drug's effects, precipitating digoxin-induced arrhythmias.

28 Correct answer — C

The most appropriate nursing diagnostic category for a patient with digoxin toxicity whose condition has been stabilized would be *Knowledge deficit*. Using the category allows the nurse to formulate an appropriate diagnosis that enables her to determine the patient's current knowledge level regarding his health status, assess the patient's cognitive and emotional readiness to learn, recognize barriers to learning, assess the patient's learning needs, establish short- and long-term goals, and encourage the patient's significant others to reinforce correct information regarding the diagnosis and therapies to the patient. The desired outcome of this diagnosis is that the patient participates in the learning process and communicates an understanding of his current health status and therapies.

29 Correct answer — C

A potassium level greater than 5 mEq/liter results in hyperkalemia, a condition represented by peaked T waves, prolonged PR intervals, and widened QRS complexes on ECG. A potassium level less than 3 mEq/

liter results in hypokalemia, a condition represented by ST-segment depression, PVCs, prominent U waves, and flattened T waves.

30 Correct answer – B

This ECG tracing represents atrial flutter, which is characterized by an atrial rate of 300 beats/minute, a sawtooth pattern of flutter waves, and normal QRS complexes. In the given strip, varying degrees of block are represented. Atrial fibrillation is characterized by an atrial rate of 350 to 600 beats/minute and indistinguishable P waves. QRS complexes are normal in configuration but occur in an irregular rhythm. Paroxysmal atrial tachycardia with block is characterized by an atrial rate of 150 to 250 beats/minute. Although P waves precede each QRS complex, they are not conducted when a block occurs. The P waves, which may be buried in preceding T waves, are often different in configuration because they arise from an ectopic focus.

31 Correct answer – C

This ECG tracing represents first-degree AV block, in which the PR interval is greater than 0.20 seconds. Prolongation of the PR interval is associated with hyperkalemia, not hypokalemia. First-degree AV block is a common finding in inferior wall MI because of AV-node ischemia. The effects of digoxin and organic heart disease can cause delayed conduction through the AV node, thus prolonging the PR interval.

32 Correct answer – A

The patient in this situation had nausea, a well-established symptom of digoxin toxicity (other symptoms include anorexia, visual disturbances, and fatigue). This ECG tracing represents ventricular bigeminy, one of several arrhythmias associated with digoxin toxicity, in which a PVC occurs after every other beat. Phenytoin, not lidocaine, is the preferred drug for treating this condition. Lidocaine would not be given because of the perfusion of PVCs; eliminating the PVCs would decrease the heart rate by 50%, severely diminishing the cardiac output. The PVCs are unifocal and therefore arise from a single ectopic focus.

33 Correct answer – B

This ECG tracing represents ventricular tachycardia. The nurse would respond appropriately by calling for help and defibrillating the patient using 200 joules. However, if the nurse had been able to detect a pulse, synchronized cardioversion would be indicated. In this case, the defibrillator would be synchronized with the cardiac monitor so that the electrical impulse is discharged on the QRS complex (depolarization) and not on the T wave, which can cause the rhythm to deteriorate.

34 Correct answer—C

If the patient goes into ventricular fibrillation, as represented in this ECG tracing, the nurse would respond correctly by immediately defibrillating the patient using 300 joules. Lidocaine or bretylium tosylate (Bretylol) may be administered after defibrillation. Because the rhythm is chaotic, without evidence of P waves or QRS complexes, synchronized cardioversion cannot be used.

35 Correct answer—C

The initial treatment of choice for symptomatic bradycardia and bradycardia associated with PVCs is administration of a 0.5-mg bolus of atropine sulfate I.V., which may be repeated every 5 minutes, as necessary, to a maximum dose of 2 mg. Afterward, treatment may include the placement of a temporary pacemaker. The patient's PVCs may be a symptom of hypoxia caused by the bradycardia. If this is the case, increasing the heart rate would eliminate the PVCs; hence, they should not be treated with an antiarrhythmic. Isoproterenol (Isuprel), which is used with or without an external pacemaker to treat symptomatic heart block that does not respond to atropine, may be used only until a pacemaker can be inserted, as isoproterenol increases myocardial oxygen consumption and predisposes the heart to life-threatening arrhythmias.

36 Correct answer—B

This ECG tracing represents second-degree AV block, Mobitz type I (Wenckebach), which is characterized by a recurring sequence in which each PR interval becomes progressively wider until a QRS complex is finally dropped. Wandering atrial pacemaker is characterized by P waves that vary in size and configuration, as well as by PR intervals that vary, depending on the distance of the pacemaker to the AV node. Second-degree AV block, Mobitz type II, is characterized by constant PR intervals and unpredictable dropping of QRS complexes. In third-degree heart block, no relationship exists between the P waves and QRS complexes. The atria and ventricles beat independently; the atrial rate may be 60 to 100 beats/minute, with regularly occurring P waves. The ventricular rate may be 20 to 60 beats/minute, depending on whether the impulse originates in the AV node or the ventricles (the rate is slowest when the impulse arises from the ventricle).

37 Correct answer — **B**

Increasing the pacemaker rate would be unsafe for a patient whose temporary pacemaker is signaling loss of capture (no ventricular complex following a pacemaker spike), as depicted in this ECG tracing. Although the pacemaker is sensing the patient's slow rate and firing appropriately, the pacing spikes are not followed by QRS complexes. Increasing the pacemaker rate will not solve the problem — it will only produce more spikes. Possible causes of capture loss include an inadequate amount of energy (measured in milliamperes [MA]) and displacement of the catheter tip. Turning up the output (MA) dial will increase the amount of electrical energy delivered by the pacemaker to the myocardium. Turning the patient on either side may cause the catheter to move back toward the endocardium. Another possible cause is disconnection of the negative terminal of the pulse generator from the distal wire of the pacing catheter. Since the distal electrode delivers the energy that paces the heart, checking the pacemaker connections would be in order.

38 Correct answer — **C**

This ECG tracing depicts loss of sensing, in which the pacemaker fails to sense the cardiac rhythm and continues to fire at a preset rate even though the patient's heart rate is higher. Pacemaker spikes normally do not appear when the patient's own rate is consistently higher than that set for the demand pacemaker. Their appearance signals that the patient's own pacemaker and the temporary pacemaker are competing for control of the heart. Pacemaker spikes that occur on T waves, which represent the repolarization (vulnerable) phase of the cardiac cycle, are dangerous because they may result in ventricular fibrillation. Runaway pacemaker, the firing of the pacemaker at a rate faster than that of the pacemaker setting, commonly results from battery depletion. The absence of pacemaker spikes will occur if an inadequate connection between the pacemaker wire and generator exists.

39 Correct answer — **C**

Aneurysms usually are described according to shape and identified according to type and location. Their shape may be *fusiform* (in which the aneurysm appears as a uniform, round arterial dilatation) or *saccular* (in which the aneurysm appears as a vascular outpouching with a small neck attached to the arterial wall). A *true* aneurysm refers to a dilatation enclosed by at least one intact arterial wall. A *false* aneurysm refers to an extravascular accumulation of blood from a disruption of all three layers of the arterial wall. A *dissecting* aneurysm is one that results from a separation of arterial layers, in

Cardiovascular Emergencies Answers

which blood accumulates in the middle layer secondary to a tear in the inner lining.

40 Correct answer—C

A patient with a proximal dissecting aortic aneurysm typically experiences anterior central chest pain that rarely radiates to the back. The patient may also have signs of a neurologic deficit (such as cerebral apoplexy, paraparesis, or peripheral neuropathy) and altered mental status. Another common finding is blood pressure variations between the arms and pulse deficits. Hypertension typically occurs in a patient with a distal dissecting aortic aneurysm.

41 Correct answer—B

The most common signs of a dissecting aortic aneurysm are an elevated lactic dehydrogenase (LDH) level, leukocytosis, and a widened aorta; therefore, the most helpful diagnostic studies include a complete blood count (CBC), an LDH level, and a chest X-ray. Other helpful diagnostic tools include ECG monitoring to detect left ventricular hypertrophy; angiography, the most definitive diagnostic procedure, to determine the location and extent of dissection and to evaluate the status of the renal, mesenteric, and iliac circulations; and emergency anteroposterior and lateral lumbosacral spinal X-ray studies or ultrasonography to determine the exact size and location of the aneurysm (if the aneurysm is small and the patient is symptomatic, ultrasound studies should be performed approximately every 6 months to monitor size and determine need for surgery).

42 Correct answer—A

The initial therapy and treatment of choice for all types of dissecting aneurysms is drug therapy, the primary objective of which is to decrease the systolic pressure to 100 to 120 mm Hg for 24 to 48 hours, thereby controlling blood pressure. Commonly prescribed agents include reserpine (Serpasil), trimethaphan camsylate (Arfonad), nitroprusside sodium (Nipride), and propranolol hydrochloride (Inderal). Another important objective of drug therapy is to decrease cardiac contractility; therefore, diuretics may be given concurrently.

Drug therapy hastens the fibrotic phase of the healing process, reduces edema, and reduces bleeding in subsequent surgery. Once pain is relieved and blood pressure controlled, aortography is performed to enable the physician to select the appropriate, definitive therapy.

43 Correct answer—**B**

Most aneurysms develop in the aorta, although they also may occur in the left ventricle after an acute MI, in the cerebral arteries, and in other central and peripheral arteries. Aortic aneurysms are categorized according to location, such as thoracic-ascending, transverse, descending, thoracoabdominal, and abdominal. Ascending thoracic aneurysms are located in the area of the aorta that is closest to the heart. Aneurysms of the transverse arch include the carotid, subclavian, and upper vertebral arteries. Aneurysms of the descending thoracic aorta are found in the proximal part of the descending aorta. Abdominal aneurysms are found below the arteries of the kidney and above the bifurcation of the iliac arteries. Thoracoabdominal aneurysms extend from immediately above the diaphragm to the area immediately below it and are typically associated with decreased blood supply to the celiac, superior mesenteric, and renal arteries.

44 Correct answer—**A**

An appropriate nursing diagnostic category for a patient with a dissecting aortic aneurysm would be *Altered tissue perfusion,* as this occurs as a result of impaired blood flow secondary to a narrowed aortic lumen.

45 Correct answer—**D**

Restlessness is a common sign of cardiac tamponade and results from hypoxia caused by a decreased cardiac output. Other common signs include narrow pulse pressure, pulsus paradoxus, and decreased amplitude of QRS complexes. Pulse pressure narrows because of a decrease in systolic pressure caused by the drop in cardiac output; diastolic pressure rises because of peripheral vasoconstriction. Pulsus paradoxus, the exaggerated decrease in systolic pressure during inspiration, is noted by the absence of heart sounds for a period greater than 10 mm Hg while the blood pressure cuff is being slowly deflated. The amplitude of the QRS complexes typically decreases as a result of fluid accumulation, which increases the distance of the heart from the chest wall, thereby interfering with ECG recording.

46 Correct answer—**B**

Preload refers to the stretching force of the ventricle immediately before contraction. According to Starling's law, an increase in the left ventricular volume will increase the volume pumped out during systole. Beyond a certain point, however, this mechanism no longer works. Therefore, increasing the circulating volume can temporarily support the patient's cardiac output until measures can be instituted

Cardiovascular Emergencies Answers

Cardiovascular Emergencies Answers

to relieve the pressure of the tamponade. Large amounts of blood are seldom lost when tamponade occurs quickly. As little as 100 ml of blood in the pericardial space is enough to cause a severe decrease in cardiac output. Patients with cardiac tamponade usually do not have pulmonary edema. They typically have normal chest X-rays, although a widened cardiac silhouette may be apparent. Afterload refers to the force against which the left ventricle must pump (peripheral vascular resistance).

47 Correct answer—C

Pericardiocentesis, the aspiration of blood or fluid through an intracardiac needle inserted into the pericardial sac, is the priority treatment for cardiac tamponade. This procedure allows the physician to withdraw a minute amount of blood to reduce myocardial compression and increase cardiac output; removing as little as 20 ml of blood may save the patient's life. After hemodynamic stability is restored, the patient may be taken for a thoracotomy, if indicated. Administration of I.V. fluids and the application of medical antishock trousers are not considered the highest priority because they increase cardiac output only temporarily.

48 Correct answer—C

Heart block is not a complication of pericardiocentesis. Ventricular perforation can occur if the needle is advanced too quickly. Pneumothorax can occur if the needle is accidentally introduced into the pleural space. Ventricular fibrillation can result from the needle making contact with the myocardium.

49 Correct answer—B

The most important nursing intervention during pericardiocentesis is to monitor the patient's ECG tracings in leads V_1 through V_6 because a precordial (V lead) lead is normally attached to the hub of the intracardiac needle. Any contact between the needle and the myocardium results in a current of injury pattern, which is represented by an ST-segment elevation on the ECG. During the procedure, an awake patient may be placed in a high Fowler's position for maximum comfort. Isoproterenol (Isuprel) and Valsalva's maneuver are not indicated in the treatment of pericardial tamponade.

50 Correct answer—B

Penetrating chest trauma is the most common cause of acute cardiac tamponade; blunt trauma, the second most common cause. Tamponade is also a rare but serious complication that can result from a transmural MI. Chronic fluid accumulation in the pericardial sac can result from various disorders, such as cancer, autoimmune disease, and uremia. Because these effusions occur chronically, the pericardium has a chance to stretch to accommodate as much as 1,500 ml of fluid. In this situation, the onset of symptoms is much more gradual and less immediately life-threatening.

51 Correct answer — A

A systolic blood pressure of 210 mm Hg would be the least important assessment finding in this situation. Hypertensive crisis is characterized by a diastolic pressure greater than 130 mm Hg. When symptoms such as headache, visual disturbances, nausea, and vomiting accompany a critically elevated diastolic pressure, hypertensive encephalopathy should be suspected. Hypertensive encephalopathy is a medical emergency and occurs when arterial spasm and cerebral edema produce neurologic symptoms. Other symptoms of this syndrome include papilledema, transient hemiparesis, disorientation, and convulsions. If untreated, hypertensive encephalopathy can lead to death.

52 Correct answer — D

In this situation, the nurse would suspect that the patient's hypertensive crisis is probably the result of increased sympathetic stimulation from the brain, resulting from the discontinuation of clonidine hydrochloride (Catapres). Clonidine lowers blood pressure by acting directly on alpha-adrenergic receptors in the central nervous system, thereby causing a decrease in sympathetic outflow from the brain. Abrupt discontinuation of this drug can cause a withdrawal reaction leading to severe rebound hypertension. This may occur within 12 to 48 hours. Clonidine does not have any effect on sodium and water balance and is not known to have any direct effect on the peripheral vasculature. Nothing in the patient's history warrants suspicion of renal failure.

53 Correct answer — B

Nitroprusside has a powerful, direct vasodilating effect on the smooth muscle of arteries and veins. This medication should always be administered through an infusion pump. Onset of action is 30 to 60 seconds. Profound hypotension can occur quickly in response to this medication; therefore, the patient's blood pressure must be closely monitored, preferably with the use of an arterial line.

54 Correct answer — D

Although various factors predispose an individual to hypertension, most patients have no known medical problems directly causing hypertension and their condition is attributed to idiopathic causes. Predisposing factors include old age, elevated cholesterol levels, heredity, obesity, and sedentary life-style. A minority of patients have secondary hypertension in which there is an identifiable cause. These include the use of tobacco, alcohol, caffeine, and certain drugs; cardiovascular disorders, such as coarctation of the aorta; endocrine disorders, such as pheochromocytoma and disorders of the adrenal cortex; neurologic disorders, such as increased intracranial pressure; kidney disorders, such as renal artery stenosis, acute or chronic renal failure, and renin-secreting tumors; and pregnancy.

55 Correct answer—A

Epinephrine hydrochloride (Adrenalin), an endogenous catecholamine with both alpha- and beta-adrenergic actions, is the drug of choice in this situation. During resuscitation, epinephrine elevates perfusion pressure generated during chest compression, improves myocardial contractility, and increases the vigor of ventricular fibrillation. It is also used in ventricular standstill in an attempt to generate electrical and mechanical activity. Recommended dose of epinephrine is 0.5 to 1 mg of a 1:10,000 solution. If an I.V. line is unavailable, 1 mg may be given endotracheally. Because of its short duration of action, it may be necessary to repeat the dose at 5-minute intervals. Epinephrine should not be added to an alkaline solution because that may result in inactivation. Depending on the circumstances, lidocaine or bretylium (or both) may be indicated after epinephrine administration. Calcium chloride is no longer recommended as an advanced life-support medication because research studies have shown no therapeutic effects from its use.

56 Correct answer—A

In this situation, the nurse should expect to administer sodium bicarbonate, an extracellular buffer responsible for controlling acid-base balance. During cardiac resuscitation, the body is in a state of ventilatory failure, which leads to respiratory acidosis and circulatory failure. Metabolic acidosis is the result of these events. Efficient lung ventilation is essential to eliminate carbon dioxide and provide adequate oxygenation. The need for therapy must be guided by evaluation of arterial blood gas studies and is appropriate only if metabolic acidosis exists. Sodium bicarbonate is administered at a dose of 1 mEq/kg. Calcium chloride, bretylium, and lidocaine are inappropriate in this situation.

57 Correct answer—B

Lidocaine is the drug of choice after termination of ventricular fibrillation or tachycardia, especially when defibrillation has been used. The use of lidocaine may terminate reentrant activity responsible for ventricular arrhythmias in ischemic zones. A common therapeutic dose is 1 mg/kg as a bolus, followed by a continuous infusion of 2 to 4 mg/minute via an infusion pump. Blood levels of lidocaine should be maintained in the effective suppressive range of 1.5 to 6 mcg/ml; blood levels above 9 mcg/ml may produce toxic effects. Lidocaine is degraded by the liver; the dosage should be reduced in patients with impaired liver function. Digoxin, verapamil hydrochloride (Isoptin), and dopamine are indicated to treat ventricular arrhythmias.

58 Correct answer — D

Bretylium possesses antiarrhythmic effects, adrenergic-blocking properties, and positive inotropic action and is beneficial in terminating ventricular fibrillation and tachycardia refractory to lidocaine. In ventricular fibrillation, 5 mg/kg of undiluted bretylium should be administered I.V. If unsuccessful, the dose can be increased to 10 mg/kg and repeated as needed. Onset of action seems to occur within a few minutes; however, in ventricular tachycardia, it may be delayed up to 20 minutes or more. In the awake patient, the bolus should be diluted and infused over 10 minutes. Bretylium is contraindicated in patients with ventricular tachycardia caused by digitalis toxicity. The most common adverse effects of bretylium are postural hypotension, nausea, and vomiting. Verapamil, calcium chloride, and epinephrine would be inappropriate in this situation.

59 Correct answer — C

The principal use for isoproterenol is in the immediate control of hemodynamically significant, atropine-refractory complete heart block until a pacemaker is made available. Isoproterenol is a pure beta-adrenergic agent possessing positive inotropic and chronotropic properties that increases cardiac output and heart rate. The recommended infusion rate is 2 to 10 mcg/minute titrated to maintain a heart rate of 60 beats/minute. Because of its cardiac-stimulating properties, isoproterenol is contraindicated when tachyarrhythmias are present. Extreme caution must be exercised when the drug is used to treat MI because isoproterenol may enlargen ischemic and infarcted areas. Dopamine, epinephrine, and propranolol hydrochloride (Inderal) are inappropriate in this situation.

60 Correct answer — D

One of the therapeutic effects of propranolol administration is prolonged AV conduction time. Propranolol is used for beta-adrenergic blockade in the treatment of angina pectoris, cardiac arrhythmias, and hypertension. Beta-blockade action is useful in controlling the ventricular response to atrial flutter or fibrillation and in preventing recurrences of paroxysmal supraventricular tachycardia, as it decreases AV conduction. Propranolol also decreases myocardial contractility, which results in decreased myocardial oxygen demand. A decrease in cardiac output would not be a therapeutic effect.

61 Correct answer — A

Dopamine, an endogenous catecholamine, is an important agent to treat various types of shock, such as hypotensive shock, because it directly increases cardiac output and renal blood flow. The hemodynamic effects depend on the dosage. At dosages less than 7 mcg/kg/minute, increases in cardiac output, myocardial contractility, and renal blood flow predominate; little or no vasoconstriction occurs. At dosages higher than 7 mcg/kg/minute, alpha-adrenergic effects predominate, leading to peripheral vasoconstriction and an increase in mean arterial pressure. Dobutamine hydrochloride (Dobutrex), isoproterenol, and epinephrine are inappropriate in this situation.

62 Correct answer — A

Dopamine should be infused through a central line by an infusion pump. This drug is contraindicated in patients with uncontrolled arrhythmias or pheochromocytoma and in those receiving monoamine oxidase inhibitors; it may cause or exacerbate cardiac arrhythmias. At high doses, dopamine increases myocardial oxygen demand and may result in the extension of ischemic areas in those with coronary artery disease.

63 Correct answer — C

Dobutamine is the preferred drug to treat severe heart failure. It produces a greater increase in cardiac output, a lessened increase in heart rate and peripheral vascular resistance, and fewer cardiac arrhythmias than equivalent doses of dopamine. Adverse effects of dobutamine include nausea, headache, dyspnea, and angina. Epinephrine and digoxin increase myocardial oxygen consumption and are therefore inappropriate in treating severe heart failure.

64 Correct answer — A

Adverse effects from the use of I.V. nitroglycerin include headache, methemoglobinemia, bradycardia, and hypotension. Hypotension is the most serious effect and can result in ischemia to organs that are dependent on perfusion pressure, such as the heart, kidneys, and brain. Hypotension can be treated with fluid administration. Bradycardia can be corrected with the use of atropine; continuous infusion is initiated at 10 to 20 mcg/minute and increased by 5 to 10 mcg/minute until desired hemodynamic or clinical results are achieved. Congestive heart failure and ventricular fibrillation are not adverse effects of I.V. nitroglycerin therapy.

65 Correct answer – B

Nitroprusside is a potent vasodilator, decreasing preload and afterload. Rapid infusion of I.V. nitroprusside results in hypotension, apprehension, restlessness, muscle twitching, palpitations, and chest and abdominal pain. Treatment consists of lowering or discontinuing the infusion rate. The dose of nitroprusside should be regulated by an infusion pump because of its potency and rapid onset of action. Thiocyanate levels should be monitored if high doses of nitroprusside are infused for longer than 48 hours. Rapid infusion of this drug does not cause hypertension, bradycardia, dyspnea, arrhythmias, syncope, or vomiting.

66 Correct answer – D

Tissue plasminogen activator (t-PA) (Activase) is indicated in the management of acute MI to dissolve thrombi obstructing coronary arteries, thereby improving blood flow; improve myocardial ventricular function and reduce the incidence of CHF; and limit the size of the infarction.

67 Correct answer – A

T-PA is not contraindicated in patients with abnormal Q waves because the appearance of Q waves does not necessarily indicate completed infarction. Reperfusion arrhythmias, a complication resulting from coronary thrombolysis, may occur within 1 hour after administration of t-PA therapy. These arrhythmias, such as sinus bradycardia, accelerated idioventricular rhythm, PVCs, and ventricular tachycardia, are not different from those often seen in the ordinary course of an acute MI and may be managed with standard antiarrhythmic measures. Lysis of coronary artery thrombi has been documented in 71% of patients treated with t-PA within 6 hours of the onset of symptoms. Because bleeding is the most common complication encountered during t-PA therapy, t-PA is contraindicated for anyone who has had recent (within 10 days) major surgery or who has any condition in which bleeding constitutes a significant hazard.

68 Correct answer – D

T-PA is intended for administration by intravenous infusion only, via a volumetric infusion pump to ensure a precise flow rate. It should be administered in a separate I.V. line with no other medications.

Cardiovascular Emergencies Answers

Heparin may be administered concomitantly with t-PA to reduce the risk of rethrombosis.

69 Correct answer—**D**

Measuring the QT interval is unnecessary because t-PA does not affect this ECG parameter. During t-PA administration, the nurse should closely monitor the patient's ECG tracings for the appearance of reperfusion arrhythmias. The nurse should remain with this patient at all time throughout the procedure to check the patient's neurologic status frequently for signs of hypotension and to inspect his skin for bruising and his urine for blood because of the increased risk of abnormal bleeding.

70 Correct answer—**A**

During the administration of t-PA, a bolus injection of lidocaine followed by an I.V. drip is initiated to help prevent the development of ventricular reperfusion arrhythmias, a common complication of t-PA therapy.

71 Correct answer—**D**

Serial ECG tracings should be monitored throughout the course of t-PA therapy. The nurse would expect to note several ECG changes if the drug has been successful, one of which is the return of ST segments to the isoelectric baseline. If the ischemia is abolished, T waves should return to their normal position. Deep Q waves are evidence of myocardial necrosis. If t-PA has been effective, the extent of myocardial necrosis may be limited; therefore, Q waves should be absent or decreased in size.

72 Correct answer—**D**

In this situation, the nurse would suspect that the patient has suffered a cardiac contusion, which commonly occurs after blunt chest trauma, such as steering wheel injuries. Myocardial edema and hemorrhage result in myocardial ischemia and necrosis. The signs and symptoms of cardiac contusion are similar to those of an MI: chest pain, shortness of breath, ECG changes (ST-segment elevation, T-wave inversion, and Q-wave formation), and cardiac enzyme elevation. However, because the precipitating event is of traumatic, rather than coronary artery, origin, the nurse would not suspect an MI.

73 Correct answer—**B**

The right ventricle is the most common area of damage after a cardiac contusion because it is situated directly behind the sternum.

74 Correct answer — A

Nitroglycerin is not indicated in the treatment of cardiac contusion because the pain is not of coronary artery origin and dilation of the coronary arteries would not relieve it. Morphine sulfate is the analgesic of choice for the pain associated with cardiac contusion. Oxygen should be given to improve the oxygen supply to the damaged myocardium. Lidocaine is indicated in the treatment of ventricular dysrhythmias associated with cardiac contusion.

75 Correct answer — C

The nurse should monitor the patient for development of CHF, one of several complications of cardiac contusion that resulta from damage to the myocardium from edema and microscopic hemorrhage. Other complications include ventricular arrhythmias, pericarditis, cardiac tamponade, and cardiogenic shock.

76 Correct answer — A

Anticoagulants, such as heparin, are contraindicated in cardiac contusion because of the microscopic hemorrhage that occurs after the trauma. Hemopericardium, or bleeding into the pericardium, may result if heparin is administered. Digoxin and dopamine may be indicated if CHF develops. Bretylium or procainamide (Pronestyl) may be indicated if the ventricular arrhythmias are not suppressed by lidocaine.

77 Correct answer — C

During the initial assessment of a patient with pericarditis, the nurse should check for pulsus paradoxus, an exaggeration of the normal physiologic response to inspiration. Further assessment typically reveals a pericardial friction rub; however, this finding does not help in evaluating the severity of the condition. An elevated temperature is not a constant finding. Kussmaul's sign, which is paradoxic inspiratory neck vein filling, is rarely seen in an acute setting. Pericarditis, or inflammation of the pericardial sac, may occur alone or with myocardial inflammation.

78 Correct answer — D

A patient with pericarditis typically exhibits dyspnea and tachypnea. The pain associated with this condition is typically augmented with deep inspiration, trunk rotation, or lying flat. Palliative measures include sitting upright or leaning forward. Pericarditis usually is evidenced by a severe pleuritic substernal chest pain with widespread ST-segment elevation on ECG.

79 Correct answer — A

Treatment for pericarditis involves the use of drug therapy to relieve pain and resolve acute inflammation. Anti-inflammatory drugs, such as aspirin, indomethacin (Indocin), or steroids, are commonly used. If pericarditis results from an infection, antibiotics, such as penicillin, would also be used. In this situation, the patient has a recent history of open-heart surgery; therefore, the pericarditis probably is an autoimmune reaction to pericardial injury, and indomethacin would be prescribed. Acetaminophen has no anti-inflammatory properties.

80 Correct answer — C

Chronic obstructive pulmonary disease is not associated with pericarditis. The causes of pericarditis are multiple. Medical histories include viral infections; inflammatory processes, such as systemic lupus erythematosus, rheumatic fever, and scleroderma; and hypersensitivity or autoimmune responses, such as postmyocardial infarction (Dressler's syndrome). Other causes of pericarditis include certain metabolic disturbances (such as uremia or myxedema), kidney disease, and blunt or penetrating trauma.

81 Correct answer — B

Monitoring ECG tracings for PVCs would be the nurse's lowest priority when assessing a patient with endocarditis because PVCs are rarely associated with infective endocarditis. Most patients with endocarditis present with sudden fever, the most essential feature of this disease, along with septicemia, and CHF. Therefore, priority nursing procedures include monitoring the patient's temperature and assessing for symptoms of CHF, which includes auscultating for S_3 heart sounds and crackles. The patient should be placed on a cardiac monitor for assessment of heart rate because the tachycardia is frequently out of proportion to the patient's temperature.

82 Correct answer — B

The nurse would expect the patient's laboratory studies to show an elevated erythrocyte sedimentation rate, the most common finding in endocarditis. Other common findings include leukocytosis (an increased white blood cell count) and anemia.

83 Correct answer — A

Blood cultures are of prime diagnostic, as well as therapeutic, importance for a patient with endocarditis. Culture specimens from several sites should be obtained as the fever is climbing. Culture media and techniques for identifying fungi and anaerobic bacteria should be used, as should the standard techniques for aerobic strains. Although a nonspecific test, measurement of the erythrocyte sedimentation rate is useful in a negative sense; that is, if the rate is not elevated, a diagnosis of bacterial endocarditis becomes most unlikely.

84 Correct answer—B

A postpartum patient may be predisposed to a venous occlusion, not an acute arterial occlusion. Patients who develop acute arterial occlusion commonly have a medical history that predisposes them to mural thrombi formation. This may occur in rheumatic valvular disease, atrial fibrillation, MI, and previous cardiac surgery, such as prosthetic valve replacement.

85 Correct answer—D

Physical examination of a patient with acute arterial occlusion typically reveals a pale or cyanotic affected extremity that is cold to the touch; nonpalpable pulses distal to the occlusion; paresthesias; and trophic changes, such as thin, shiny, hairless skin. Swelling and tenderness in the affected extremity and a positive Homans' sign are symptoms of a venous occlusion.

86 Correct answer—C

In this situation, administering an infusion of heparin, as ordered, would be an appropriate action. Other appropriate nursing interventions for a patient with acute arterial occlusion include providing warm environmental temperature to relieve arterial spasms (heat is never applied to the extremity) and elevating of the head of the bed or stretcher on 8- to 10-inch (20- to 25-cm) blocks so that gravity will augment flow of blood to the ischemic extremity (the affected extremity should never be elevated).

87 Correct answer—A

The nurse would not anticipate preparing the patient for an arteriovenous shunt. Such a shunt may be surgically placed in a patient requiring hemodialysis. The nurse would anticipate preparing the patient for possible embolectomy, thrombolytic infusion, or extraction of emboli with a balloon-tipped catheter.

CHAPTER 3

Eye, Ear, Nose, and Throat Emergencies

1 A 5-year-old child who recently underwent adenotonsillectomy is brought to the ED because of profuse bleeding from the nose and mouth. The child is weak, pale, tachycardic, and hypotensive. Which nursing action holds the highest priority?

A. Clearing any blood clots from the nose and mouth
B. Placing a postnasal packing
C. Drawing a blood sample for hemoglobin and hematocrit testing and a type and cross-match
D. Administering I.V. lactated Ringer's solution

SITUATION

A 22-year-old woman with a recent history of an upper respiratory tract infection is being examined in the emergency department (ED). She complains of hoarseness that has lasted 3 days, along with pain on speaking, nasal congestion, and dysphagia. Assessment findings reveal a purulent nasal discharge, erythematous posterior oropharynx, and a temperature of 101° F (38.3° C).

Questions 2 to 4 refer to the above situation.

2 Which condition is indicative of the patient's assessment findings?

A. Acute laryngitis
B. Chronic laryngitis
C. Laryngeal carcinoma
D. Vocal cord polyps

3 Which instructions would the nurse include in the discharge plan for this patient?

A. Voice rest, with whispering permitted
B. Complete voice rest
C. Swishing and gargling with an alcohol-based astringent
D. Gargling with aspirin and salt water

4 Which nursing action would be most effective in providing patient comfort?

A. Administering metaproterenol (Alupent)
B. Applying an icebag to the patient's throat
C. Instructing the patient to gargle with an antiseptic solution
D. Instructing the patient to swish and swallow a topical anesthetic solution of lidocaine (Xylocaine) before eating

---

SITUATION

An 18-year-old man arrives at the ED complaining of being suddenly awakened by a feeling of something moving in his ear. On physical examination, the nurse notes a large, live cockroach in his external auditory canal.

Questions 5 and 6 refer to the above situation.

5 The nurse would anticipate the initial treatment for this patient to include:

A. Removing the insect with forceps
B. Spraying lidocaine 10% in the auditory canal
C. Irrigating the ear with warm water
D. Instilling warm mineral oil into the ear

6 After the insect is successfully removed from the ear, subsequent management would include:

A. Administering 500 mg of ampicillin (Amcill) orally to prevent infection
B. Irrigating the ear canal with peroxide and applying a dry, sterile dressing
C. Packing the ear canal with iodoform gauze
D. Instilling antibacterial drops into the ear and packing the ear canal with ¼″ gauze strips

---

SITUATION

A 65-year-old man with a history of chronic obstructive pulmonary disease and laryngeal carcinoma is being examined in the ED. He is currently undergoing radiation therapy and has symptoms of acute respiratory distress. Assessment reveals inspiratory stridor, dyspnea, increasing apprehension, and facial flushing.

Questions 7 and 8 refer to the above situation.

7 The most appropriate nursing action would be to:

A. Obtain samples for arterial blood gas evaluation and administer 100% oxygen via face mask
B. Prepare for a tracheotomy
C. Prepare for intubation
D. Call for a chest X-ray

8 If the immediate action is unsuccessful, the nurse would expect to:

A. Obtain a smaller endotracheal tube
B. Assemble necessary equipment for a tracheotomy
C. Obtain a cricothyroidotomy tray
D. Order an X-ray of the patient's lateral neck

SITUATION

A 40-year-old man is brought to the ED after a mugging incident with blood oozing from his left ear. The physician diagnoses a ruptured tympanic membrane.

Questions 9 and 10 refer to the above situation.

9 The nurse anticipates the initial treatment for this patient to include:

A. Removing blood clots and packing the ear canal
B. Administering antibacterial otic drops
C. Administering 50 mg of ampicillin orally
D. Administering tetanus toxoid

10 During discharge teaching, the nurse would stress the importance of:

A. Gentle nose blowing
B. Avoiding heavy lifting
C. Rinsing the ear canal with warm water daily
D. Retaining packing in the ear canal for 1 week

SITUATION

A 6-year-old child is examined in the ED for complaints of ear pain. She has a 2-day history of itchiness in her ear, diminished hearing, and fever. Her mother informs the physician that the child had been swimming in a public pool during the previous week.

Questions 11 to 16 refer to the above situation.

11 Based on the above findings, which condition would the nurse suspect the child to have?

A. Acute otitis externa
B. Acute otitis media
C. Ruptured tympanic membrane
D. Ear canal cellulitis

Eye, Ear, Nose, and Throat Emergencies Questions

12 The treatment plan for this patient includes all of the following *except:*

A. Administration of acetaminophen (Tylenol)
B. Administration of an oral antibiotic
C. Administration of an otic antibiotic
D. Application of ice packs to the ear

13 The nurse is aware that a patient with acute otitis externa commonly demonstrates:

A. Upper respiratory tract infection
B. An elevated temperature above 102° F (38.9° C)
C. Otalgia
D. Periauricular lymphadenopathy

14 Which otic emergency is more common in children than adults?

A. Acute otitis externa
B. Acute otitis media
C. Ménière's disease
D. Bullous myringitis

15 If otitis media is not treated aggressively, all of the following serious complications may result *except:*

A. Meningitis
B. Ototoxicity
C. Mastoiditis
D. Permanent hearing loss

16 Which procedure is *not* warranted for the patient with acute otitis media?

A. Myringotomy
B. Tympanocentesis
C. Caloric test
D. Blood cultures

SITUATION

A 54-year-old man with a history of alcohol abuse is examined by the triage nurse. He complains of having difficulty breathing through his nose after having fallen the previous night. His symptoms include a lacerated bridge of the nose, periorbital edema, and dried blood in his nares.

Questions 17 to 20 refer to the above situation.

Eye, Ear, Nose, and Throat
Emergencies Questions

17 The most serious cause of this patient's breathing difficulty can be attributed to:

A. Blood clots in the nares
B. Edema of the nose
C. Deviated septum
D. Septal hematoma

18 Which nursing intervention is appropriate in caring for this patient?

A. Asking the patient to blow his nose to help loosen and remove the clot
B. Inserting an intranasal packing
C. Examining the nasal bone for mobility
D. Administering tetanus toxoid, as ordered

19 Treatment for a linear fracture with nasal bleeding may include:

A. Nasal packing and establishment of an I.V. line
B. Administration of a decongestant and a vasoconstrictor
C. Application of a cold pack to the bridge of the nose
D. All of the above

20 Which nursing action is inappropriate for a patient with an anterior epistaxis?

A. Pinching the patient's nose for 4 to 5 minutes
B. Alleviating patient apprehension
C. Placing the patient in a semirecumbent position with his head tilted forward
D. Administering I.V. fluids

SITUATION

A 19-year-old man is brought to the hospital by emergency medical service after an automobile accident. He has multiple facial lacerations, nasal deformity, and cheek flattening, as well as diplopia and difficulty opening his mouth.

Questions 21 to 25 relate to the above situation.

Eye, Ear, Nose, and Throat
Emergencies Questions

21 The nurse suspects that, based on the assessment findings, the patient has a:

A. Mandibular fracture
B. Maxillary fracture
C. Zygomatic fracture
D. Temporomandibular joint dislocation

22 An inappropriate nursing action during the immediate care of this patient would be to:

A. Prepare the patient for definitive treatment of fracture by the physician
B. Observe for potential airway obstruction
C. Assess the patient's level of consciousness
D. Evaluate the patient for cervical or spinal trauma

23 Which nursing action is considered unsafe when assisting the patient to maintain optimal airway clearance?

A. Positioning the patient on his side
B. Inserting a nasopharyngeal airway
C. Placing the patient in semi-Fowler's position
D. Having tracheotomy equipment available

24 After assessment of this patient, which diagnostic procedure would the nurse expect the physician to order?

A. Water's view X-rays
B. Submental-vertex X-rays
C. Cervical spine X-rays
D. All of the above

25 After the patient's condition stabilizes and the physician rules out spinal injury and neurologic deficits, the nurse would expect to ensure the patient's comfort by performing all of the following *except:*

A. Administering narcotics or analgesics, as ordered
B. Positioning the patient with the head of the bed elevated
C. Applying cold compresses to the fracture site
D. Taping the bridge of the patient's nose to stabilize the bones

81

SITUATION

A 25-year-old male carpenter is assessed by the triage nurse. He complains of severe right eye pain, a gritty sensation in the eye, and sensitivity to light. He angrily claims that his symptoms began suddenly while he was hammering a nail and states that he is going to sue his boss.

Questions 26 and 27 refer to the above situation.

26 Which question is of least priority when obtaining a history from this patient?

A. "Describe your visual acuity before this incident; did you have any previous eye disease?"

B. "Were you wearing goggles or glasses and did any damage occur to them?"

C. "What caused the injury, and what was its trajectory and distance to your head?"

D. "Are you currently seeing halos around lights?"

27 Which nursing action would least effectively relieve the patient's pain?

A. Instilling a fluorescein stain

B. Applying topical analgesics

C. Covering the eye with an occlusive patch

D. Irrigating the eye with normal saline solution

SITUATION

A 60-year-old woman is examined by the triage nurse after having sustained blunt trauma to her right eye during a fall. Her only complaint is blurred vision in the right eye. The physician diagnoses hyphema.

Questions 28 to 30 refer to the above situation.

28 Which is the most important information to collect from this patient during the initial assessment?

A. The mechanism of injury

B. The patient's history of ocular disorders

C. The patient's symptoms before her arrival at the ED

D. The patient's use of medications, especially aspirin

Eye, Ear, Nose, and Throat Emergencies Questions

29 Which nursing action should be included in the plan of care for this patient?

A. Maintaining the patient in a supine position
B. Patching the patient's eyes during the acute phase
C. Irrigating the eye frequently with normal saline solution during the acute phase
D. Applying gentle finger massage to the eye

30 Which instruction should *not* be included in patient teaching before discharge?

A. Avoid coughing and performing Valsalva's maneuver
B. Remain on bed rest for 2 weeks
C. Elevate the head of the bed to a 30-degree angle
D. Reduce stress and physical strain

SITUATION

A 29-year-old man is brought to the hospital via ambulance after sustaining a chemical burn to his eyes. He had been involved in a fight during which lye was thrown in his face.

Questions 31 to 33 refer to the above situation.

31 Which nursing action has the *highest* priority for this patient?

A. Checking the pH of the patient's eyes with litmus paper
B. Instilling antibiotic otic drops
C. Flushing the eyes with a sodium bicarbonate solution
D. Continuously irrigating the eyes with copious amounts of normal saline solution

32 All of the following statements regarding chemical burns of the eye are true *except:*

A. Alkaline burns are the most destructive
B. Acid burns are extremely irritating
C. An acid substance continues to dissolve soft tissue in the eye until it is removed
D. The principles of management for alkaline and acid burns are similar

33 What is the best indication that treatment has been effective for this patient?

A. Slight evidence of corneal whitening
B. A pH value of 7.0 on a litmus paper reading
C. Extraocular movements
D. Visual acuity limited to light perception

Answer Sheet

	A	B	C	D			A	B	C	D
1	○	○	○	○		31	○	○	○	○
2	○	○	○	○		32	○	○	○	○
3	○	○	○	○		33	○	○	○	○
4	○	○	○	○						
5	○	○	○	○						
6	○	○	○	○						
7	○	○	○	○						
8	○	○	○	○						
9	○	○	○	○						
10	○	○	○	○						
11	○	○	○	○						
12	○	○	○	○						
13	○	○	○	○						
14	○	○	○	○						
15	○	○	○	○						
16	○	○	○	○						
17	○	○	○	○						
18	○	○	○	○						
19	○	○	○	○						
20	○	○	○	○						
21	○	○	○	○						
22	○	○	○	○						
23	○	○	○	○						
24	○	○	○	○						
25	○	○	○	○						
26	○	○	○	○						
27	○	○	○	○						
28	○	○	○	○						
29	○	○	○	○						
30	○	○	○	○						

Eye, Ear, Nose, and Throat Emergencies Answer Sheet

1 Correct answer — **A**

Bleeding after adenotonsillectomy must be treated with utmost urgency. Priority action always includes clearing any blood clots from the nose and mouth to ensure a patent airway. I.V. fluids, such as lactated Ringer's or normal saline solution, should be started promptly because children become hypovolemic much faster than adults, and the patient must be ready to go to the operating room immediately. Tonsillar sponges may be used to apply pressure to the tonsils, but a physician must place postnasal packing to control adenoidal bleeding.

2 Correct answer — **A**

A recent history of an upper respiratory tract infection, hoarseness, fever, and erythematous oropharynx are indicative of acute laryngitis. Patients with vocal cord polyps have hoarseness but no upper respiratory tract infection, whereas those with laryngeal cancer may have hoarseness and difficulty breathing only if the lesion is large. Laryngeal cancer usually occurs in older men with a long history of smoking and alcohol abuse.

3 Correct answer — **B**

Treatment for acute laryngitis involves complete voice rest, with no whispering permitted. Smoking, alcohol, and aspirin may cause further irritation, inflammation, edema, and pain; therefore, gargling with an alcohol-based astringent or a mixture of aspirin and salt water is never recommended. Saline solution gargles and topical anesthetics, however, may be helpful.

4 Correct answer — **B**

The most effective comfort measure for the patient with acute laryngitis is the application of an icebag to the throat. Metaproterenol (Alupent) treatments and antiseptic gargles are inappropriate. Swishing and swallowing an anesthetic solution before eating is unsafe because aspiration may occur.

5 Correct answer — **B**

Recent studies indicate that insects may be removed from the ear by spraying a topical neurostimulant, such as lidocaine, into the external auditory canal. If this is unavailable, the insect should be immobilized and drowned in mineral oil, then removed with minute forceps. Irrigation with water may cause the insect's body to swell or may push the insect closer to the tympanic membrane.

Eye, Ear, Nose, and Throat
Emergencies Answers

6 Correct answer—**D**

Subsequent management would include instilling antibacterial drops into the ear and packing the ear canal with ¼″ gauze strips. Because insects are potential disease carriers, a topical otic antibiotic may be used prophylactically to prevent infection caused by bites or scratches. Attempts to remove foreign objects from the ear produce trauma, which may result in further swelling and even bleeding of the ear canal walls. Bleeding may be controlled by a light packing of gauze strips. Oral antibiotics and iodoform gauze are unnecessary.

7 Correct answer—**C**

The most appropriate nursing action would be to prepare the patient for immediate intubation to establish an airway. Patients undergoing radiation therapy to the head and neck are subject to complications, including edema of the upper airway, severe dryness of the oral cavity, and skin burns. Arterial blood gas studies are not an immediate priority in this situation. A patient with chronic obstructive pulmonary disease should not receive 100% oxygen. Administration of oxygen higher than 30% is contraindicated in a patient with COPD, as the patient breathes on an oxygen drive and higher levels would decrese the respiratory rate. Tracheotomy should not be performed in a patient with laryngeal cancer because this may lead to stomal carcinoma via direct extension of the tumor.

8 Correct answer—**C**

If the immediate action, intubation, is unsuccessful, the next step would be to obtain a cricothyroidotomy tray for an emergency cricothyroidotomy. This procedure is indicated when the patient's edema or tumor is so great that an endotracheal tube cannot be passed initially and subsequent attempts would cause further swelling.

9 Correct answer—**A**

When a patient has a ruptured tympanic membrane and basal skull fracture has been ruled out, bleeding from the ear may be controlled by removing blood clots and packing the ear canal. The packing may be removed when bleeding has stopped. Tympanic membrane rupture does not require antibiotics; a healthy exposed middle ear mucosa is especially vulnerable to ototoxicity from ear drops. The tympanic membrane should heal in 1 to 2 weeks.

10 Correct answer — B

During discharge teaching, the patient must be encouraged to avoid heavy lifting and straining from Valsalva's maneuver for 1 to 2 weeks. Other activities to avoid include nose blowing, swimming, and any activity that might involve exposing the ear canal to water. Packing should be retained in the ear canal until the bleeding has stopped.

11 Correct answer — A

Swimming in a public pool is a common source of contamination, especially for the ears, producing an inflammatory disorder of the auricle and external auditory canal known as acute otitis externa. It is most commonly caused by bacterial or fungal infections, particularly *Pseudomonas.* Predisposing factors include moisture in the ear canal, which may occur in a warm, moist climate or as a result of swimming, and trauma resulting from attempts to clean or scratch an itchy ear.

12 Correct answer — D

Applying ice packs to the ear is inappropriate in this situation. Appropriate treatment includes administering analgesics, antibiotics (oral, otic, or topical), and antipyretics and applying hot, moist compresses to the affected ear.

13 Correct answer — D

Periauricular lymphadenopathy is a common manifestation in patients with acute otitis externa. A history of an upper respiratory tract infection, a temperature of 102° F (38.8° C) or higher, and otalgia that increases with prone position are manifestations of acute otitis media.

14 Correct answer — B

Acute otitis media is more common in children than adults because of children's narrower eustachian tubes, which are prone to occlusion. The condition is commonly preceded by an upper respiratory tract infection or childhood disease, such as measles or scarlet fever. This is because of the proximity and connection of the eustachian tube to the upper respiratory tract.

15 Correct answer — B

Ototoxicity is an adverse reaction to salicylates or antibiotics, such as kanamycin (Kantrex) and streptomycin; it is not a complication of otitis media. Common complications that result when otitis media is

Eye, Ear, Nose, and Throat
Emergencies Answers

not treated aggressively include meningitis, mastoiditis, intracranial abscess, and permanent hearing loss.

16 Correct answer — C

The caloric test is used in neurologic examinations to assess cranial nerve function and is not warranted for a patient with acute otitis media. The procedures usually performed for such a patient include pneumatic otoscopy, hearing test, and blood cultures if the patient's temperature is 102.2° F (39° C) or higher. Tympanocentesis, aspiration of the middle ear, may be required for effusion, and myringotomy may be performed if the tympanic membrane is bulging.

17 Correct answer — D

In nasal trauma, a collection of blood develops under the septal mucosa, forming a septal hematoma — a bulging mass that causes serious breathing difficulty in both nares. Blood clots in the nares, edema of the nose, and a deviated septum also may cause breathing difficulty, but these are less serious conditions.

18 Correct answer — D

Because the patient sustained a nasal laceration, the appropriate nursing action would be to administer a tetanus toxoid, a routine precaution for any open wound. Further treatment involves cleaning the nose with such agents as povidone-iodine solution and peroxide, followed by an irrigation with normal saline solution. Before applying intranasal packing or blowing the nose, cerebrospinal fluid (CSF) rhinorrhea must be ruled out. This is accomplished by observing for drainage from the nose and testing any drainage for glucose (60% of CSF is serum glucose).

19 Correct answer — D

Treatment for a linear nasal facture with nasal bleeding includes packing the nasal cavity, establishing an I.V. line, administering decongestants and vasoconstrictors, and applying cold packs to the bridge of the nose to decrease bleeding. Establishing an I.V. line is necessary to infuse fluids because of lost blood volume.

20 Correct answer — D

Administering I.V. fluids to a patient with an anterior epistaxis would be inappropriate. Active bleeding from an anterior epistaxis can be controlled temporarily by pinching the nose for 4 to 5 minutes. If bleeding persists, cauterization with silver nitrate sticks or electrocautery should be attempted. If bleeding still is not controlled, the physician will anesthetize the nasal chamber and insert nasal packing. Whenever nasal packing of any sort is used, the patient should be placed on broad-spectrum antibiotics until packs are removed. Alleviating the patient's apprehension and placing the patient in a semirecumbent position with his head tilted forward are appropriate measures.

21 Correct answer—C

Nasal deformity, cheek flattening, difficulty in opening the mouth, and diplopia most likely indicate a zygomatic fracture. This type of facial fracture is associated with asymmetry of the face, painful jaw movement, limited movement of lower jaw, and visual disturbances. Zygomatic fractures are most commonly caused by automobile accidents and fights and are frequently associated with orbital floor fractures, also referred to as "blow-out fractures."

22 Correct answer—A

The immediate management of a patient who sustained a zygomatic fracture would not include preparation for definitive treatment of the fracture by a physician. Definitive treatment may require semi-open reduction, open reduction, or internal wire fixation, which may be performed later. Appropriate immediate nursing actions aim to maintain a patent airway by examining for potential obstruction from blood clots, saliva, and loose teeth. The nurse should also assess the patient's level of consciousness to establish a baseline by which deterioration in neurologic status from associated head trauma can be recognized. The patient also should be evaluated for possible cervical or spinal trauma. Subsequent actions include controlling bleeding from facial lacerations and applying cold compresses to prevent facial edema. Prompt application of compresses will permit fractures to be tended sooner.

23 Correct answer—B

Nursing interventions to ensure airway patency are of the utmost importance in a patient with a zygomatic fracture. However, the insertion of a nasopharyngeal airway is inappropriate and unsafe in such a patient because of the risk of further trauma and bleeding. Appropriate interventions include placing the patient in a side-lying or semi-Fowler's position for optimal airway clearance and having emergency suction equipment on hand. Aspiration of teeth, bony fragments, blood clots, and vomitus must be prevented. Emergency intubation or tracheotomy equipment should also be accessible to ensure the immediate establishment of an airway, if necessary.

Eye, Ear, Nose, and Throat
Emergencies Answers

24 Correct answer—D

Diagnostic procedures are essential for determining the extent of injuries and formulating a plan of care based on the patient's needs. Water's view X-rays permit evaluation of malar or zygoma eminence, and submental-vertex view permits evaluation of the zygomatic arch. Cervical spine X-rays, which are in many cases neglected because the facial deformities are not striking, must be obtained to evaluate fractures or dislocations that may result from the trauma.

25 Correct answer—D

Taping the bridge of the patient's nose is not indicated. Appropriate interventions to ensure patient comfort include administering narcotics or analgesics as ordered, elevating the head of the bed, and applying cold compresses to the fracture site to decrease edema.

26 Correct answer—D

Asking the patient whether he sees halos around lights is the least important information to elicit at this time. This symptom usually is associated with glaucoma, not extraocular foreign body emergencies. Because this type of trauma may be associated with future compensation, the nurse must conduct a comprehensive interview. Information obtained must include the time elapsed since the occurrence; the circumstances of the injury; the type and condition of safety apparatus worn at the time of injury; treatment before arrival; the patient's medical history, including his current medications, the date of his last tetanus immunization, any known allergies, and his visual status before the accident; and the time the patient last took any food or fluid by mouth.

27 Correct answer—A

Instilling a fluorescein stain into the eye is a diagnostic procedure; it would be the least effective measure to relieve the patient's pain. Effective pain-relief interventions include irrigating the eye gently with a normal saline solution and applying topical analgesics. Photosensitivity is common in ocular injuries; therefore, the eye should be covered with an occlusive patch.

28 Correct answer—D

The most important information to collect from the patient during the initial interview is the patient's use of medications, especially aspirin. Hyphema is a condition in which the blood vessels in the iris bleed into the anterior chamber of the eye. Prior use of any medications that may increase bleeding and decrease clotting time must be known; if bleeding is not minimized, severe ocular problems and loss of vision may ensue. Other important information to gather during the interview includes the nature of the specific injury; the mechanism by which the injury occurred; the time elapsed since the occurrence; the patient's symptoms and treatment before arrival in the ED; any changes in the patient's clinical status, such as visual changes; the patient's description of the pain; and the patient's history of ocular disorders.

29 Correct answer — B

Patching the patient's eyes during the acute phase is part of the initial treatment for a patient with hyphema. To minimize recurrent bleeding, the patient's activities are restricted. Typically, the patient is put on bed rest in a semi-Fowler's position, with bathroom privileges only. Sedation may be given judiciously. Hyphema usually clears in 5 to 6 days.

30 Correct answer — B

Discharge teaching for the patient with hyphema would not include remaining on bed rest for 2 weeks, as this has no therapeutic importance. Appropriate discharge instructions would include telling the patient to avoid coughing and performing the Valsalva's maneuver because these activities increase intraocular pressure, to maintain the head of the bed at a 30-degree angle to decrease intraocular pressure, and to try to reduce stress and physical strain during the recovery period.

31 Correct answer — D

The highest priority in this situation would be to continuously irrigate the eyes with copious amounts of normal saline solution, preferably with a continuous irrigation setup. Checking the pH of the eye with litmus paper and instilling antibiotic drops are appropriate after complete irrigation. Steroids are also applied after irrigation, to reduce local inflammation. Flushing the eyes with sodium bicarbonate is inappropriate because of the bicarbonate's alkalinity.

32 Correct answer — C

An acid substance does not continue to dissolve soft tissue in the eye until it is removed. Acid chemicals cause a coagulation necrosis of the cornea; the extent of damage to the eye is limited by the coagulation formed in the process. Alkaline burns are the most destructive and are therefore considered an ocular emergency. The most destructive chemicals to enter the eye are alkaline substances, which include lye, ammonia, and plaster. Alkaline chemicals cause necrosis of the

Eye, Ear, Nose, and Throat
Emergencies Answers

conjunctiva and cornea, which will continue to react with ocular tissues, producing severe damage. All traces of the chemical must be removed to halt its corrosive action. Acid burns are usually not as devastating to the eye as are alkaline burns. Similar principles of management apply to alkaline and acid burns of the eye.

33 Correct answer—B

A pH value of 7.0 on a litmus paper reading is the best indication that treatment has been effective. This finding verifies adequate irrigation and absence of chemical in the eye. Whitening of the cornea and visual acuity limited to light perception result from ocular tissue damage, which produces varied degrees of vision loss.

Eye, Ear, Nose, and Throat
Emergencies Answers

CHAPTER 4

Environmental Emergencies

1 A patient is brought to the emergency department (ED) complaining of burning, tingling, and numbness of the fingers of both hands after an afternoon of shoveling snow. On examination, the nurse notes that the tissue is soft and the fingers fail to "pink up" after blanching. These assessment findings are characteristic of which condition?

A. Raynaud's phenomenon
B. Superficial frostbite
C. Deep frostbite
D. Chilblains

2 When planning the care of a hypothermic patient, the nurse should keep in mind that the major areas of heat loss from the body are the:

A. Hands and feet
B. Head and back of the neck
C. Head and chest
D. Exposed chest and abdomen

SITUATION

A 38-year-old man who spent the night in a snowbank after becoming intoxicated from alcohol is brought to the ED. He is conscious and protesting. The fingers of both hands, the toes of both feet, and both ears are whitish yellow, cold, and solid to the touch. His rectal temperature is 92° F (33.3° C).

Questions 3 to 6 refer to the above situation.

3 The nurse knows that frostbite is a traumatic condition caused by ice crystals forming and expanding in the:

A. Extracellular space
B. Intracellular space
C. Intravascular space
D. Subcutaneous tissues

4 The burned appearance of frostbitten tissue is a sign of:

A. Tissue destruction by the ice crystals
B. Histamine release with decreased capillary permeability
C. Red blood cell (RBC) aggregation and microvascular occlusion
D. Rewarming

5 Which nursing intervention would be most appropriate to rewarm frostbitten digits?

A. Giving the patient alcohol to promote vasodilation
B. Rubbing the affected areas with crushed ice to promote circulation
C. Allowing the digits to thaw indoors, spontaneously and gradually
D. Rewarming the digits rapidly in a water bath at 100° to 105° F (38° to 40.5° C)

6 Which information should be included in the discharge teaching for a patient with frostbite?

A. Smoking is permissible
B. Children and elderly people are at a lower risk for frostbite
C. Any insulating effect is diminished when clothing becomes wet
D. The new insulating fabrics, such as those in a down jacket, are better than multiple clothing layers

SITUATION

A woman is brought to the ED by her husband. She had been burned when a pot of boiling water spilled down the front of her body. The patient weighs 120 lb (54.4 kg).

Questions 7 to 15 refer to the above situation.

7 Which nursing action would be inappropriate for this patient?

A. Removing all of the patient's jewelry
B. Removing the patient's wet clothing and covering her with sterile towels
C. Flushing the burned areas with cool water
D. Applying ice to the burned areas

8 After ensuring airway patency, obtaining baseline vital signs, and establishing an I.V. of lactated Ringer's solution, the patient's condition stabilizes. Because airway obstruction may still occur, the nurse must assess frequently for airway patency. How long after injury should frequent airway assessments be made?

A. 12 hours
B. 24 hours
C. 36 hours
D. 48 hours

9 Admission assessment of this patient shows first- and second-degree (partial-thickness) and third-degree (full-thickness) burns over one half the anterior chest and abdomen, the perineal area, and the anterior aspect of both legs and feet. Based on the Rule of Nines, the closest estimate of total body-surface area (BSA) involved would be:

A. 18%
B. 28%
C. 40%
D. 50%

10 Which solution would the nurse most expect to be used during the first 24 hours to prevent hypovolemic shock in a severely burned patient?

A. Dextrose 5% in water
B. Colloid
C. Lactated Ringer's
D. Normal saline

11 Based on the standard fluid replacement formula, approximately how much fluid should the patient receive over the first 24 hours?

A. 2,460 ml
B. 6,100 ml
C. 13,400 ml
D. 61,100 ml

12 Which parameter is commonly used as a guideline for adequate fluid replacement?

A. Half the fluid should be given in the first 8 hours
B. Airway should be patent after 24 hours
C. Urine output should be between 30 and 50 ml/hour
D. Pulse rate should be less than 100 beats/minute

13 After the shock phase of a burn injury, the capillaries seal and electrolytes remobilize with the fluid. At this time, the nurse should assess the laboratory results for:

A. Elevated hematocrit (hemoconcentration)
B. Elevated red blood cell count and hypokalemia
C. Hypernatremia and hypokalemia
D. Hyponatremia and hyperkalemia

14 Which statement best describes the rationale for keeping this patient from ingesting food or liquids (NPO status) while in the ED?

A. A danger of esophageal edema exists because of the burn injury
B. Keeping the patient NPO will prevent aspiration from nausea and vomiting
C. Burn patients are prone to developing paralytic ileus
D. Keeping the patient NPO will prevent bowel infarction

15 Cold, pain, apprehension, and septic episodes potentiate a catabolic state in the burn patient. The nursing care plan should address appropriate nutritional support, which requires large amounts of:

A. Sodium
B. Lipids
C. Protein
D. Glucose

SITUATION

A 72-year-old man is admitted to the ED after an automobile accident. He had been trapped in the wreckage for 3 hours; the air temperature was 30° F (-1° C). Although his fingers and toes were not frostbitten, he is stuporous. His pulse rate is 52 beats/minute; his respiratory rate, 8 breaths/minute. His core temperature is 81° F (27.2° C).

Questions 16 to 22 refer to the above situation.

16 Elderly people are at risk for hypothermia because of:

A. Impaired hypothalamic function
B. Impaired thyroid function
C. Impaired circulation
D. Higher use of vasoactive medications

17 An appropriate nursing diagnosis for this patient would be:

A. Fluid volume excess related to increased antidiuretic hormone secretion
B. Decreased cardiac output related to impaired myocardial contractility and risk of arrhythmias
C. Decreased cardiac output related to hypermetabolic state
D. Potential fluid volume deficit related to hemorrhage

18 Which statement regarding hypothermia is *false?*

A. The myocardium is depressed and irritable, which may cause arrhythmias

B. Decreased retention of water and sodium causes generalized dehydration (cold diuresis)

C. Insulin release is increased

D. Hepatic function (for example, handling of substrates or drugs) is altered

19 Which of the following would *not* be indicated for this patient?

A. Electrocardiographic monitoring, taking core temperature and urine output measurements, and performing a neurologic check

B. Warming I.V. fluids, checking the blood pressure frequently, and monitoring arterial blood gas measurements

C. Monitoring serum electrolyte and glucose measurements

D. Repositioning the patient frequently to enhance rewarming

20 Which body temperature extremes are compatible with human life?

A. 77° to 113° F (25° to 45° C)

B. 78.8° to 108° F (26° to 42.2° C)

C. 87.8° to 104° F (31° to 40° C)

D. 89.6° to 105.8° F (32° to 41° C)

21 After treatment is initiated, the nurse evaluates the hypothermic patient for afterdrop or afterfall, which refers to:

A. Drooping of the fingers or toes after rewarming

B. Temporary gait impairment after rewarming of the lower extremities

C. Continued drop of core temperature after the cause of hypothermia has been removed

D. Microcirculatory sludging, which may result in renal or hepatic failure

22 Which rewarming method is least effective for a hypothermic patient?

A. Applying hypothermia blankets to the entire body

B. Administering warm peritoneal dialysis

C. Administering warm enemas and I.V. infusions

D. Administering warm saturated oxygen

SITUATION

The nurse has just received word that the rescue team is about to arrive with a victim of radiation exposure who has associated injuries.

Questions 23 to 29 refer to the above situation.

23 In preparation for the patient's arrival, which nursing action should be performed?

A. The hospital probably has no established procedure because of the rarity of radiation exposure; therefore, the best action would be to protect other patients and personnel from exposure as best as possible

B. Prepare any available treatment room to isolate the patient, and cover the floor with newspaper or nonskid plastic

C. Notify maintenance to shut off the air circulation system to any one available treatment area and to cover the floor in that room with nonskid plastic

D. Notify maintenance to shut off the air circulation system; use only a room with a lead-lined shield or an X-ray room; and gather the following equipment: Geiger counter, water, scrub brushes, soap, lead-lined containers for disposal, dosimeters, and protective garb for personnel who will care for the patient

24 Which nursing intervention should be done after the patient arrives in the ED and his breathing and circulation have been stabilized?

A. Remove all of the patient's clothing and jewelry, disposing of them properly; scrub the patient with soap and water

B. Assess the amount of external radiation with a Geiger counter; if radiation is detected, cover the patient with a plastic sheet and move him to the treatment room

C. Assess and treat any serious associated injuries

D. Debride open wounds or radiation burns

25 Which patient is *least* likely to have been exposed to radiation?

A. A cancer patient complaining of fatigue, vomiting, and diarrhea

B. A firefighter who suffered smoke inhalation 2 days ago during a warehouse fire and now complains of vomiting

C. A nuclear power plant worker who complains of weakness and epistaxis but who was not involved in a plant accident

D. A 55-year-old female bank employee with fever, chills, and malaise

26 Which finding would the nurse expect to occur in a patient exposed to 100 to 2,000 rad?

A. Tremors
B. Nausea and vomiting
C. Convulsions
D. Death

27 After the decontamination process, the Geiger counter readings show no reduction in the amount of external radiation. The nurse would interpret these findings to mean that:

A. The patient may have internal contamination
B. Convulsions and death will soon follow
C. This is a common and normal reaction
D. The patient should receive additional body scrubs

28 After radiation exposure, leukopenia and thrombocytopenia may be detected:

A. Immediately
B. Anywhere from 1 to 5 weeks after exposure, depending on the amount of exposure
C. 2 months after exposure
D. None of the above

29 Which two nursing diagnoses would be appropriate for a patient with leukopenia and thrombocytopenia?

A. Potential for infection related to diminished immunity and Potential for fluid volume deficit related to bleeding
B. Impaired gas exchange related to decreased oxygen-carrying capacity of the blood and Altered microcirculatory tissue perfusion related to enhanced coagulation
C. Decreased cardiac output related to impaired myocardial contractility and Potential for injury related to seizures
D. Altered cerebral tissue perfusion related to thrombotic event and Potential for injury related to seizures

SITUATION

The nurse is assessing several patients in the ED who had attended or participated in an annual Fourth of July marathon. The physician diagnoses heatstroke.

Questions 30 to 34 refer to the above situation.

30 Which finding would the nurse expect when assessing a patient with heatstroke?

A. Anxiety
B. Elevated temperature above 106° F (41.1° C)
C. Blood pressure of 160/110 mm Hg
D. Respiratory rate of 8 breaths/minute

31 The nurse assesses two runners and an 83-year-old man who had been observing the race; all of them have signs and symptoms of heatstroke. Which differences would the nurse expect to note between the runners and the elderly man?

A. The runners will continue to sweat
B. The runners' skin will be hot and flushed
C. The runners will have bradycardia
D. The runners will have lower temperatures than the elderly man

32 Which laboratory finding would the nurse expect for a patient with heatstroke?

A. Elevated serum glucose
B. Low serum blood urea nitrogen
C. Respiratory acidosis
D. Elevated hematocrit

33 All of the following nursing interventions are appropriate in caring for a patient with heatstroke *except:*

A. Applying ice packs to the axillae and groin
B. Instituting measures to prevent shivering
C. Stopping all cooling measures when the patient's body temperature reaches 100° F (37.8° C)
D. Instituting ice baths

34 The nurse explains to one runner how to prevent heatstroke when participating in future marathons. Which response indicates that the patient understands the information given?

A. "Running in the rain is good because it will keep me cool"
B. "I should keep hydrated by drinking beer before the race"
C. "I should run shorter distances in the same weather for several days before the race so that my body is prepared"
D. "I should try to run sprints during the race so that I don't have to run so long"

Answer Sheet

	A B C D		A B C D
1	○ ○ ○ ○	31	○ ○ ○ ○
2	○ ○ ○ ○	32	○ ○ ○ ○
3	○ ○ ○ ○	33	○ ○ ○ ○
4	○ ○ ○ ○	34	○ ○ ○ ○
5	○ ○ ○ ○		
6	○ ○ ○ ○		
7	○ ○ ○ ○		
8	○ ○ ○ ○		
9	○ ○ ○ ○		
10	○ ○ ○ ○		
11	○ ○ ○ ○		
12	○ ○ ○ ○		
13	○ ○ ○ ○		
14	○ ○ ○ ○		
15	○ ○ ○ ○		
16	○ ○ ○ ○		
17	○ ○ ○ ○		
18	○ ○ ○ ○		
19	○ ○ ○ ○		
20	○ ○ ○ ○		
21	○ ○ ○ ○		
22	○ ○ ○ ○		
23	○ ○ ○ ○		
24	○ ○ ○ ○		
25	○ ○ ○ ○		
26	○ ○ ○ ○		
27	○ ○ ○ ○		
28	○ ○ ○ ○		
29	○ ○ ○ ○		
30	○ ○ ○ ○		

1 Correct answer—**B**

Burning, tingling, and numbness of digits that are soft and fail to "pink up" after blanching are signs and symptoms of superficial frostbite. Deep frostbite is characterized by whitish tissue that is cold and solid to the touch and that turns pink or purplish blue and causes pain. Blisters typically form after thawing. Raynaud's phenomenon is characterized by intermittent attacks of pallor and cyanosis after exposure to cold or emotional stimuli. Chilblains, which results from intermittent exposure to temperatures ranging from 33° to 60° F (1° to 15° C), is characterized by edematous tissue with reddish-blue patches that itch and burn.

2 Correct answer—**B**

The major areas of heat loss from the body are the head and the back of the neck because of the large amount of blood flowing near the surface of these areas. The other areas mentioned are considered minor areas of heat loss.

3 Correct answer—**A**

Frostbite occurs when ice crystals enlarge in the extracellular space, compressing the cells and resulting in cell membrane rupture.

4 Correct answer—**C**

As ice crystals enlarge and cells rupture, enzymatic and metabolic activity becomes interrupted. Such interruption results in histamine release and increased capillary permeability with resultant red blood cell aggregation and microvascular occlusion, which causes the burned appearance of frostbitten tissue. Rewarming frostbitten tissue has nothing to do with its burned appearance.

5 Correct answer—**D**

The treatment of choice for rewarming frostbitten digits is rapid rewarming in a water bath, no warmer than 106° F (41° C). No mechanical friction, such as rubbing, should be used, nor should the affected part touch the bottom of the basin. Analgesics may be used to control pain. Nurses should use sterile technique, administer tetanus prophylaxis, and provide a bed cradle to prevent pressure and friction, as thawed tissue is extremely sensitive to trauma and infection. Giving the patient alcohol, rubbing the affected areas with crushed ice, and allowing the digits to thaw spontaneously and gradually are inappropriate measures that were formerly used but found to be ineffective in preserving tissue.

6 Correct answer – **C**

When preparing discharge teaching for a patient with frostbite, the nurse should mention that cold conduction is enhanced by wet clothing and that any insulating effect is diminished when clothing becomes wet. The patient should be warned to take extra garments whenever he expects to be in the cold for an extended period. Multiple layers of clothing offer more effective insulation than a single garment, even a down jacket. Smoking causes peripheral vasoconstriction, resulting in decreased blood flow. Vasoconstriction promotes the development of frostbite because blood is less available to keep the extremities warm. Children, with a smaller body mass, and elderly persons with peripheral vascular disease are at increased risk for frostbite.

7 Correct answer – **D**

Applying ice to already compromised tissue would be inappropriate because this could cause frostbite. Appropriate nursing actions in a burn situation would be to remove all of the patient's jewelry as soon as possible and to cover the patient with sterile towels or sheets to conserve heat that is paradoxically lost from damaged microcirculation. Covering burned areas also protects exposed nerves and minimizes the risk of wound infection. Flushing the burned areas with cool water may be necessary if the skin is still hot from the burn or from hot jewelry.

8 Correct answer – **D**

Frequent airway assessments are necessary during the first 48 hours after injury. Although a burn victim may not suffer mechanical airway obstruction as a result of the burn, the patient will have edema as fluid shifts from plasma to the interstitial spaces. This shifting occurs because of endothelial cellular swelling and disruption of the capillaries, which allows escape of colloidal and isotonic fluid. Fluids must be replaced during the first 24 to 48 hours to prevent hypovolemic shock. Such fluid replacement can add to the edema, thereby decreasing lung compliance. After about 48 hours, a burn patient enters the diuretic phase, characterized by increased urine output and decreased edema, and the danger of airway obstruction decreases. If burn injuries occur in an enclosed environment, the toxic products of combustion can cause deterioration of pulmonary function.

9 Correct answer – **B**

Using the Rule of Nines, a method of estimating the body-surface area (BSA) of a burn patient in which the total BSA equals 100%, the estimated area of involvement would be 28%: the anterior chest and abdominal area is 18% , so one half equals 9%; the perineal area equals 1%; the anterior aspect of one full leg is 9%, so two legs equal 18%.

10 Correct answer—C

Lactated Ringer's solution, which contains no dextrose and closely approximates the composition of extracellular fluid, should be infused during the first 24 hours after a severe burn injury. In the severely burned patient, dextrose significantly increases the blood glucose level and produces osmotic diuresis. Normal saline solution may be used selectively in patients with electrolyte imbalances. Colloids are not used at this stage except in small children or in patients with burns covering 50% of BSA, because the albumin will leak into the tissue.

11 Correct answer—B

Using the standard fluid replacement formula, the approximate amount of fluid that a 120 lb (54.4 kg) patient should receive is 6,100 ml. The standard fluid replacement formula is:

4 ml lactated Ringer's × body weight (kg) × % BSA burned
= the amount of fluid given in 24 hours.

Therefore:

4 ml × 54.4 kg × 28 = 6,093 or 6,100 ml.

12 Correct answer—C

A urine output of 30 to 50 ml/hour is the parameter commonly used as a guideline for adequate fluid replacement. Because evaporative losses from wounds are difficult to estimate, fluid replacement is titrated so that the patient achieves a serum sodium level of 135 to 145 mEq/liter, a urine output of 30 to 50 ml/hour, a pulse rate between 60 and 140 beats/minute, a systolic blood pressure between 100 and 140 mm Hg, and a clear sensorium. The goal is to perfuse vital organs as fully as possible without overloading the circulatory system and causing cardiac and respiratory complications. Half the fluid usually is given over the first 8 hours; however, this does not always indicate adequate fluid placement. A patent airway and a pulse rate under 100 beats/minute do not reflect adequate fluid status.

13 Correct answer—C

After the initial shock phase of a burn injury, the nurse should assess for hypernatremia and hypokalemia. Hypernatremia can result because interstitial fluid, with its high sodium content, now shifts intravascularly, resulting in evaporative losses at the wound site. Hypokalemia occurs because of potassium losses incurred from damaged tissue and destroyed RBCs along with the selective renal excretion of potassium that occurs with high aldosterone levels. Hemoconcentration and sludging of RBCs occur with the early fluid shift to interstitial tissues, resulting in decreased intravascular volume and slowed blood flow. Hemodilution occurs with a drop in hematocrit and RBC count.

14 Correct answer – C

Patients with massive burns frequently develop gastric distention and paralytic ileus from the stress of the injury; therefore, the patient should be prevented from ingesting food or liquids (NPO status) while in the ED. A nasogastric tube should be inserted, and gastric output should be measured and recorded. The aspirate should be checked for occult blood, and pH should be measured every 2 hours. Cimetidine (Tagamet) or ranitidine (Zantac) may be ordered. A sliding-scale antacid coverage may be ordered for a gastric pH less than 5.0. If the pH is 3.0, then 60 ml of an antacid is given; if pH is 4.0, then 30 ml of an antacid is given.

15 Correct answer – C

Nutritional support for a burn patient requires large amounts of protein. Extensive burns produce a hypermetabolic response, which increases caloric and protein requirements to two and one-half times the patient's preburn state. A positive nitrogen balance is maintained by an intake of 6,000 to 10,000 calories per day, depending on the burn size and the presence of any associated trauma. Sodium may need to be replaced as needed. Lipids usually are administered once daily to maintain adequate fat intake. Glucose is necessary for caloric intake to prevent further protein breakdown.

16 Correct answer – A

Elderly people have impaired hypothalamic function, presumably because of atherosclerotic changes. They are at risk for hypothermia even without any predisposing causes, such as impaired thyroid function or circulation, or the use of vasoactive medications.

17 Correct answer – B

An appropriate nursing diagnosis for this patient would be *Decreased cardiac output related to impaired myocardial contractility and risk of arrhythmias* because ventricular tachycardia and fibrillation are common arrhythmias in hypothermic patients. The other nursing diagnoses would be inappropriate because the patient is more at risk for fluid volume deficit than overload because of sodium and water loss; however, he has no evidence of trauma and is not at risk for hemorrhage. Also, the patient is in a hypometabolic state, not a hypermetabolic one.

18 Correct answer – C

Insulin release is suppressed in hypothermia; as a result, the serum glucose level may be elevated to 500 to 600 mg/dl. However, glucose uptake and insulin secretion return to normal during rewarming.

19 Correct answer – D

To prevent ventricular fibrillation, extreme caution must be used when moving, transporting, manipulating, and intubating a hypothermic patient because defibrillation is ineffective below 86° F (30° C), and, at 85° F (29.4° C), the heart will not respond to drug therapy. Therefore, repositioning the patient frequently to enhance rewarming would be contraindicated. Appropriate nursing interventions would include electrocardiographic monitoring, recording of core temperature, taking blood pressure readings, performing neurologic checks, and monitoring urine output, serum electrolyte and glucose levels, vital signs, and arterial blood gas measurements. Warming I.V. fluids before administering them is also therapeutic.

20 Correct answer – A

The extreme temperature range compatible with human life is 77° to 113° F (25° to 45° C). Hypothermia, a core temperature of 95° F or below (35° C), is categorized as follows: *mild* hypothermia, 95° F, shivering, sluggish, and decreased coordination; *moderate* hypothermia, 89.6° F (32° C), muscular rigidity, stupor, and dilated pupils; *severe* hypothermia, 78.8° to 82.4° F (26° to 28° C), pulse and respirations undetectable, ventricular fibrillation likely, electroencephalogram likely to be flat, and death imminent.

21 Correct answer – C

Afterdrop is a common phenomenon in postoperative patients in whom the core temperature continues to drop about 2 F degrees (1.1 C degrees) after the cause of hypothermia is removed. Vasodilation and increased muscular activity return peripherally sequestered cold blood to the central circulation. Microcirculatory sludging does occur, but this is not referred to as afterdrop. Drooping of the fingers and toes and temporary gait impairment do not occur after rewarming.

22 Correct answer – A

Applying hypothermia blankets to the entire body is the least effective method of rewarming a hypothermic patient. Unlike administering warm I.V. fluids, enemas, peritoneal dialysis, and saturated oxygen, this external method does not result in core rewarming and an even return to a normothermic state.

23 Correct answer — D

The most appropriate nursing action would be to notify maintenance to shut off the air circulation system and to prepare a room with a lead-lined shield or an X-ray room in which to treat the patient. Necessary equipment, including a Geiger counter, water scrub, brushes, soap, lead-lined containers for disposal, and protective garb for personnel who will care for the patient, should be gathered and assembled in the room. The floor of the room should be covered with newspaper or nonskid plastic. These actions prevent radiation contamination of the hospital personnel and environment. Following an emergency plan for a radiation disaster is essential. Using any treatment room that is not lined with lead would cause radiation leakage through the walls.

24 Correct answer — B

After the patient arrives in the ED and his breathing and circulation have been stabilized, the nurse should use a Geiger counter to determine the patient's level and extent of radiation exposure. Documentation of this level serves as a baseline for comparison after the patient has been decontaminated. Covering the patient with a plastic sheet protects against further contamination. Removing and disposing the patient's clothing and jewelry and scrubbing the patient with soap and water are part of the decontamination process. After decontamination, reassessment with a Geiger counter is necessary. Assessing and treating injuries may be indicated next, with possible debridement of wounds if necessary.

25 Correct answer — D

The bank employee with fever, chills, and malaise is least likely to have been exposed to radiation. All of the other patients should be ruled out carefully, since they show signs of radiation exposure (vomiting, diarrhea, bleeding from mucous membranes, and weakness) and have a likely source of contamination. For example, the firefighter may have been exposed to radiation during a fire, the nuclear power plant worker may have become contaminated at work, and the cancer patient may have received radiation as a form of therapy.

26 Correct answer — B

Mild to severe nausea and vomiting are associated with most cases of radiation exposure, regardless of the amount of exposure. Tremors, convulsions, and death are associated with severe contamination (exposure to more than 2,000 rad).

27 Correct answer—A

If the Geiger counter readings do not show a reduction in the amount of external radiation after the decontamination process, the patient probably has internal contamination. Additional body scrubs will not help. Body fluids (saliva, blood, and waste) must be tested. Gastric lavage, cathartics, or emetics may be administered, as well as chelating or blocking agents, which prevent uptake of radioactive iodine by the thyroid gland. Convulsions and death can still be avoided if appropriate treatment is instituted promptly.

28 Correct answer—B

Leukopenia (a decreased white blood cell count) and thrombocytopenia (a decreased platelet count) always occur in patients exposed to radiation and manifest anywhere from 1 to 5 weeks after the incident, depending on the amount of exposure. In cases of mild exposure (100 rad), these symptoms typically manifest 4 to 5 weeks later; moderate exposure (300 to 600 rad), 3 weeks later; and high exposure (more than 600 rad), 1 to 3 weeks later.

29 Correct answer—A

The two most appropriate nursing diagnoses for a patient with leukopenia and thrombocytopenia would be *Potential for infection related to diminished immunity* and *Potential for fluid volume deficit related to bleeding.* Such a patient would have decreased protection against infection because of fewer white blood cells and would be at increased risk for bleeding because of fewer platelets. Anemia would be associated with *Impaired gas exchange related to decreased oxygen-carrying capacity of the blood.* A low platelet count would not enhance coagulation or increase the risk of thrombosis. Seizures and impaired myocardial contractility are not associated with leukopenia or thrombocytopenia.

30 Correct answer—B

When assessing a patient with heatstroke, the nurse would expect him to have a temperature above 106° F (41.1° C). Other common signs include tachypnea, hypotension, and lethargy or coma.

31 Correct answer—A

Exertional heatstroke, which is common in athletes, occurs with exercise during periods of high heat or humidity. Nonexertional heatstroke, which is not associated with activity, may also occur during periods of high heat and humidity or with overuse of a hot tub or sauna. Since exertional heatstroke, manifests differently than nonexertional heatstroke, the nurse would expect the runners with exertional heatstroke to continue to sweat and their skin to appear moist and clammy. A patient with nonexertional heatstroke will have hot, flushed skin, but will not sweat. Both forms of heatstroke cause variations in pulse rate and either elevated or severely elevated temperatures.

32 Correct answer — D

The nurse would expect a patient with heatstroke to have an elevated hematocrit and blood urea nitrogen level from hemoconcentration. Other laboratory findings typically include a decreased serum glucose level, from depletion of glucose stores, and respiratory alkalosis, from hyperventilation — a compensatory method of increasing heat elimination from the body.

33 Correct answer — C

Stopping all cooling measures, such as the application of ice packs to the axillae and groin and the institution of ice baths, when the patient's body temperature reaches 100° F (37.8° C) is inappropriate because the body temperature will continue to drop even after the measures have been removed. Such measures should be stopped after the body temperature reaches 102° F (38.9° C). The patient should be prevented from shivering because this mechanism increases heat production, which increases the body temperature.

34 Correct answer — C

"I should run shorter distances in the same weather for several days before the race so that my body is prepared" indicates that the runner understands the nurse's instructions on ways to prevent heatstroke. Running shorter shorter distances in the same type of weather for several days before a race acclimatizes the body to the need for increased sweat production. Running in the rain or in high humidity would be inappropriate becuase this decreases heat elimination from the body. Drinking alcohol before a race is also inappropriate because this promotes vasodilation, thereby decreasing heat elimination. Sprinting should also be avoided because this increases heat production, thereby raising the body temperature.

CHAPTER 5

Facial Emergencies

SITUATION

A 22-year-old man is bleeding profusely from a facial laceration when brought to the emergency department (ED). A part of his nose is missing. As the patient screams for help, he shows the nurse the missing nose part in his hand.

Questions 1 to 7 refer to the above situation.

1 The priority nursing intervention at this time would be to:

A. Apply direct digital pressure to the bleeding vessels
B. Obtain arterial blood gas measurements to assess airway patency
C. Question the patient about cause of the trauma
D. Evaluate the amputated nose part for possible reimplantation

2 The nurse's next appropriate step would be to take the amputated part and:

A. Place it in a jar of sterile normal saline solution
B. Wrap it in a saline-dampened cloth and place it in a plastic bag
C. Place it on dry ice
D. Discard it because noses are always contaminated

3 Before the patient's facial lacerations are treated, the nurse should:

A. Irrigate the wounds with normal saline solution
B. Scrub the wounds vigorously
C. Apply an aerosol anesthetic
D. Provide a mirror for the patient to assess the injury

4 One of the patient's lacerations extends through his left eyebrow. The nurse responds appropriately by:

A. Shaving the eyebrow
B. Applying adhesive skin closures
C. Leaving the eyebrow intact
D. Assessing for injury to the first cranial nerve

5 When suturing the patient's lacerations, the physician orders lidocaine with epinephrine. However, when anesthetizing the nose wound, the physician requests lidocaine without epinephrine because:

A. Epinephrine is a vasodilator and will cause further bleeding
B. Epinephrine will cause further nasal discharge and contaminate the wound
C. Epinephrine is a vasoconstrictor and may cause tissue ischemia
D. Administering epinephrine so close to the respiratory tract may cause bronchospasms

6 After the patient's lacerations are sutured, the nurse questions the patient and learns he received a tetanus booster 8 months ago. Based on this information, the nurse would:

A. Not administer a tetanus prophylaxis because it is unnecessary
B. Administer half the usual dose of tetanus toxoid
C. Administer 0.5 ml of absorbed tetanus toxoid
D. Suggest that the patient have two tetanus booster shots 3 months apart

7 During the discharge instructions, the nurse should tell the patient to:

A. Keep the incision moist with a wet dressing
B. Ignore any redness or swelling because this is normal
C. Return to the hospital in 4 to 5 days for suture removal
D. Avoid touching the incision because scarring will occur

SITUATION

A 35-year-old woman is admitted to the ED with ecchymotic areas over her face, malocclusion, and complaints of pain. She withdraws when the nurse attempts to palpate the mandible.

Questions 8 to 12 refer to the above situation.

8 Based on the patient's reaction, the nurse suspects a mandibular fracture. Which assessment finding is consistent with a mandibular fracture?

A. Subscleral hematoma
B. Numbness of the lower lips
C. Diplopia
D. Epistaxis

Facial Emergencies Questions

9 The patient claims that her injury resulted from falling in the bathtub. However, the nurse suspects that the patient's history is inaccurate because mandibular fractures most commonly result from:

A. Heavy weights or objects falling on the chin
B. Contact sports and diving accidents
C. Penetrating wounds from sharp instruments
D. Interpersonal altercations and vehicle accidents

10 The priority nursing diagnosis for a patient with a mandibular fracture would be:

A. Pain related to broken bones and altered tissue integrity
B. Body image disturbance related to facial trauma
C. Knowledge deficit related to wound care
D. Ineffective airway clearance related to aspiration

11 The patient is being prepared for emergency surgery. The nurse attempts to control any preoperative pain by:

A. Performing range-of-motion exercises and providing a quiet environment
B. Providing multiple distractions, including music
C. Administering narcotics, as ordered, and encouraging verbalization
D. Applying ice packs and administering analgesics, as ordered

12 After the patient is sent to the operating room for a reduction and fixation, the nurse calls the medical-surgical unit to prepare for the patient's arrival. Which item should the ED nurse suggest that the unit have on hand?

A. A blender
B. Mouthwash
C. Wire cutters
D. A tilt bed

SITUATION

A 40-year-old man arrives at the ED with severe midfacial trauma. He had been sitting in the front passenger seat of an automobile that crashed into a tree at 60 miles/hour.

Questions 13 to 18 refer to the above situation.

13 Because of the severe facial trauma and the report of the vehicular accident, the nurse's first priority would be to:

A. Call the patient's family to come to the hospital
B. Notify the police about the accident
C. Perform a drug screening on the patient
D. Maintain alignment of the spine

14 During the physical assessment, the nurse notes clear drainage from the patient's nose. The nurse should:

A. Report the finding on the assessment form
B. Test the nasal drainage for cerebrospinal fluid (CSF)
C. Assume that the patient has a respiratory infection
D. Suction the nose gently using a circular motion

15 The physician orders Water's view X-rays to determine:

A. The presence of orbital floor fractures
B. The extension of fracture to the mastoid process
C. Whether external manipulation will fixate the fracture
D. The extension of the fracture to the mental protuberance

16 The radiologist reports that the patient's X-rays reveal a Le Fort II fracture, which involves:

A. The nasomaxillary segments of the zygomatic and orbital portions of the face
B. Displacement of facial bones from the cranium
C. A horizontal fracture line that separates the maxillary alveolus from the upper face
D. Compression of temporal bone fragments and lacrimal tears

17 The nurse assesses for function of the first cranial nerve by:

A. Observing the patient's facial expression
B. Asking the patient whether he recognizes a familiar odor
C. Asking the patient to follow finger movements
D. Checking for bilateral corneal reflexes

Facial Emergencies
Questions

18 The orthopedic surgeon examines the patient and determines that an open reduction and internal fixation is required. When communicating the news to the patient's family, the nurse should:

A. Emphasize that the procedure will take several hours
B. Warn them that the surgical incision will be disfiguring
C. Reassure them that the patient will be able to talk soon
D. Discourage them from asking questions because the outcome cannot be predicted

SITUATION

A 16-year-old boy is admitted to the ED after being hit across the face with a baseball bat. He is complaining of pain, and bright red blood is draining from his nose.

Questions 19 to 25 refer to the above situation.

19 The physician determines that the patient has a zygomatic fracture. Which assessment findings are consistent with this type of fracture?

A. Restricted eye movement and a retinal tear
B. Periorbital ecchymosis and inferior orbit rim tenderness
C. Malocclusion and inability to close the mouth
D. Craniofacial detachment

20 The nurse documents that the patient also has trismus, which is characterized by:

A. Swelling over the fracture site
B. Purging in the ear when changing position
C. Toxic contractions of the mastication muscles
D. Infraorbital hypoesthesia with loss of sensation

21 The patient continues to bleed through the left nare. The nurse prepares a nasal packing tray by assembling all of the following *except*:

A. A catheter with a 30-cc balloon
B. Oxytetracycline-coated gauze
C. Gauze packing
D. Sterile gloves

22 The nurse informs the patient that the nasal packing will be removed after 24 to 48 hours. The purpose of removing the packing at that time would be to:

A. Assess the degree of edema
B. Prevent scab formation
C. Obtain clear nasal X-rays
D. Prevent infection

23 After the surgeon informs the patient that an open reduction is necessary, the patient becomes agitated. The nurse responds appropriately by:

A. Obtaining an order for a minor tranquilizer
B. Listening to the patient's concerns to determine the source of anxiety
C. Restraining the patient to prevent removal of the nasal packing
D. Requesting that the surgery be postponed until a later time

24 When caring for a patient with a zygomatic fracture, the nurse should assess for a possible orbital floor fracture, which is indicated by:

A. Subcutaneous emphysema
B. Trismus
C. Vertical diplopia
D. Malocclusion

25 To evaluate the effectiveness of nursing care for the patient with a zygomatic fracture, the nurse would:

A. Check the X-ray report to determine bone alignment
B. Ask the patient to repeat the treatment plan
C. Observe patient to determine independent functioning
D. Compare the patient's length of stay in the ED with that of other patients treated for zygomatic fractures

Facial Emergencies Questions

SITUATION

The nurse is examining a 35-year-old man who is complaining of ear pain and pain on attempting to clench his teeth. The nurse notes that the patient cannot close his mouth completely and hears a click when he opens his mouth fully. The patient states that he recently stopped smoking and admits to frequent gum chewing as a substitute.

Questions 26 to 28 refer to the above situation.

26 Based on the assessment findings, the nurse suspects that the patient has:

A. Acute odontalgia
B. Temporomandibular joint (TMJ) dislocation
C. Bilateral malocclusion
D. Dental abscess of a wisdom tooth

27 A manual reduction of the patient's jaw is indicated. Which nursing intervention would best facilitate this procedure?

A. Administering diazepam (Valium) I.V.
B. Spraying a topical anesthetic on the mucous membranes of the mouth
C. Giving atropine sulfate I.M. to reduce oral secretions
D. Holding hot compresses to each side of the patient's face

28 Discharge instructions for this patient should stress the importance of:

A. Frequent mouth exercises to strengthen muscles
B. Wearing a jaw brace while sleeping
C. Eating a soft diet for 3 to 4 days
D. Daily compliance with muscle relaxant therapy

SITUATION

A 40-year-old woman arrives at the ED with unilateral flaccid facial paralysis of acute onset. Physical examination reveals a lag on the affected side when closing the eyes, decreased lacrimation, and drooping of the mouth. The physician diagnoses Bell's palsy.

Questions 29 and 30 refer to the above situation.

29 To prevent development of corneal abrasions, the nurse should:

A. Administer 1% methylcellulose to the affected eye
B. Place an adhesive skin closure to maintain closure of the affected eye
C. Rinse the eyes with an antibiotic irrigating solution
D. Apply eye patches bilaterally until treatment is instituted

30 Discharge teaching for this patient should include instructions regarding:

A. Facial massage, exercises, and application of moist heat to the face
B. Techniques for corneal protection
C. Therapy with analgesics and steroids
D. All of the above

Answer Sheet

	A	B	C	D
1	○	○	○	○
2	○	○	○	○
3	○	○	○	○
4	○	○	○	○
5	○	○	○	○
6	○	○	○	○
7	○	○	○	○
8	○	○	○	○
9	○	○	○	○
10	○	○	○	○
11	○	○	○	○
12	○	○	○	○
13	○	○	○	○
14	○	○	○	○
15	○	○	○	○
16	○	○	○	○
17	○	○	○	○
18	○	○	○	○
19	○	○	○	○
20	○	○	○	○
21	○	○	○	○
22	○	○	○	○
23	○	○	○	○
24	○	○	○	○
25	○	○	○	○
26	○	○	○	○
27	○	○	○	○
28	○	○	○	○
29	○	○	○	○
30	○	○	○	○

Facial Emergencies
Answer Sheet

1 Correct answer—**A**

Because exsanguination is possible with facial artery lacerations, the priority nursing intervention in this situation would be to apply direct digital pressure to the bleeding vessels. Obtaining arterial blood gas measurements is unnecessary because the patient has a patent airway, as evidenced by his screaming. Questioning the patient about the cause of trauma and evaluating the amputated part for possible reimplantation are not priority interventions at this time; they should be included in the nurse's assessment once the bleeding is controlled.

2 Correct answer—**B**

The next appropriate step would be to rinse the amputated part with normal saline solution, wrap it in a saline-dampened cloth, place the wrapped part in a plastic bag, then place the bag on ice. Placing an amputated part directly in saline solution or on ice will macerate the tissue. Amputated parts should never be discarded until the surgeon has had time to evaluate any injury to the part and the amputated site.

3 Correct answer—**A**

Before treating a facial laceration, the nurse should irrigate the wounds with normal saline solution until clean. If the area is large or extremely dirty, the lacerations may be irrigated with direct, hydraulic force, using a 30-ml syringe and a 22G needle. Scrubbing should be avoided if at all possible because mechanical force can further traumatize the tissue. Because repair of facial lacerations is painful, local anesthetics are injected into the involved area. Patients are typically distressed at the possibility of disfigurement after facial injuries. The visualization of the trauma site before suturing would not provide an accurate assessment of potential scarring and may further distress the patient.

4 Correct answer—**C**

A lacerated eyebrow should be left intact. It should never be shaved, as it may not grow back properly. Also, the eyebrows serve as important landmarks for proper alignment when suturing. In this situation, the patient's wound is bleeding severely and requires suturing; therefore, adhesive skin closures would probably be inadequate. Assessment of the first cranial nerve is not specific to this injury, as injuries to this nerve typically occur with midface trauma.

Facial Emergencies
Answers

5 Correct answer—**C**

Epinephrine is a vasoconstrictor used on facial lacerations for hemostatic purposes; however, it would not be used in the nose because it may cause tissue ischemia. When administered with lidocaine, epinephrine produces localized effects, not the systemic effects needed to achieve the degree of anesthesia required for suturing a severe nose injury.

6 Correct answer—**A**

According to guidelines established by the American College of Surgeons, tetanus prophylaxis is unnecessary in an immunized person who has received a booster within the previous year. The usual dose for a patient who has never been immunized is 0.5 ml of tetanus toxoid.

7 Correct answer—**C**

During discharge instructions, the nurse should tell the patient to return to the hospital in 4 to 5 days, as facial sutures usually can be removed at that time. Until then, the patient should try to keep the wound clean and dry. Any sign of infection, such as heat, redness, and swelling, should be reported. Infection may increase the possibility of scarring; however, advising the patient to avoid touching the incision is no guarantee that scarring will not occur.

8 Correct answer—**B**

Assessment findings consistent with a mandibular fracture include paresthesia and numbness of the lower lip, swelling, sublingual edema, and tearing of gingival tissue with bleeding around the teeth. Subscleral hematoma, diplopia, and epistaxis are signs of a zygomatic fracture. Although the patient may experience epistaxis with a mandibular fracture, it typically results from other facial trauma and not the fracture itself.

9 Correct answer—**D**

Mandibular fractures most commonly result from interpersonal altercations involving direct blows to the mandible with a blunt object or fist and from vehicular accidents. Although falling in a bathtub could result in a mandibular fracture, the person would have to fall directly forward onto the chin to incur such an injury. Also, such a fall would probably result in bruises to the body; such bruises were not evident in this situation.

10 Correct answer—D

A patient with a mandibular fracture is at risk for aspirating teeth, bone fragments, blood, and vomitus; maintaining a patent airway takes priority over every other problem. Therefore, the priority nursing diagnosis would be *Ineffective airway clearance related to aspiration.* Appropriate interventions would include maintaining the patient in a side-lying position, having suction equipment ready, and being prepared to intubate if necessary.

11 Correct answer—D

Mandibular fractures are painful injuries. Preoperative pain-control measures typically include the application of ice packs to control swelling and reduce discomfort and the administration of analgesics (particularly narcotics), as ordered, to decrease pain sensation. Because any movement of the fracture part will increase the pain, exercise and verbalization should not be encouraged. Although music may be an appropriate distraction, the nurse should keep in mind that a patient in pain typically cannot tolerate multiple stimuli or distractions; the environment should be quiet and restful.

12 Correct answer—C

The ED nurse should suggest that the medical-surgical unit have wire cutters on hand. These should be kept at the patient's bedside at all times and carried by the patient as long as the jaw is wired shut. Keeping wire cutters on hand is a necessary precaution in the event that suctioning does not remove airway secretions and the patient goes into respiratory distress; the nurse would have to cut the wires and institute emergency intubation. A blender is unnecessary in this situation because, initially, the patient will be on a clear liquid diet; blenderized foods are not indicated until after discharge. Most mouthwashes are contraindicated in patients with wiring of fractures. To prevent infection, patients are instructed to rinse with half-strength peroxide and water while wires are in place. After discharge, the patient may use mouthwash, water, or salt water to rinse the mouth. A tilt bed is unnecessary; a side-lying position is adequate to prevent aspiration.

13 Correct answer—D

The nurse's first priority in this situation would be to maintain alignment of the patient's spine. A patient with a severe midfacial injury probably has suffered a maxillary fracture. Such a fracture, when combined with a high-speed vehicular deceleration accident, may be accompanied by cervical spine injury. Alignment of the spine is necessary to prevent possible cord damage until cervical fractures are ruled out.

14 Correct answer—B

Any rhinorrhea noted during assessment of a patient with midfacial trauma should be checked for cerebrospinal fluid (CSF) because the patient may have a fracture of the cribriform plate, resulting in CSF leakage. The nurse can check for CSF as it contains glucose and respiratory secretions do not. After assessing for CSF, the nurse should report the finding on the assessment form. Nasal suctioning should be avoided; the nose may no longer be attached to other bones and suctioning may produce further trauma to the area. If the patient has bloody drainage from the nose, the nurse should check for a clot with a yellow ring (halo sign), indicating CSF.

15 Correct answer—A

Water's view X-rays enable the physician to visualize the frontal, supraorbital, orbital floor, zygomatic, maxillary, and nasal areas. Although the physician may use these views to determine the extension of a maxillary fracture, injuries to the mastoid and mandible (common in midfacial trauma) are not extensions of a maxillary fracture and cannot be seen with these views.

16 Correct answer—A

All midfacial fractures are classified according to the Le Fort classification system. A Le Fort II fracture is one involving the nasomaxillary segments of the zygomatic and orbital portions of the face, which cause the nose to move with the dental arch. A Le Fort I fracture involves a horizontal fracture line that separates the maxillary alveolar process from the upper face. A Le Fort III fracture involves total displacement of the facial bones from the cranium. Temporal fractures do not involve the midface and, therefore, are not classified as Le Fort fractures.

17 Correct answer—B

Trauma to the midface sometimes reults in damage to the first cranial nerve, known as the olfactory nerve. The nurse would assess for function of this nerve by asking the patient to identify a pungent odor. Assessment of the seventh cranial nerve, the facial nerve, involves observing the patient's facial expression and checking his sense of taste. Ocular movement is controlled by three cranial nerves—the third (oculomotor), fourth (trochlear), and sixth (abducens)—which may be assessed by asking the patient to follow finger movements.

Damage to the fifth cranial (trigeminal) nerve, which controls corneal function, may be assessed by checking for bilateral corneal reflexes.

18 Correct answer—A

Facial reconstruction procedures for Le Fort II fractures are complex, requiring internal wiring and bone grafting. When communicating news of the surgery to the patient's family, the nurse should emphasize that the procedure will take several hours. Aesthetic effects of the surgical incision are usually good, as the incisions are made along the skin folds of the lower eyelids. The patient's jaw will be wired during the procedure, making talking and eating difficult; therefore, reassuring the family that the patient will be able to talk soon would be inappropriate. Families should never be discouraged from asking questions or expressing their concerns. Although no absolute predictions can be made, the patient's expected outcome can be discussed.

19 Correct answer—B

Periorbital ecchymosis and tenderness over the inferior orbital rim are two of the most common clinical findings in a zygomatic fracture. Restricted eye movement does not result from a zygomatic fracture itself, but rather from other coexisting problems. Retinal tears do not occur with this type of fracture. Malocclusion and inability to close the mouth are indications of temporomandibular joint dislocation, not a zygomatic fracture. Craniofacial detachment is consistent with a midface fracture, not a zygomatic fracture.

20 Correct answer—C

Trismus, which is characterized by tonic contractions of the mastication muscles, is a common assessment finding in patients with a zygomatic fracture as well as other types of trauma.

21 Correct answer—D

Wearing gloves is a necessary precaution whenever body fluids are handled. However, because nasal packing is considered a medically aseptic, not surgically aseptic, procedure, sterile gloves are unnecessary. When preparing a nasal packing tray, the nurse should include gauze packing with string, a catheter with a 30-cc balloon, oxytetracycline-coated gauze, forceps, and silk sutures. At the time of the packing, the physician decides whether to pack the nares with the oxytetracycline-coated gauze or the catheter.

22 Correct answer — D

Nasal packing should never be left in place for over 48 hours because of the risk for infection and the possibility of compression necrosis. Edema can be assessed and X-rays taken with the packing in place.

23 Correct answer — B

The idea of surgery, especially one that is unplanned, may be particularly distressing. Because the cause of distress will vary from patient to patient, the nurse must listen to the patient's concerns to determine the source of anxiety and intervene appropriately. The patient's anxiety may stem from fear of additional pain, fear of anesthesia, fear of separation from loved ones, or fear of the unknown. Before obtaining an order for a mild tranquilizer, the nurse should reassure the patient, provide honest and accurate explanations about the procedure, and attempt to strengthen the patient's coping skills. If the anxiety becomes severe, a mild tranquilizer may be used as an adjunctive therapy. Restraining the patient to protect himself from injury should always be a last resort. Postponing the surgery may be impractical or impossible; however, during the preoperative period, the nurse should attempt to prepare the patient physically and psychologically for the surgery.

24 Correct answer — C

Vertical diplopia, the imposition of one image above another, occurs when a patient suffers a blowout fracture of the orbital floor. It is most apparent when the patient looks upward. Other common signs of orbital floor fracture include exophthalmos and depression of the eye globe. Local swelling, not subcutaneous emphysema, may occur from a traumatic injury that results in a fracture. Malocclusion does not occur with orbital floor fractures. Trismus, which occurs when a bone fragment from the zygomatic arch impinges on the temporalis muscle and the coronoid process of the jaw, is a common finding with zygomatic fractures and does not occur with orbital floor fractures.

25 Correct answer — B

To evaluate the effectiveness of nursing care in this situation, the nurse should ask the patient to repeat the treatment plan. The nurse should never assume that the patient has understood explanations or instructions; traumatic stress and anxiety over the immediate future may interfere with the patient's ability to learn. Having the patient repeat the treatment plan allows the nurse to evaluate the patient's comprehension and identify knowledge deficits. Checking the X-ray report to determine bone alignment would be an appropriate measure to evaluate orthopedic surgical care, not nursing care. Independent functioning is a long-term patient goal, not an immediate, realistic goal applicable to ED nursing. A patient's length of stay in the ED is affected by multiple factors and is an inappropriate evaluation criterion of nursing care.

26 Correct answer—**B**

Based on the assessment findings, this patient probably has temporomandibular joint (TMJ) dislocation, a condition characterized by jaw displacement in which spasms of jaw muscles prevent the condyles from returning to their normal position. TMJ dislocation, which may be unilateral or bilateral, usually is caused by trauma or opening the mouth too widely. It also may occur in individuals in high-stress occupations or constant chewers. On assessment, the patient typically cannot close his mouth completely and has referred pain to his teeth, temples, or ears.

27 Correct answer—**A**

The administration of diazepam (Valium) I.V. facilitates manual reduction of the jaw by alleviating tension and anxiety, relaxing facial muscles, and increasing patient cooperation during the procedure. After the procedure, postreduction X-rays are necessary.

28 Correct answer—**C**

Discharge instructions for a patient with TMJ dislocation should stress the importance of adhering to a soft diet for 3 to 4 days. A soft diet enables the patient to avoid excessive chewing or opening the mouth widely, which could place additional stress on the joint. Other important discharge information should include specific instructions on adhering to the medication regimen, if analgesics are prescribed. Frequent mouth exercises could precipitate a TMJ dislocation and therefore would not be included in the discharge plan.

29 Correct answer—**A**

Appropriate nursing interventions to help prevent the development of corneal abrasions include administering a 1% methylcellulose (artificial tears) solution to the affected eye; performing gentle, manual closure of the eyelid periodically; instructing the patient to wear sunglasses; and applying an eye patch to the affected eye.

30 Correct answer—**D**

Appropriate discharge teaching for a patient with Bell's palsy should include specific instructions on therapeutic aids, such as facial massage, facial muscle exercises, and the application of moist heat to

Facial Emergencies
Answers

the face, to speed recovery. Because Bell's palsy is thought to result from polyneuritis, steroids are beneficial; they decrease edema and inflammation. Analgesics may be given to decrease pain. Specific instructions on medication, such as analgesics and steroids, are essential to foster patient compliance. Techniques that promote corneal protection, such as wearing eyepatches or sunglasses, should also be stressed.

CHAPTER 6

General Medical Emergencies

SITUATION

A 70-year-old man was admitted to the hospital 2 months ago with a diagnosis of pulmonary embolism. He had been treated with heparin and discharged on warfarin sodium (Coumadin) therapy after the embolism resolved. Earlier today, he became confused and ingested 100 mg of warfarin. He is now being readmitted with hematemesis and bright-red rectal bleeding.

Questions 1 to 8 refer to the above situation.

1 During the initial assessment of this patient, the emergency department (ED) nurse should be particularly alert for:

A. Facial flushing
B. Petechiae
C. Pruritus
D. Hypertension

2 The nurse knows that a patient on long-term anticoagulant therapy must be carefully monitored for potential hemorrhagic complications that most commonly affect the:

A. GI tract
B. Genitourinary tract
C. Respiratory tract
D. Capillary vasculature

3 Which therapy would the nurse expect the physician to order for this patient?

A. Peritoneal dialysis
B. Administration of vitamin K
C. Ethylenediaminetetraacetic acid (EDTA) chelation
D. Plasmapheresis

4 Which therapy would be inappropriate for a patient with hemorrhagic complications from oral anticoagulants?

A. Volume replacement
B. Administration of whole blood
C. Administration of fresh frozen plasma
D. Administration of protamine sulfate

5 The nurse would normally instruct a patient receiving anticoagulant therapy to:

A. Avoid excessive alcohol intake
B. Avoid using an electric shaver
C. Avoid using soft-bristled toothbrushes
D. Trim corns and calluses weekly

6 An appropriate nursing intervention for a patient receiving heparin therapy for deep vein thrombosis of the left calf would include:

A. Observing for hypertensive crisis and hematemesis
B. Monitoring the patient's prothrombin time (PT) to maintain therapeutic anticoagulant blood levels
C. Testing the patient's urine and stool for blood
D. Administering aspirin for leg pain, as needed

7 Which nursing action is inappropriate when administering heparin subcutaneously?

A. Changing the injection site with each dose
B. Using the iliac crest or abdominal fat layer as an injection site
C. Massaging the area after injection to facilitate absorption
D. Observing for bleeding at the injection site

8 Which statement regarding heparin administration is *true?*

A. Partial thromboplastin time (PTT) must be checked after each dose
B. Larger heparin doses are required during continuous infusion
C. Major bleeding episodes are more common with continuous I.V. infusions than with intermittent I.V. infusions
D. During continuous infusion, the drip rate must be accurately calculated and controlled

SITUATION

A 4-year-old boy is admitted to the ED with a sudden high fever. His mother notes that he has been weak and dyspneic and has had generalized pain and recurrent infections. He is found to have an elevated white blood cell count, anemia, thrombocytopenia, and tachycardia. The physician diagnoses acute lymphocytic leukemia.

Questions 9 to 12 refer to the above situation.

General Medical Emergencies
Questions

9 After which age is acute lymphocytic leukemia considered uncommon?
A. 20
B. 30
C. 40
D. 50

10 Which nursing diagnosis would be appropriate for this patient?
A. Altered tissue perfusion related to enhanced coagulation from thrombocytosis
B. Altered tissue perfusion related to increased blood viscosity from polycythemia vera
C. Potential for infection related to immunosuppression
D. Potential for injury related to seizures

11 The nurse would expect to treat a leukemic patient with an elevated temperature with:
A. Aspirin
B. Acetaminophen (Tylenol)
C. Azathioprine (Imuran)
D. Antibiotics

12 The nurse explains to the patient, in age-appropriate terms, that chemotherapy is used to treat leukemia because it:
A. Destroys abnormal leukemic cells
B. Causes bone marrow recovery
C. Increases the patient's immunologic defense mechanisms
D. Produces granulocytosis

SITUATION

A 17-year-old girl is admitted to the ED 10 days after an abortion. She continues to have heavy bleeding and lower abdominal pain. The physician suspects retained products of conception. While the patient is in the ED, her laboratory studies reveal a prolonged PT and PTT. The physician diagnoses disseminated intravascular coagulation (DIC).

Questions 13 to 17 relate to the above situation.

13 Which assessment finding is most significant in a patient with DIC?

A. Leukopenia
B. Maculopapular rash
C. Abnormal bleeding
D. Severe hypertension

14 The nurse would expect to observe bleeding from which site in a patient with DIC?

A. Mucous membranes
B. Venipuncture sites
C. GI tract
D. All of the above

15 Which obstetric incident leads to the development of DIC?

A. Thromboembolism resulting from bed rest and microemboli formation
B. Activation of the clotting mechanism by placental and fetal tissue
C. Hemolysis of red blood cells (RBCs) resulting from fetal enzyme release
D. Thrombocytopenic state, which normally occurs during pregnancy

16 Which statement does *not* support the rationale for heparin administration in the treatment of DIC?

A. The antithrombin activity of heparin neutralizes free-circulating thrombin
B. Heparin permits normalization of clotting test results
C. Heparin prevents fibrinogenesis
D. Heparin increases hemorrhagic manifestations

17 Which laboratory finding would indicate successful treatment of this patient?

A. Platelet count of 40,000/mm³
B. PTT of 76 seconds
C. Fibrin degradation products of 10 μg/ml
D. Hemoglobin level of 7 g/dl

General Medical Emergencies
Questions

SITUATION

A 10-year-old boy is brought to the ED after injuring his right knee in a bicycle accident. He is known to have hemophilia A and presents symptoms indicating hemarthrosis of the right knee.

Questions 18 to 22 relate to the above situation.

18 Hemophilia A and hemophilia B are bleeding disorders that can be distinguished only by laboratory studies. Which statement about these disorders is *true?*

A. Hemophilia B is caused by a deficiency of Factor VIII
B. Hemophilia A is caused by a deficiency of Factor IX
C. Hemophilia A is more common than hemophilia B
D. Almost all of the individuals with hemophilia A are female

19 Hemarthrosis, especially of the knees, elbows, and ankles, is a common assessment finding in hemophilia. Other common assessment findings include:

A. Bruising and bleeding gums
B. Neuropathy and paresthesia
C. Pain and hematuria
D. All of the above

20 The most common cause of death in a patient with hemophilia occurs from bleeding of the:

A. GI tract
B. Heart
C. Cranium
D. Larynx

21 Diagnosis is typically based on the patient's bleeding pattern, family history, and physical examination. Confirming diagnostic studies indicate:

A. Factor VIII or Factor IX deficiency
B. Prolonged PT and PTT
C. Increased fibrinogen level
D. Decreased platelet count

22 Priority nursing care of this patient would include all of the following *except:*

A. Immobilizing the right leg
B. Stopping local bleeding
C. Preventing deformity
D. Assisting with immediate aspiration of hemarthroses

SITUATION

A 40-year-old man with a history of alcohol abuse is admitted to the ED with hematemesis. His blood pressure is 88/56 mm Hg; temperature, 99° F (37.2° C); hemoglobin, 8.4 g/dl; and hematocrit, 24%.

Questions 23 to 26 refer to the above situation.

23 The patient's blood is typed and cross-matched for transfusion; his blood type is designated as group AB. Which statement about group AB is *true?*

A. The plasma contains both A and B antibodies
B. The plasma contains both A and B antigens
C. The red cell membrane contains both A and B antigens
D. This blood group possesses neither A nor B antigens

24 Packed RBCs are recommended for transfusion. Which statement regarding packed RBCs and whole blood is *true?*

A. Both packed cells and whole blood cause the hemoglobin and hematocrit to increase at the same rate
B. Fresh packed cells provide all of the necessary blood components, including platelets and coagulation factors
C. Packed cells decrease the risk of anaphylactic reaction
D. Packed cells are indicated for massive hemorrhage and hypovolemia

25 The nurse who administers the transfusion of packed RBCs to this patient must be cognizant of standard transfusion practices. Which statement about blood transfusions is *true?*

A. Lactated Ringer's and normal saline are the only solutions used when administering blood products
B. During a blood transfusion, the nurse must assess the patient's vital signs before and after the transfusion only
C. When using a blood warmer, the temperature should not exceed 103.1° F (38.5° C)
D. An 18G or 20G catheter may be used during a blood transfusion

26 One hour after the transfusion has been initiated, the patient complains of chills and headache. The nurse checks his vital signs and notes that his temperature has increased to 103.1° F (39.5° C). Based on these findings, the nurse determines that the patient is probably experiencing a:

A. Febrile, nonhemolytic transfusion reaction
B. Hemolytic transfusion reaction
C. Delayed hemolytic transfusion reaction
D. Bacterial transfusion reaction

SITUATION

A 60-year-old man with thrombocytopenia is admitted to the ED because of rectal bleeding.

Questions 27 and 28 relate to the above situation.

27 The nurse knows that thrombocytopenia does not result from:

A. Chlorothiazide (Diuril) therapy
B. Zidovudine (AZT) therapy
C. Splenectomy
D. Viral infection

28 The nurse would expect a thrombocytopenic patient's platelet count to return to normal levels within what time after discontinuation of quinidine therapy?

A. 24 hours
B. 72 hours
C. 1 week
D. 2 weeks

SITUATION

A 28-year-old black man with a history of sickle-cell disease is admitted to the ED. During assessment, the nurse notes the following symptoms: severe abdominal and back pain, aching joint pain, fever, vomiting, and dyspnea.

Questions 29 to 33 refer to the above situation.

General Medical Emergencies
Questions

29 All of the following are forms of sickle-cell crisis *except:*

A. Aplastic crisis
B. Sequestration crisis
C. Painful crisis
D. Anemic crisis

30 Which nursing diagnosis would be inappropriate for this patient?

A. Altered tissue perfusion related to increased blood viscosity
B. Pain related to ischemia from impaired blood flow
C. Impaired gas exchange related to dysfunctional RBCs
D. Decreased cardiac output related to impaired myocardial contractility

31 During the nursing history, the nurse would question the patient about all of the following factors that may precipitate a crisis *except:*

A. Cigarette smoking
B. Infection
C. Increased fluid intake
D. A strenuous game of tennis

32 One of the treatments for this patient in sickle-cell crisis involves hydration, which may be achieved by:

A. Inserting the smallest-possible-gauge I.V. catheter and infusing dextrose 5% in ½ normal saline solution at 100 ml/hour
B. Inserting a large-gauge I.V. catheter and infusing normal saline solution at 150 ml/hour
C. Inserting a large-gauge I.V. catheter and infusing lactated Ringer's solution at 300 ml/hour
D. Having the patient drink 4 to 6 quarts (about 4 to 6 liters) of liquid within the following 24 hours

33 Which analgesic would the nurse *not* expect to administer to a patient in a painful crisis?

A. Meperidine hydrochloride (Demerol) I.M.
B. Morphine sulfate I.V.
C. Aspirin
D. Codeine

General Medical Emergencies
Questions

SITUATION

A 33-year-old man with a positive history of human immunodeficiency virus (HIV) is brought to the ED complaining of dyspnea and a productive cough. He has been taking zidovudine, also known as azidothymidine or AZT (Retrovir), for the past year.

Questions 34 to 37 refer to the above situation.

34 Which assessment finding is characteristic of a patient with acquired immunodeficiency syndrome (AIDS)?

A. Oral candidiasis
B. Hairy leukoplakia
C. Purplish skin lesions
D. All of the above

35 Which laboratory finding would the nurse expect for a patient with a depressed immune system resulting from AIDS?

A. Hemoglobin of 8 g/dl
B. High T4:T8 lymphocyte ratio
C. Platelet count of 40,000/mm³
D. T lymphocyte count of 150/mm³

36 The nurse knows that zidovudine is classified as an:

A. Antiviral agent used to decrease the replication of HIV
B. Antibiotic used to treat *Pneumocystis carinii* pneumonia
C. Antitubercular agent
D. Antifungal used to treat oral candidiasis

37 The physician orders aerosolized pentamidine isethionate (Pentam 300) for this patient. Which statement about pentamidine therapy is *false?*

A. Pentamidine should be administered in a well-ventilated room
B. Respiratory (acid fast bacilli [AFB]) precaution measures should be used during the administration of pentamidine
C. Pregnant nurses or those who are trying to become pregnant should avoid administering pentamidine
D. Pentamidine should be administered only via intermittent positive-pressure breathing

General Medical Emergencies
Questions

SITUATION

A 5-year-old boy is transferred to the ED by ambulance from his pediatrician's office with a suspected diagnosis of Reye's syndrome.

Questions 38 to 40 refer to the above situation.

38 When obtaining the nursing history from the child's mother, the nurse should inquire about a recent history of:

A. Chicken pox
B. Diarrhea
C. Measles
D. Insect bites

39 Which laboratory finding supports the diagnosis of Reyes syndrome?

A. Elevated serum glucose level
B. Elevated serum potassium level
C. Low WBC count
D. Elevated serum ammonia level

40 The physician is having difficulty establishing a peripheral I.V. line and considers inserting an intraosseous catheter. When the mother asks which bone will be used, the nurse responds appropriately that the most common insertion site is the:

A. Iliac crest
B. Sternum
C. Tibia
D. Femur

SITUATION

A 17-year-old female model arrives at the ED complaining of generalized cramps and numbness in her fingers. When asked about her medical history, she informs the nurse that she has been on a high-protein diet for about 6 weeks. The nurse establishes an I.V. line and draws blood for laboratory studies. The patient's serum calcium level is 5.5 mg/dl.

Questions 41 to 43 relate to the above situation.

General Medical Emergencies
Questions

41 When assessing a patient for hypocalcemia, the nurse attempts to elicit Chvostek's sign by:

A. Applying a blood pressure (BP) cuff to the upper arm, inflating the cuff, and observing for carpopedal spasm
B. Tapping a finger on the skin above the supramandibular portion of the parotid gland and observing for twitching of the upper lip on the side opposite the stimulation
C. Tapping a finger on the skin above the supramandibular portion of the parotid gland and observing for twitching of the upper lip on the same side as the stimulation
D. Having the patient hyperventilate (expelling more than 30 breaths/minute) to produce carpopedal spasm caused by respiratory alkalosis

42 The nurse would assess a patient with hypocalcemia for which electrocardiogram (ECG) changes?

A. Shortened PR intervals
B. Prolonged PR intervals
C. Prolonged QT intervals
D. Appearance of U waves

43 The nurse would assess a hypocalcemic patient for all of the following potential complications *except:*

A. Seizures
B. Oliguria
C. Laryngeal stridor
D. Bleeding abnormalities

SITUATION

A 71-year-old woman is brought to the ED because of fatigue and a change in mental status. Assessment findings reveal a rectal temperature of 96.8° F (36° C); a BP of 110/74 mm Hg; a pulse rate of 48 beats/minute; a respiratory rate of 12 breaths/minute; periorbital edema; and a yellowish skin pigmentation. The patient's daughter relates a history of thyroid problems and noncompliance with medical therapy. The physician diagnoses myxedema coma.

Questions 44 to 47 refer to the above situation.

44 The nurse would assess a patient admitted with myxedema coma (hypothyroid crisis) for which electrolyte abnormality?

A. Hyponatremia
B. Hypernatremia
C. Hyperglycemia
D. Hypocalcemia

45 Which acid-base imbalance would the nurse expect this patient to have?

A. Respiratory acidosis
B. Respiratory alkalosis without compensation
C. Metabolic alkalosis
D. Respiratory alkalosis with compensation

46 Which signs would the nurse expect to note during the assessment of this patient?

A. Increased urine output and hyperactive bowel sounds
B. Oliguria and abdominal distention
C. Diarrhea and hyperglycemia
D. Polycythemia and hypothermia

47 Which I.V. fluid is most likely to be used in the treatment of this patient?

A. Dextrose 5% in water (D_5W)
B. Dextrose 10% in water
C. Dextrose 5% in normal saline solution
D. 0.3% sodium chloride

SITUATION

A 78-year-old woman arrives at the ED complaining of abdominal cramping. She states that she has had diarrhea and has felt tired for about 1 week. She has a history of diabetes mellitus and chronic renal failure. The nurse establishes an I.V. line and draws blood for laboratory studies. The serum potassium level is 6 mEq/liter. The physician diagnoses hyperkalemia.

Questions 48 to 51 relate to the above situation.

General Medical Emergencies
Questions

48 The nurse would anticipate pharmacologic management of hyperkalemia to include administration of all of the following *except:*

A. Lactulose enemas
B. Dextrose 50% and regular insulin
C. Sodium bicarbonate
D. Calcium chloride

49 The nurse would assess a patient with hyperkalemia for which ECG change?

A. Prolonged QT intervals
B. Peaked T waves
C. Prominent U waves
D. Shortened PR intervals

50 Which signs would the nurse expect to note during the physical assessment of a patient with hyperkalemia?

A. Apathy and absent bowel sounds
B. Ascending muscle weakness and bradycardia
C. Descending muscle weakness and tachycardia
D. Hyperactive bowel sounds and polyuria

51 Which acid-base imbalance is characteristic of a hyperkalemic patient?

A. Respiratory acidosis
B. Metabolic alkalosis
C. Respiratory alkalosis
D. Metabolic acidosis

SITUATION

A 52-year-old man with newly diagnosed multiple myeloma is admitted to the ED with back pain. He informs the nurse that he fell against a bookcase at home. X-rays reveal a rib fracture; electrolyte studies reveal a serum calcium level of 12.7 mg/dl. The physician diagnoses hypercalcemia.

Questions 52 to 55 refer to the above situation.

52 The nurse is aware that hypercalcemia occurs in multiple myeloma as a result of:

A. Mobilization of calcium from the bones
B. Release of calcium from lesions into the plasma
C. Increased tubular reabsorption of calcium
D. Increased intestinal reabsorption of calcium secondary to excessive vitamin D intake

53 The nurse assesses the patient for signs of hypercalcemia, including:

A. Flank or thigh pain and polyuria
B. Anuria or oliguria and constipation
C. Diarrhea and metabolic alkalosis
D. Constipation and metabolic acidosis

54 Which ECG change is characteristic of a patient with hypercalcemia?

A. Prolonged PR intervals
B. Prolonged QT intervals
C. Shortened ST segments
D. Appearance of U waves

55 The nurse would expect the treatment for this patient to include the administration of:

A. Normal saline solution and loop diuretics
B. Normal saline solution and thiazide diuretics
C. Sodium polystyrene sulfonate (Kayexalate) enemas
D. Hemodialysis, glucose, and insulin

SITUATION

A 64-year-old man is admitted to the ED with altered mental status, jaundice, and increased abdominal girth. He has a medical history of cirrhosis. The nurse establishes an I.V. line and draws blood for laboratory studies. Liver enzyme levels (serum aspartate aminotransferase, serum alanine aminotransferase, and bilirubin) are elevated. The physician diagnoses hepatic encephalopathy.

Questions 56 to 59 relate to the above situation.

General Medical Emergencies
Questions

56 The nurse would assess a patient with hepatic failure for signs of:

A. Hypercalcemia
B. Hyperproteinemia
C. Hypokalemia
D. Free-water depletion

57 The nurse knows that respiratory alkalosis, a common acid-base imbalance in patients with hepatic failure, is a result of:

A. A high blood ammonia level, which acts as a respiratory stimulant
B. Hypocalcemia, which causes neuromuscular irritability
C. Hypokalemia, which causes hyperventilation
D. Hypomagnesemia, which causes hypoventilation

58 Aldosterone-blocking agents, such as spironolactone (Aldactone), may be administered to a patient with hepatic failure. The nurse would evaluate the effectiveness of these agents by assessing for:

A. Increased serum sodium levels and decreased serum potassium levels
B. Decreased serum sodium levels and increased serum potassium levels
C. Decreased serum sodium levels and increased serum magnesium levels
D. Decreased serum sodium and potassium levels

59 The nurse would anticipate the physician to order all of the following measures to treat hepatic failure *except:*

A. Administration of sodium polystyrene sulfonate enemas to remove excess potassium
B. Limiting the administration of hypotonic solutions
C. Decreasing or eliminating the patient's dietary protein intake
D. Decreasing the patient's dietary sodium intake

SITUATION

A 28-year-old woman is admitted to the ED after a house fire. She has second- and third-degree burns over approximately 30% of her body-surface area, including her face. Endotracheal intubation is performed, and I.V. lines are established.

Questions 60 to 63 refer to the above situation.

60 The goals of I.V. therapy for this patient would be based on all of the following *except:*

A. Sex and medical history
B. Depth and percentage of the burns
C. Urine output and urine specific gravity measurements
D. Hemoglobin and hematocrit values

61 During the initial treatment phase, fluid replacement at 4 ml/kg/ percent of burns is given over the first 24 hours. The calculated amount of solution is divided so that:

A. One-third of the solution is given every 8 hours
B. One-half of the solution is given in the initial 8 hours, one-half in the next 16 hours
C. One-half of the solution is given in the first 12 hours, one-half in the next 12 hours
D. One-half of the solution is given in the first 16 hours, one-half in the next 8 hours

62 During the initial stages (first 3 days) of a burn injury, the nurse would expect the patient to show signs of:

A. Jugular venous distention and hypernatremia
B. Edema and hyperkalemia
C. Jugular venous distention and hyponatremia
D. Jugular venous distention and hypokalemia

63 During the later stages (after the first 3 days) of a burn injury, the nurse would expect the patient to show signs of:

A. Jugular venous distention and hypokalemia
B. Edema and hypokalemia
C. Oliguria and hypokalemia
D. Edema and hyponatremia

SITUATION

A 40-year-old man is admitted to the ED with lethargy and tachypnea. His skin is dry and flushed, and he has a fruity breath odor. An I.V. line is started and blood is drawn for laboratory studies. His blood glucose level is 840 mg/dl, and his urinalysis reveals +3 glucose, +3 ketones. The physician diagnoses diabetic ketoacidosis.

Questions 64 to 67 refer to the above situation.

64 The nurse would expect to note all of the following physiologic abnormalities during the assessment of this patient *except:*

A. Jugular venous distention
B. Hyperkalemia
C. Hyperventilation
D. Poor skin turgor

65 The nurse's first priority in caring for this patient would be to:

A. Administer insulin I.V.
B. Administer insulin S.C.
C. Administer volume replacement fluids and insulin I.V.
D. Establish an airway and monitor its patency

66 Which I.V. solution would the nurse expect to use in the initial treatment of this patient?

A. Isotonic saline solution
B. Hypotonic saline solution
C. Hypertonic saline solution
D. Hypotonic dextrose solution

67 During therapy, evaluation of this patient's serum potassium level is likely to demonstrate which pattern?

A. An initially elevated level, followed by gradually decreasing levels
B. An initially decreased level, followed by gradually increasing levels
C. An increased level that remains generally elevated
D. A decreased level that remains generally low

SITUATION

A 12-year-old boy arrives at the ED complaining of difficulty breathing. His parents inform the nurse that the family has a long history of asthma and that the child has suffered previous wheezing episodes but none this severe. Arterial blood gas (ABG) studies performed while the patient is breathing room air (21% oxygen) reveal pH, 7.21; PO_2, 65 mm Hg; PCO_2, 62 mm Hg; and HCO_3^-, 24 mEq/liter.

Questions 68 to 70 refer to the above situation.

68 This patient's ABG measurements would be interpreted as:

A. Metabolic acidosis
B. Metabolic alkalosis
C. Respiratory acidosis
D. Respiratory alkalosis

69 Which action would be the nurse's lowest priority when caring for this patient?

A. Oxygen therapy
B. Inhaled bronchodilator therapy
C. Continuous cardiac monitoring
D. Preparation for possible tracheotomy

70 The nurse knows that, if therapy is not implemented immediately, this patient could suffer:

A. Respiratory arrest
B. Gastric aspiration
C. Adult respiratory distress syndrome
D. Acute renal failure

Questions 71 and 72 continue the previous situation.

The patient stops breathing shortly after the nurse institutes inhaled bronchodilator therapy, as ordered. After initial ventilation with a bag-valve-mask device, the patient achieves good bilateral chest rising. He is then intubated with an orotracheal tube, and ventilation is continued. A repeat ABG analysis indicates pH, 7.12; PCO$_2$, 55 mm Hg; PO$_2$, 33 mm Hg; and HCO$_3$$^-$, 25 mEq/ liter. No loss of vital signs is noted. The patient is then given 100 mEq of sodium bicarbonate. Ten minutes later, ABG analysis indicates pH, 7.55; PCO$_2$, 35 mm Hg; PO$_2$, 425 mm Hg; and HCO$_3$$^-$, 36.5 mEq/liter.

71 Based on the latest ABG results, the nurse knows that the patient is exhibiting signs of:

A. Metabolic acidosis
B. Metabolic alkalosis
C. Respiratory acidosis
D. Respiratory alkalosis

General Medical Emergencies Questions

72 The nurse should have anticipated the correct treatment after the patient stopped breathing to have included:

A. Hyperventilation with a bag-valve-mask device
B. Administration of 1 mEq/kg of sodium bicarbonate I.V. push
C. Admministration of 40% oxygen via a high flow oxygen (Venturi) mask
D. Administration of 0.5 to 1 mg of epinephrine I.V.

SITUATION

A 37-year-old woman arrives at the ED after having ingested ten 5-mg methamphetamine hydrochloride (Desoxyn) tablets about 2 hours ago. She appears excited and nervous. Her blood pressure is 145/70 mm Hg; pulse rate, 124 beats/minute; respiratory rate, 44 breaths/minute; and temperature, 99.5° F (37.5° C). She complains of circumoral tingling and numbness as well as tingling in her hands and feet. An ABG analysis, which is taken while the patient is receiving 28% oxygen by face mask, indicates pH, 7.60; PCO_2, 15 mm Hg; PO_2, 140 mm Hg; and HCO_3^-, 22 mEq/liter.

Questions 73 to 76 refer to the above situation.

73 This patient's ABG results may be interpreted as:

A. Metabolic acidosis
B. Metabolic alkalosis
C. Respiratory acidosis
D. Respiratory alkalosis

74 The goal of treatment for this patient would be to increase:

A. Oxygenation
B. Ventilation
C. HCO_3^- level
D. CO_2 retention

75 All of the following statements about this patient are correct *except:*

A. After treatment in the ED, the patient will require follow-up care
B. The patient is having an anxiety attack
C. Emergency treatment for this patient should include rebreathing exhaled CO_2
D. Emergency treatment for this patient should include the administration of sodium bicarbonate I.V.

General Medical Emergencies Questions

76 The nurse suspects that the patient is experiencing numbness and tingling because:

A. Alkalosis causes vasodilation and paresthesia
B. Hypocapnia causes vasoconstriction and decreases calcium levels
C. Diazepam causes these symptoms
D. None of the above

SITUATION

A 78-year-old, 155-lb (70-kg) man was transported from a nursing home to the ED about 4 hours ago, complaining of difficulty voiding. His temperature upon arrival was 104.5° F (40.3° C). He is now demonstrating labored respirations and tachycardia. ABG analysis reveals pH, 7.01; PO_2, 125 mm Hg (28% O_2); PCO_2, 42 mm Hg; and HCO_3^-, 10 mEq/liter.

Questions 77 to 80 refer to the above situation.

77 The nurse would correctly interpret the patient's ABG results as an indication of:

A. Metabolic acidosis
B. Metabolic alkalosis
C. Respiratory acidosis
D. Respiratory alkalosis

78 The bicarbonate deficit in this situation would be:

A. 10 mEq/liter
B. 14 mEq/liter
C. 24 mEq/liter
D. 30 mEq/liter

79 The nurse correctly calculates that the amount of sodium bicarbonate required to correct this abnormality to be:

A. 44 mEq
B. 88 mEq
C. 100 mEq
D. 245 mEq

80 Which laboratory studies are likely to provide essential information necessary for the treatment of this patient's acid-base imbalance?

A. Complete blood count and reticulocyte count
B. Creatine phosphokinase isoenzyme and serum amylase levels
C. Lactate level and anion gap
D. Electrolyte studies and acetone level

SITUATION

The nurse is in the process of resuscitating a 45-year-old man in the ED. ABG measurements (obtained 5 minutes ago) indicate pH, 7.15; PO_2, 50 mm Hg; PCO_2, 68 mm Hg; and HCO_3^-, 18 mEq/liter.

Questions 81 to 83 refer to the above situation.

81 The nurse correctly interprets the ABG results to mean that the patient has:

A. Fully compensated respiratory acidosis
B. Fully compensated metabolic acidosis
C. Partially compensated respiratory alkalosis
D. Mixed metabolic and respiratory acidosis

82 The nurse anticipates that the best initial therapy for this patient would be to:

A. Improve oxygenation and ventilation
B. Defibrillate immediately
C. Administer sodium bicarbonate
D. Administer epinephrine

83 Which blood gas abnormalities, if unreversed, can seriously compromise this patient's myocardial function?

A. Hypoxemia and a low bicarbonate level
B. Acidosis and hypoxemia
C. Acidosis and a low bicarbonate level
D. Acidosis and hypercapnia

SITUATION

A family of five arrives at a small, rural ED complaining of headaches, malaise, nausea, and vomiting. This occurs during the winter, and toxic ingestion or inhalation is suspected. The father's ABG analysis indicates pH, 7.25; PCO_2, 47 mm Hg; PO_2, 97 mm Hg; O_2 saturation, 75%; and HCO_3^-, 15 mEq/liter. Other family members have similar results.

Questions 84 to 87 refer to the above situation.

84 This family's symptoms suggest:

A. Viral syndrome
B. CO_2 narcosis
C. Carbon monoxide poisoning
D. Radon poisoning

85 The nurse anticipates the initial treatment for this family to include:

A. Breathing into a paper bag
B. Administration of 100% O_2 via a nonrebreather mask
C. Acetylcysteine (Mucomyst) inhalant therapy
D. I.V. bronchodilator therapy

86 If initial treatment is unsuccessful, the nurse would prepare each patient for:

A. Hyperbaric therapy
B. Exploratory laparotomy
C. Cariopulmonary bypass surgery
D. Hemodialysis

87 After appropriate treatment, when all family members are stabilized, the nurse formulates a nursing diagnosis of:

A. Ineffective family coping related to guilt
B. Noncompliance related to financial status
C. Powerlessness related to current health situation
D. Knowledge deficit related to medical diagnosis of carbon monoxide poisoning

---

SITUATION

A 22-year-old man is unconscious when brought to the ED. The nurse notes that he is breathing rapidly and deeply. Although his skin is warm and dry, his pulse is 130 beats/minute and weak, and his blood pressure is 92/60 mm Hg. The nurse draws blood for ABG and electrolyte studies and sends the specimens to the laboratory.

Questions 88 to 106 relate to the above situation.

88 The nurse would expect the physician to order the administration of which drugs at this time?

A. Dextrose 50% and naloxone (Narcan)
B. Regular insulin and sodium bicarbonate
C. NPH insulin and potassium
D. Activated charcoal and naloxone

89 While awaiting the laboratory findings, the nurse learns from the patient's parents that the patient has a 10-year history of Type I diabetes mellitus. The ABG results reveal pH, 7.03; PO_2, 98 mm Hg; PCO_2, 28 mm Hg; and HCO_3^-, 12 mEq/liter. Other laboratory studies indicate the following serum levels: sodium, 140 mEq/liter; potassium, 5 mEq/liter; chloride, 104 mEq/liter; CO_2, 18 mEq/liter; blood urea nitrogen (BUN), 40 mg/dl; and glucose, 592 mg/dl. The physician diagnoses diabetic ketoacidosis (DKA). Which treatment would the nurse expect the physician to order now?

A. Dextrose 50% and naloxone
B. Regular insulin and sodium bicarbonate
C. NPH insulin and potassium
D. Activated charcoal and naloxone

90 Which I.V. fluid would be most appropriate for this patient?

A. 0.45% saline solution
B. 0.9% (normal) saline solution
C. Dextrose 5% in 0.45% saline ($D_5\frac{1}{2}NS$) solution
D. Dextrose 5% in normal saline solution

91 The nurse anticipates that the physician will order the preferred initial insulin treatment by preparing to administer:

A. I.V. boluses of regular insulin 10 to 20 units/hour
B. An I.V. bolus of 20 units regular insulin followed by a continuous infusion of 4 to 8 units/hour
C. 10 units of regular insulin I.V. and 20 units of NPH insulin S.C.
D. 10 units of regular insulin I.V. and 10 units of regular insulin S.C.

92 Which history finding is considered a precipitating factor in the development of DKA?

A. Omission of or resistance to insulin in a patient with diabetes mellitus
B. Surgery or trauma in a patient with diabetes mellitus
C. Pancreatitis
D. All of the above

93 Which patient with insulin-dependent diabetes mellitus would the nurse determine is most at risk for DKA?

A. A child with otitis media
B. A child who participates in a gym class
C. A child who requires insulin twice a day
D. A child who self-administers insulin

94 The nurse knows that signs and symptoms of DKA may also occur in a child with:

A. Hypoglycemia
B. Appendicitis
C. Seizures
D. Upper respiratory tract infection

95 Which ECG abnormality may be assessed initially in a patient with DKA?

A. Sinus bradycardia
B. Appearance of U waves
C. ST-segment depression
D. Tall T waves

96 The nurse should assess for which electrolyte abnormality in a patient with DKA?

A. Hypomagnesemia
B. Hypophosphatemia
C. Hyperchloremia
D. Hypercalcemia

97 All of the following physical findings are characteristic of a patient with DKA *except:*

A. Acetone breath and slow respirations
B. Altered level of consciousness and Kussmaul's respirations
C. Polyuria and signs of dehydration
D. Tachycardia and possible hypotension

98 Which assessment findings would *not* support a diagnosis of DKA?

A. Decreased PCO_2, pH, and HCO_3^-
B. Elevated serum potassium level and decreased bicarbonate level
C. Elevated urine specific gravity and elevated BUN level
D. Decreased serum potassium level and decreased hematocrit

99 Which assessment finding is considered the most obvious sign of DKA?

A. Elevated serum potassium level
B. Elevated blood pH
C. Hypertension
D. Polyuria

100 The priority nursing diagnostic category for a patient with DKA would be:

A. Altered nutrition: Less than body requirements
B. Ineffective breathing pattern
C. Impaired gas exchange
D. Fluid volume deficit

101 After instituting the appropriate treatment, the nurse should assess the patient for which potential treatment-related complication?

A. Hyperosmolar nonketotic syndrome (HNKS)
B. Acute renal failure
C. Cerebral edema
D. Respiratory acidosis

102 Which other potential complication may occur in a patient treated for DKA?

A. Shock
B. Oliguria
C. Hypercalcemia
D. Hypokalemia

103 Which diabetic patient is considered at highest risk for hypovolemic shock from DKA?

A. A child
B. An adolescent
C. An elderly patient
D. A cardiac patient

104 Six hours after admission, the patient's serum glucose level decreases to 243 mg/dl. Which fluid therapy would the nurse expect the physician to order now?

A. 0.45% saline solution
B. Normal saline solution
C. $D_5\frac{1}{2}NS$ solution
D. Lactated Ringer's solution

105 Which parameter is most appropriate for determining a DKA patient's response to insulin therapy in the ED?

A. Laboratory studies of serum glucose levels
B. Laboratory studies of serum ketone levels
C. Bedside urine glucose measurements
D. Bedside capillary glucose measurements with a glucometer

106 All of the following treatments are appropriate for a patient with DKA *except:*

A. Continuous administration of NPH insulin at 4 to 8 units/hour
B. Rapid administration of fluids, initially 1,000 ml/hour
C. Infusion of $D_5\frac{1}{2}NS$ solution when serum glucose levels decrease to 250 mg/dl
D. Infusion of potassium as ketosis decreases and insulin therapy is begun

SITUATION

A 68-year-old woman is brought to the ED by her son, who informs the nurse that his mother has been experiencing weakness, polydipsia, and polyuria for the past few days. Initial laboratory studies reveal a serum glucose level of 2,000 mg/dl; no ketones are detected in the urine. The physician diagnoses HNKS.

Questions 107 to 110 relate to the above situation.

107 Which assessment finding would result in a change in the level of consciousness in a patient with HNKS?

A. Serum osmolarity of 380 mOsm/liter
B. BUN level of 50 mg/dl
C. Serum sodium level of 125 mEq/liter
D. Nonketotic state

108 Which nursing action is *not* a priority during the initial management of a patient with HNKS?

A. Administering insulin
B. Administering hypotonic saline solution
C. Monitoring the patient's rectal temperature and notifying the physician if the temperature rises above 101° F (38.3° C)
D. Assessing the patient's neurologic status

109 The nurse would expect the management of a patient with HNKS to differ from that of a patient with DKA because the patient with HNKS requires:

A. Hypertonic fluid replacement and less insulin and potassium than that needed for a patient with DKA
B. Hypotonic fluid replacement and less insulin and potassium than that needed for a patient with DKA
C. Hypotonic fluid replacement and no insulin or potassium
D. Isotonic replacement fluid and more insulin and potassium than that needed for a patient with DKA

110 All of the following nursing diagnoses would be appropriate for a patient with HNKS *except:*

A. Fluid volume deficit related to osmotic diuresis
B. Potential for injury related to altered level of consciousness
C. Altered peripheral tissue perfusion related to decreased cardiac output
D. Ineffective breathing pattern related to hyperventilation

SITUATION

A 47-year-old man is brought to the ED. His family reports that he had become confused over the past 72 hours and suffered a seizure while on the way to the hospital. Upon arrival, the patient is minimally responsive. His respiratory rate is 32 breaths/minute; pulse rate, 110 beats/minute; and blood pressure, 120/90 mm Hg. Immediate laboratory work reveals an abnormal sodium level of 117 mEq/liter. The patient's chest X-ray reveals a mass in the right midlung field.

Questions 111 to 116 relate to the above situation.

111 The nurse suspects that the underlying factor responsible for this patient's change in mental status is related to:

A. Lung cancer with cerebral metastatis
B. Syndrome of inappropriate antidiuretic hormone (SIADH) secretion
C. Seizures associated with meningitis
D. Possible subarachnoid hemorrhage

112 Which patient would not be considered at risk for developing SIADH?

A. A 20-year-old patient who is transferred from a skilled nursing facility where he received prolonged positive-pressure ventilation
B. A 36-year-old patient receiving phenytoin sodium (Dilantin)
C. A 64-year-old patient with chronic obstructive pulmonary disease complicated by pneumonia
D. A 70-year-old patient with a lung carcinoma

113 The nurse knows that an increase in antidiuretic hormone (ADH) secretion may result from:

A. Chlorpropamide (Diabinese) therapy
B. Head trauma
C. Viral respiratory infection
D. All of the above

114 Which laboratory finding is characteristic of a patient with SIADH?

A. Serum sodium level of 120 mEq/liter
B. Serum potassium level of 6 mEq/liter
C. Serum osmolarity of 350 mOsm/liter
D. Urine specific gravity of 1.003

115 The nurse would expect the initial treatment of this patient to include all of the following *except:*

A. Administration of furosemide (Lasix)
B. Administration of 3% hypertonic saline solution
C. Fluid restriction
D. Administration of demeclocycline hydrochloride (Declomycin) 300 mg P.O.

116 Prevention of which potential complication is the goal of nursing care for a patient with SIADH?

A. Tetany
B. Seizures
C. Hypotension
D. All of the above

SITUATION

A 16-year-old boy is brought to the ED by his parents because he has been experiencing polydipsia and polyuria. His medical history reveals no significant findings. Immediate laboratory studies indicate a serum sodium concentration of 160 mEq/liter and a urine osmolarity of 250 mOsm/liter. The physician diagnoses diabetes insipidus. Vasopressin tannate therapy is initiated.

Questions 117 to 121 relate to the above situation.

117 Which patient is most likely to develop diabetes insipidus?

A. An elderly man receiving thiazides and clofibrate (Atromid-S)
B. A young woman with severe pneumonia
C. A middle-aged man receiving vasopressin tannate for esophageal varices
D. A young man with a skull fracture resulting from a head trauma

118 Which laboratory finding would support a diagnosis of diabetes insipidus?

A. Decreased serum sodium level
B. Decreased serum osmolarity
C. Increased urine osmolarity
D. Urine specific gravity of 1.001

119 The priority nursing intervention in this situation would be to:

A. Assess for signs and symptoms of hypovolemic shock
B. Institute seizure precautions
C. Auscultate lung fields for crackles
D. Monitor the patient for cardiac arrhythmias

120 The nurse notes that the patient is not responding to vasopressin tannate (Pitressin Tannate) therapy. This may be caused by:

A. Administration of vasopressin with calcium channel blockers
B. Mixing vasopressin with normal saline solution
C. Inadequate warming or agitation of the medication vial
D. Failure to keep medication refrigerated

121 The nurse would question administering vasopressin tannate to a patient who has:

A. Liver dysfunction
B. Brain tumor
C. Angina pectoris
D. Undergone kidney transplantation

SITUATION

A 25-year-old man is brought to the ED by a friend. The patient had been complaining of blurred vision, headache, slurred speech, and weakness. He is now comatose. Earlier in the morning, he had been playing tennis. Immediate laboratory studies indicate a serum glucose level of 34 mg/dl.

Questions 122 and 123 refer to the above situation.

122 The nurse suspects that this patient's symptoms resulted from:

A. Neuroglycopenia
B. Glycopenia
C. Decreased liver glycogenolysis
D. Decreased response of the sympathetic nervous system

General Medical Emergencies
Questions

123 The nurse knows that emergency management of a comatose patient with hypoglycemia includes:

A. Measurement of fasting blood sugar levels and administration of sweetened orange juice via a nasogastric tube
B. Measurement of fasting blood sugar levels and administration of 50 ml of dextrose 5% in water (D_5W) I.V.
C. Administration of 50 ml of dextrose 50% I.V.
D. Infusion of 1 liter of dextrose 10% in water followed by measurement of blood glucose levels

SITUATION

A 66-year-old woman is brought to the ED by paramedics. Her blood pressure is 104/58 mm Hg; pulse rate, 44 beats/minute; respiratory rate, 14 breaths/minute; and temperature, 92.4° F (33.6° C). No medical history is available, except for the patient's statement of not feeling well for the past month. Physical examination reveals a lethargic, thin woman with dry skin and periorbital and facial edema. Bilateral pulmonary congestion is noted. ECG monitoring shows sinus bradycardia. The physician diagnoses impending myxedema coma.

Questions 124 to 128 refer to the above situation.

124 Which statement regarding myxedema coma is *true?*

A. It is an extremely advanced form of hypothyroidism
B. It does not occur in all patients with hypothyroidism
C. All patients who have myxedema coma are in a hypothyroid state
D. All of the above

125 Which electrolyte imbalance would the nurse expect this patient to have?

A. Hyponatremia
B. Hypernatremia
C. Hypokalemia
D. Hyperkalemia

126 The patient remains hypothermic, with a temperature of 95° F (35° C). An appropriate nursing intervention would be to:

A. Apply a hypothermia blanket
B. Rewarm the patient with blankets
C. Administer a glycerin suppository every 4 hours as needed
D. All of the above

127 The nurse would anticipate the treatment for this patient to include all of the following *except:*

A. Fluid restriction
B. Thyroid hormone replacement
C. Electrolyte replacement
D. Diuretic administration

128 The nurse draws blood for arterial blood gas analysis. Measurements reveal pH, 7.28; PO_2, 50 mm Hg; PCO_2, 64 mm Hg; and HCO_3^-, 20 mEq/liter. Based on these findings, the nurse would expect to:

A. Administer dextrose 5% in lactated Ringer's solution I.V. at 150 ml/hour
B. Administer 35% oxygen via a high flow oxygen (Venturi) mask
C. Measure the patient's serum electrolyte levels immediately
D. Prepare for endotracheal intubation

SITUATION

An obese patient with an 8-year history of Addison's disease is transferred to the ED after ambulatory surgery. The paramedics report that the patient has a fever; pallor; rapid, weak pulse; signs of dehydration; headache; confusion; restlessness; and a blood pressure of 90/50 mm Hg. Laboratory findings reveal a serum potassium level of 6.5 mEq/liter; white blood cell count, 15,000/mm³; serum glucose level, 55 mg/dl; and serum sodium level, 124 mEq/liter. The physician diagnoses adrenal crisis.

Questions 129 to 135 refer to the above situation.

129 The nurse suspects that this patient's adrenal crisis probably resulted from:

A. Obesity
B. Decreased exercise
C. Increased appetite
D. Fasting status before surgery

130 Nursing care of this patient should focus on the prevention of which life-threatening aspect of adrenal crisis?

A. Hypokalemia
B. Hyperglycemia
C. Vascular collapse
D. Hypernatremia

General Medical Emergencies
Questions

131 Which diagnostic test is the best indicator of this patient's condition?

A. Plasma carcinoembryonic antigen level
B. 24-hour urine 17-hydroxycorticosteroid level
C. Plasma cortisol level
D. Adrenocorticotropic hormone (ACTH) infusion test

132 Which fluid replacement method would the nurse expect to administer to this patient?

A. Dextrose 5% in lactated Ringer's solution at 100 ml/hour
B. 1 liter of dextrose 5% in normal saline in 2 hours
C. D_5W at 200 ml/hour
D. 1 liter of 0.45% saline solution in 6 hours

133 Which medication should the nurse prepare for immediate administration?

A. 0.1 mg of levothyroxine sodium (Synthroid)
B. 200 mg of dexamethasone (Decadron)
C. 200 mg of hydrocortisone (Cortef)
D. 0.1 mg of fludrocortisone acetate (Florinef)

134 The nurse would assess for hyperkalemia by observing for which ECG change?

A. T-wave depression with prolonged QT intervals
B. Peaked T waves, wide QRS complexes, and prolonged PR intervals
C. Q-wave inversion and shortened PR intervals
D. Bradycardia and bundle branch block

135 The clinical signs and symptoms of acute adrenal crisis are caused by:

A. Decreased aldosterone and cortisol levels
B. Decreased ADH and cortisol levels
C. Increased ADH and cortisol levels
D. Increased aldosterone and cortisol levels

General Medical Emergencies
Questions

A 55-year-old woman is admitted to the ED with a temperature of 105° F (40.5° C); blood pressure, 180/110 mm Hg; pulse rate, 120 beats/minute; and respiratory rate, 36 breaths/minute. She shows signs of dehydration and states that she has been experiencing muscle weakness and bone pain for the past week. She has a history of Graves' disease. The physician diagnoses thyroid crisis.

Questions 136 to 140 refer to the above situation.

136 The nurse would assess this patient for signs of:

A. Hypocalcemia and hypoglycemia
B. Hyperglycemia and hyponatremia
C. Hypernatremia and hypokalemia
D. Metabolic alkalosis

137 The nurse learns that the patient is iodine-sensitive. Based on this information, which drug would the nurse expect to be included in the treatment plan?

A. ACTH
B. Levothyroxine sodium (Synthroid)
C. Lithium carbonate (Lithobid)
D. Phenytoin (Dilantin)

138 Which nursing measure would be inappropriate in controlling this patient's pyrexia?

A. Administration of aspirin
B. Administration of muscle relaxants to control shivering
C. Application of ice packs to the axillae and groin
D. Use of a hypothermia blanket with a rectal probe

139 Which of the following would *not* be useful in assessing the patient's thyroid function?

A. Serum protein-bound iodine
B. Radioactive iodine uptake
C. Thyroid-stimulating hormone
D. Urine 17-ketosteroids

140 The patient begins to complain of bone pain and thirst. The nurse notes a decreased level of consciousness and hypotonicity of muscles. Which laboratory findings should be monitored in this situation?

A. Blood urea nitrogen
B. Serum potassium
C. Serum sodium
D. Serum calcium

SITUATION

A 65-year-old woman is brought to the ED by ambulance after fainting. Physical examination reveals central-type obesity with a fatty buffalo hump in the neck; hirsutism; thin, fragile extremities with ecchymotic areas; hypertension; and mild congestive heart failure. She informs the nurse that she has experienced extreme weakness and fatigue during the past month and that her sleep patterns have become altered.

Questions 141 to 145 refer to the above situation.

141 The nurse realizes that the patient's signs and symptoms are characteristic of:

A. Conn's syndrome
B. Cushing's syndrome
C. Diabetes insipidus
D. Myxedema coma

142 Which statement regarding the pathophysiology of the patient's condition is *true?*

A. It is caused by removal of the pituitary gland
B. It is a disorder of the posterior lobe of the pituitary gland and caused by vasopressin deficiency
C. The clinical manifestations reflect excessive adrenocortical activity
D. The clinical manifestations reflect deficient adrenocortical activity

143 The nurse would expect to assess this patient for signs of:

A. Hypernatremia
B. Hypokalemia
C. Hyperglycemia
D. All of the above

General Medical Emergencies
Questions

165

144 The patient's condition produces anti-inflammatory effects. Which nursing diagnosis best reflects this assessment?

A. Potential for injury related to decreased protein catabolism
B. Potential for infection related to altered metabolism
C. Altered body image related to physical appearance
D. Sleep pattern disturbance related to anxiety

145 Which assessment finding would a patient with increased mineralocorticoid and glucocorticoid levels exhibit?

A. Increased heart rate with atrial premature complexes
B. Decreased serum osmolarity
C. Elevated calcitonin levels
D. Chvostek's sign

Answer Sheet

	A B C D		A B C D		A B C D		A B C D
1	○ ○ ○ ○	31	○ ○ ○ ○	61	○ ○ ○ ○	91	○ ○ ○ ○
2	○ ○ ○ ○	32	○ ○ ○ ○	62	○ ○ ○ ○	92	○ ○ ○ ○
3	○ ○ ○ ○	33	○ ○ ○ ○	63	○ ○ ○ ○	93	○ ○ ○ ○
4	○ ○ ○ ○	34	○ ○ ○ ○	64	○ ○ ○ ○	94	○ ○ ○ ○
5	○ ○ ○ ○	35	○ ○ ○ ○	65	○ ○ ○ ○	95	○ ○ ○ ○
6	○ ○ ○ ○	36	○ ○ ○ ○	66	○ ○ ○ ○	96	○ ○ ○ ○
7	○ ○ ○ ○	37	○ ○ ○ ○	67	○ ○ ○ ○	97	○ ○ ○ ○
8	○ ○ ○ ○	38	○ ○ ○ ○	68	○ ○ ○ ○	98	○ ○ ○ ○
9	○ ○ ○ ○	39	○ ○ ○ ○	69	○ ○ ○ ○	99	○ ○ ○ ○
10	○ ○ ○ ○	40	○ ○ ○ ○	70	○ ○ ○ ○	100	○ ○ ○ ○
11	○ ○ ○ ○	41	○ ○ ○ ○	71	○ ○ ○ ○	101	○ ○ ○ ○
12	○ ○ ○ ○	42	○ ○ ○ ○	72	○ ○ ○ ○	102	○ ○ ○ ○
13	○ ○ ○ ○	43	○ ○ ○ ○	73	○ ○ ○ ○	103	○ ○ ○ ○
14	○ ○ ○ ○	44	○ ○ ○ ○	74	○ ○ ○ ○	104	○ ○ ○ ○
15	○ ○ ○ ○	45	○ ○ ○ ○	75	○ ○ ○ ○	105	○ ○ ○ ○
16	○ ○ ○ ○	46	○ ○ ○ ○	76	○ ○ ○ ○	106	○ ○ ○ ○
17	○ ○ ○ ○	47	○ ○ ○ ○	77	○ ○ ○ ○	107	○ ○ ○ ○
18	○ ○ ○ ○	48	○ ○ ○ ○	78	○ ○ ○ ○	108	○ ○ ○ ○
19	○ ○ ○ ○	49	○ ○ ○ ○	79	○ ○ ○ ○	109	○ ○ ○ ○
20	○ ○ ○ ○	50	○ ○ ○ ○	80	○ ○ ○ ○	110	○ ○ ○ ○
21	○ ○ ○ ○	51	○ ○ ○ ○	81	○ ○ ○ ○	111	○ ○ ○ ○
22	○ ○ ○ ○	52	○ ○ ○ ○	82	○ ○ ○ ○	112	○ ○ ○ ○
23	○ ○ ○ ○	53	○ ○ ○ ○	83	○ ○ ○ ○	113	○ ○ ○ ○
24	○ ○ ○ ○	54	○ ○ ○ ○	84	○ ○ ○ ○	114	○ ○ ○ ○
25	○ ○ ○ ○	55	○ ○ ○ ○	85	○ ○ ○ ○	115	○ ○ ○ ○
26	○ ○ ○ ○	56	○ ○ ○ ○	86	○ ○ ○ ○	116	○ ○ ○ ○
27	○ ○ ○ ○	57	○ ○ ○ ○	87	○ ○ ○ ○	117	○ ○ ○ ○
28	○ ○ ○ ○	58	○ ○ ○ ○	88	○ ○ ○ ○	118	○ ○ ○ ○
29	○ ○ ○ ○	59	○ ○ ○ ○	89	○ ○ ○ ○	119	○ ○ ○ ○
30	○ ○ ○ ○	60	○ ○ ○ ○	90	○ ○ ○ ○	120	○ ○ ○ ○

Answer Sheet

	A	B	C	D
121	○	○	○	○
122	○	○	○	○
123	○	○	○	○
124	○	○	○	○
125	○	○	○	○
126	○	○	○	○
127	○	○	○	○
128	○	○	○	○
129	○	○	○	○
130	○	○	○	○
131	○	○	○	○
132	○	○	○	○
133	○	○	○	○
134	○	○	○	○
135	○	○	○	○
136	○	○	○	○
137	○	○	○	○
138	○	○	○	○
139	○	○	○	○
140	○	○	○	○
141	○	○	○	○
142	○	○	○	○
143	○	○	○	○
144	○	○	○	○
145	○	○	○	○

1 Correct answer — **B**

In this situation, the nurse should be particularly alert for signs and symptoms of anticoagulant overdose, including petechiae, tachycardia, hypotension, hematuria, epistaxis, bleeding gums, ecchymoses, tarry stools, and coffee-ground vomitus. Pruritus and facial flushing are clinical signs of an allergic drug reaction.

2 Correct answer — **A**

A patient on long-term anticoagulant therapy is at risk for serious hemorrhagic complications, most commonly involving the intracranial compartment and GI tract. GI hemorrhage is typically associated with underlying lesions, such as ulcers. Minor bleeding, as evidenced by epistaxis or hematuria, may occur as a result of capillary rupture. Bleeding of the genitourinary or respiratory tract rarely occurs in patients on long-term anticoagulant therapy but may result from instrumentation.

3 Correct answer — **B**

The nurse would expect the physician to order administration of vitamin K, the treatment of choice for warfarin overdose. Because the patient ingested a large amount of warfarin, which has a half-life of 48 to 72 hours, the physician would need to reverse the effects rather than allow them to wear off gradually, as gradual wearing off may prolong the bleeding. Administering vitamin K, either orally or parenterally, antagonizes warfarin, thereby reversing its effects. Peritoneal dialysis, ethylenediaminetetraacetic acid (EDTA) chelation therapy, and plasmapheresis are not indicated in this situation because warfarin's effects can be easily reversed with vitamin K.

4 Correct answer — **D**

Administration of protamine sulfate would be inappropriate for a patient with hemorrhagic complications from oral anticoagulant therapy. Protamine sulfate neutralizes the effects of parenterally administered heparin and is therefore used to treat heparin overdose. Therapy for hemorrhagic complications from oral anticoagulants includes fluid volume replacement, clotting factor replacement, administration of vitamin K, and infusion of fresh frozen plasma and whole blood.

5 Correct answer — **A**

A patient receiving anticoagulant therapy should be instructed to avoid excessive alcohol intake because prolonged usage destroys liver cells, causing impaired coagulation from lack of clotting factors. Such

General Medical Emergencies
Answers

a patient should also be cautioned to wear gloves while gardening, to use an electric shaver rather than one with a straight-edged blade, to use a soft-bristled toothbrush, and to avoid trimming corns and calluses, as these measures help prevent trauma and decrease the risk of bleeding. A medical-alert bracelet or necklace is recommended for all patients receiving anticoagulant therapy.

6 Correct answer—C

An appropriate nursing intervention for a patient receiving heparin therapy would be to test the patient's urine and stool for blood. The nurse also should observe for other signs and symptoms of GI hemorrhage, including tachycardia, hypotension, and hematemesis. The partial thromboplastin time (PTT), not the prothrombin time (PT), is normally monitored to maintain therapeutic anticoagulation in heparin therapy; the therapeutic range should be 1.5 to 2.5 times the patient's control. PT is normally monitored during warfarin therapy. A patient receiving anticoagulant therapy should avoid aspirin because it aggravates bleeding tendencies.

7 Correct answer—C

Massaging an area before or after a subcutaneous injection of heparin is inappropriate because it increases the risk of trauma and hematoma formation at the injection site. Appropriate nursing actions would include changing the injection site with each dose to prevent massive hematoma formation; using the iliac crest or abdominal fat layer because injecting these sites produces minimal trauma to subcutaneous tissues; and observing the site for prolonged bleeding.

8 Correct answer—D

To prevent overdosage and the risk of prolonged bleeding during continuous administration, the drip rate must be accurately calculated and controlled. The PTT must be checked just before the next scheduled dose to ensure that clotting times are not dangerously prolonged. Larger doses and frequent injections are required during intermittent infusion to maintain therapeutic prolonged clotting times. Major bleeding episodes occur more commonly with intermittent I.V. infusion than with continuous I.V. infusion because larger doses must be given.

9 Correct answer—A

Acute lymphocytic leukemia, a malignant disease of the bone marrow and lymphatic system that affects the hematologic cells and causes a proliferation of nonfunctional white blood cells and possibly the destruction of red blood cells and platelets, primarily affects young children; it is uncommon after age 20. Approximately 80% of all patients with this disease are between ages 2 and 5.

10 Correct answer — C

An appropriate nursing diagnosis for a patient with acute lymphocytic leukemia would be *Potential for infection related to immunosuppression* because infection uncontrolled by dysfunctional white blood cells is a serious complication and a leading cause of death in acute cases. Other major causes of death include chemotherapeutic side effects, bleeding resulting from anemia, and thrombocytopenia. Infection is commonly caused by gram-negative sepsis. Frequent cultures are necessary, and treatment with appropriate antibiotics is required. The patient may require placement in a protected environment. Because anemia and thrombocytopenia occur, *Altered tissue perfusion related to enhanced coagulation from thrombocytosis* and *Altered tissue perfusion related to increased blood viscosity from polycythemia vera* would be inappropriate diagnoses. Seizures rarely occur in this disease; therefore, *Potential for injury related to seizures* would be an inappropriate diagnosis.

11 Correct answer — B

The nurse would expect to treat a leukemic patient with an elevated temperature with acetaminophen. Fever is perhaps the most important sign of infection in such a patient; judicious use of analgesic and antipyretic medications is appropriate. Granulocytosis and inflammation are commonly absent; therefore the presence of a fever is an important indicator of the onset of infection. Frequent use of analgesics or antipruritics may mask fever. Bleeding is another major complication; therefore, aspirin must be used cautiously because of its antiplatelet activity and the risk of Reye's syndrome. Azathioprine and antibiotics are inappropriate for treating fever.

12 Correct answer — A

Chemotherapy destroys abnormal leukemic cells, causes bone marrow depression, and depresses the patient's immunologic defense mechanisms. Chemotherapy produces granulocytopenia, so the patient must be observed for the first signs of infection.

13 Correct answer — C

The most significant clinical finding in a patient with disseminated intravascular coagulation (DIC) is abnormal bleeding — such as hemoptysis, petechiae, or hematuria — without a history of a serious bleeding disorder. Other signs and symptoms include a prolonged PT and PTT, decreased fibrinogen levels, decreased platelet count, increased fibrin degradation products, and an elevated blood urea nitrogen level. Leukopenia, maculopapular rash, and severe hypertension are not symptoms of DIC.

14 Correct answer — D

Bleeding may occur from mucous membranes, venipuncture sites, and the GI and genitourinary tracts. In DIC, widespread clotting occurs in small blood vessels, leading to the consumption of clotting factors and platelets and the development of a bleeding disorder.

15 Correct answer — B

Activation of the clotting mechanism via fetal and placental tissue may lead to the development of DIC. In pregnancy, a normally hypercoagulable (not thrombocytopenic) state, amniotic fluid causes clot-promoting activities. However, because dead fetal and placental tissues also cause clot-promoting activities, such conditions as retained dead fetus and abruptio placentae may release clots into the maternal circulation that can lead to DIC. Under these conditions, the incidence of DIC approaches 50%. Treatment involves blood factor replacements and removal of fetal material. Hemolysis of red blood cells does not occur from fetal enzyme release. Although thromboembolism may occur in a postpartum patient, it does not cause DIC.

16 Correct answer — D

Because heparin therapy retards the coagulation process, it decreases hemorrhagic manifestations and permits normalization of clotting test results. Its antithrombin activity neutralizes free-circulating thrombin, thus preventing proliferation of thrombin (which leads to the formation of fibrin) and further blood clotting.

17 Correct answer — C

A fibrin degradation products result of 10 ug/ml is considered normal and therefore reflects a successful treatment outcome. A platelet count of 40,000/mm³ is still quite low, and a PTT of 76 seconds is still prolonged; both indicate a state of impaired coagulation. A hemoglobin level of 7 g/dl is low, reflecting blood loss.

18 Correct answer — C

Hemophilia A (a deficiency of Factor VIII) is five times more common than hemophilia B (a deficiency of Factor IX). Both types are inherited as X-linked traits; therefore, almost all affected individuals are male.

General Medical Emergencies
Answers

The mothers and some sisters of hemophiliacs may be asymptomatic carriers of the disorder.

19 Correct answer — **D**

Bleeding near peripheral nerves causes neuropathy, pain, paresthesia, and muscle atrophy. Bleeding gums and hematuria, unrelated to trauma, are common. Abnormal bleeding occurs through the absence or deficiency of a specific clotting factor. About one-half of all hemophiliacs have severe, spontaneous bleeding into joints, which can lead to crippling and deformity.

20 Correct answer — **C**

The most common cause of death in a patient with hemophilia occurs from bleeding of the cranium. Intracerebral hemorrhage may also lead to shock and death. Other less common bleeding sites include the GI and genitourinary tracts, pharynx, and heart.

21 Correct answer — **A**

Confirming diagnostic studies in hemophilia indicate a Factor VIII or Factor IX deficiency, a prolonged PTT and normal PT, a normal fibrinogen level, and a normal platelet count.

22 Correct answer — **D**

Assisting with immediate aspiration of hemarthroses would be inappropriate in this situation, as hemarthroses should not be aspirated unless the patient is feeling acute pain and pressure; aspiration may cause infection and additional bleeding. Treatment should focus on preventing crippling deformities and prolonging life expectancy. Joint bleeding is initially managed by immobilizing the affected limb and applying ice packs to diminish swelling and reduce pain. Because the plasma level of the deficient factor must be raised, an immediate infusion of cryoprecipitate (Factors VIII, XIII, and fibrinogen) may be necessary. Hemarthroses are not associated with von Willebrand's disease.

23 Correct answer — **C**

In the four main blood groups of the ABO system — A, B, AB, and O — the antigens are located on the red cell membrane and match the blood group designation. Therefore, in a patient with group AB blood, the red cell membrane contains both A and B antigens. The antibodies of the ABO system are located in the serum; they do not correspond to the antigens on the red cell membrane because antibodies cannot be produced against antigens present. The table below lists the antigens and antibodies of the ABO system.

ABO Blood Typing

Type	Red Cell Antigens	Serum Antibodies
0	None	Anti-A, anti-B
A	A	Anti-B
B	B	Anti-A
AB	A, B	None

24 Correct answer—C

Packed red blood cells (RBCs) decrease the risk of anaphylactic reaction. A unit of whole blood, which contains all the necessary blood components, including platelets and coagulation factors, is centrifuged to separate the RBCs from the plasma. Packed cells consist of the same RBC mass as whole blood with only small amounts of plasma, leukocytes, and platelets. Because only a small amount of plasma is present, the risk of plasma protein reaction, which may cause an anaphylactic reaction, decreases. A transfusion of packed RBCs causes the hemoglobin and hematocrit levels to rise faster than a whole blood transfusion does. In the average patient, the hemoglobin rises 1 g/dl, and the hematocrit rises 2% to 3%. With a whole blood transfusion, a similar increase will be seen; however, it typically occurs 24 hours after administration. Packed RBCs restore or maintain oxygen-carrying capacity and are indicated in anemia or surgical blood loss or to increase RBC mass. Whole blood is indicated when massive hemorrhage occurs.

25 Correct answer—D

When administering a blood transfusion, an 18- or 20-G catheter may be used. To prevent hemolysis, 18-G catheters are recommended for most blood transfusions. However, 20-G catheters are acceptable for average transfusion rates. Only normal saline solution may be used when administering blood products. Lactated Ringer's solution causes agglutination, and dextrose 5% in water (D_5W) causes hemolysis. During a blood transfusion, the patient's vital signs should be assessed before initiating the transfusion, 15 minutes after initiation, and after the transfusion is completed. Assessing the vital signs at these times enables the nurse to detect any adverse effects. It is particularly important to assess the vital signs 15 minutes after the initiation of the transfusion, because this is when most severe reactions occur. When using a blood warmer, the temperature should not exceed 98.6° F (37° C); RBCs heated above this temperature may hemolyze.

26 Correct answer—A

Based on these signs and symptoms, the nurse would determine that the patient is experiencing a febrile, nonhemolytic transfusion reaction, the most common of the immediate reactions. This type of reaction, which typically occurs in patients who have received multiple transfusions, is characterized by fever, chills, headache, hypotension, lumbar pain, palpitations, and malaise. The fever typically occurs 1 to 6 hours after the transfusion has been initiated. A hemolytic transfusion reaction, the most acute and most dreaded adverse effect of a transfusion, occurs because of ABO blood group incompatibility. It is characterized by the immediate onset of a fever that may exceed 104.9° F (40.5° C), facial flushing, chills, lumbar pain, hypotension, headache, chest pain, dyspnea, oliguria, and shock. A delayed hemolytic transfusion reaction, which typically occurs 2 or more days after a transfusion, most commonly occurs in patients who have received previous transfusions. It is characterized by continued anemia, decreased hemoglobin level, hemoglobinuria, and bilirubinuria. A bacterial transfusion reaction, a rare occurrence, is caused by bacterial contamination of the blood product. It is characterized by high fever, severe hypotension, dry flushed skin, pain in the abdomen and extremities, vomiting, and bloody diarrhea.

27 Correct answer—C

The nurse knows that thrombocytopenia (a decreased number of thrombocytes) does not result from a splenectomy, which would cause the platelet count to increase. The spleen collects one-third of all the platelets, and its removal eliminates the site of platelet antibody production, thus decreasing platelet destruction. Chlorothiazide may cause thrombocytopenia because of platelet antibody formation. Both chlorothiazide and zidovudine (AZT) suppress thrombocyte production because of bone marrow depression. A viral infection may cause thrombocytopenia because the virus can destroy circulating platelets or impair platelet production.

28 Correct answer—C

The nurse would expect the platelet count to return to normal levels within 1 week after discontinuation of quinidine therapy. Thrombocytopenia, which occurs in only 1 in 100,000 persons taking quinidine, develops as a result of an idiosyncratic reaction to platelet antibody formation. It may develop within 12 hours after quinidine therapy is started and typically recedes within 24 hours after discontinuation of the drug. A normal platelet count and even mild thrombocytosis should occur within 1 week.

29 Correct answer—**D**

Anemic crisis is not a form of sickle-cell crisis. Sickle-cell crisis, the initiation of sickling of red blood cells leading to severe hemolytic anemia, may take on one of three forms: aplastic, sequestration, or painful. In aplastic crisis, the bone marrow stops producing RBCs and the hemoglobin level drops. In sequestration crisis, which is caused by splenic blockage, the patient has a sudden, large pooling of blood in the spleen. In painful crisis, the most common form of sickle-cell crisis, sickled cells occlude the blood vessels, decreasing blood flow and producing ischemia and infarction.

30 Correct answer—**D**

Sickle cell anemia usually does not result in impaired myocardial contractility; therefore a diagnosis of *Decreased cardiac output related to impaired myocardial contractility* would be inappropriate. The other nursing diagnoses are appropriate for a patient with sickle-cell anemia. Increased blood viscosity (from clumping of sickled cells) may decrease the blood flow to the organs and extremities. Impaired blood flow causes tissue ischemia and pain. Because sickled cells are dysfunctional, and occluded peripheral vessels prevent oxygen delivery to tissues, impaired gas exchange occurs.

31 Correct answer—**C**

Increased fluid intake will prevent sickle-cell crisis by preventing dehydration; therefore, it would not be considered a precipitating factor. Cigarette smoking, infection, and such physically demanding activities as tennis may precipitate a painful episode of sickle-cell crisis. Cigarette smoking contributes to sickle-cell crisis by interfering with oxygen exchange. Although infection is considered a precipitating factor, the precise relationship between infection and sickle-cell crisis has not been identified; researchers are uncertain whether the decreased oxygen state is caused by infection or whether the crisis encourages infection. Physically demanding activities, such as tennis, lead to overexertion and dehydration. The dehydration potentiates the sickling process, thereby causing a crisis.

32 Correct answer—**A**

Inserting the smallest-possible-gauge I.V. catheter and infusing dextrose 5% in ½ normal saline solution ($D_5\frac{1}{2}NS$) at 100 ml/hour would be the best way to maintain hydration in this patient. Inserting a small-gauge I.V. catheter, such as a 21G or 23G catheter, will minimize trauma and reduce tissue scarring. Patients with sickle-cell anemia have a lifelong illness in which venous access must be preserved. The recommended I.V. solutions for hydration of patients in sickle-cell crisis include dextrose 5% in water (D_5W), $D_5\frac{1}{2}NS$, and lactated Ringer's solution. To avoid fluid overload and congestive heart failure, the recommended rate of infusion is 100 to 150 ml/hour. Patients with sickle-cell anemia should normally consume 4 to 6 quarts (about 4 to 6 liters) of liquid every 24 hours. In sickle-cell crisis, adequate hydration is critical because it assists in halting the sickle cycle by decreasing blood viscosity. In this situation, however, the patient has been vomiting and probably would not be able to tolerate oral fluids.

33 Correct answer—B

Morphine sulfate I.V. is not the ideal medication for providing analgesia to patients in a painful crisis because it may produce respiratory depression. However, morphine that is administered orally or subcutaneously is considered safe for such patients. Meperidine I.M., aspirin, and codeine also may provide analgesia for these patients. The analgesic used varies with the severity of the crisis; typically, oral analgesics are ordered before I.M. or I.V. agents.

34 Correct answer—B

Hairy leukoplakia, or a hairy covering on the tongue, is characteristic only of the immunodepression seen in acquired immunodeficiency syndrome (AIDS). Oral candidiasis (thrush) is characteristic of the immunodepression that occurs with various illnesses. Purplish skin lesions are associated with Kaposi's sarcoma, an immunosuppressed condition that may be unrelated to AIDS.

35 Correct answer—D

A T lymphocyte count of 150/mm³ reflects a depressed immune system; normal counts range from 600 to 1,000/mm³. Because T4 cells are the lymphocytes affected in AIDS, the nurse would expect a a low T4:T8 ratio. Platelets and hemoglobin levels are not reflective of a person's immune status.

36 Correct answer—A

Zidovudine (AZT), classified as an antiviral agent used to decrease the replication of human immunodeficiency virus (HIV), is the only FDA-approved medication for AIDS. It may be given to those with a positive HIV status to prevent the development of AIDS. Co-trimoxasole (Bactrim) is the antibiotic most useful in treating *Pneumocystis carinii* pneumonia. Rifampin and isoniazid are antitubercular agents. Clotrimazole (Mycelex) is an antifungal agent effective against oral candidiasis.

37 Correct answer—D

Pentamidine is administered via a nebulizer. Because it is unknown whether the patient has tuberculosis, which is contagious, or *Pneumocystis carinii* pneumonia, which is not considered a threat to someone with an intact immune system, and because aerosolized pentamidine stimulates coughing, pentamidine should be administered in a well-ventilated room, using acid fast bacilli (AFB) respiratory measures. Such measures include placing the patient in a closed room with special ventilation to prevent the spread of tuberculosis. Administering this drug in a well-ventilated room while wearing a mask reduces the nurse's exposure to the drug, which may cause irritation to the eyes and throat. Because researchers do not know whether pentamidine causes fetal damage, pregnant nurses and those who are trying to become pregnant should avoid administering the drug.

38 Correct answer—A

The nurse should inquire about a recent history of chicken pox, influenza, and salicylate (aspirin) ingestion, which have been associated with the development of Reye's syndrome. Diarrhea, measles, and insect bites have no bearing in this situation.

39 Correct answer—D

Because liver dysfunction occurs with Reyes syndrome, an elevated serum ammonia level is considered indicative of this disease. Other common findings include increased aspartate aminotransferase, alanine aminotransferase, and lactic dehydrogenase (LDH) levels. Hypoglycemia (decreased glucose levels) may also occur as glucose stores become depleted because of the stress, anorexia, and vomiting associated with this disease.

40 Correct answer—C

The anterior aspect of the tibia below the knee is the most common site for insertion of an intraosseous catheter. Although the iliac crest may sometimes be used, it is a difficult site to maintain for catheterization; it also decreases the patient's mobility. The sternum and femur are not used for intraosseous catheterization.

General Medical Emergencies
Answers

41 Correct answer—C

A positive Chvostek's sign is indicative of hypocalcemia because a decrease in ionized calcium causes an increase in neuromuscular excitability. To elicit Chvostek's sign, the nurse would tap a finger on the skin above the supramandibular portion of the parotid gland and observe for twitching of the upper lip on the same side as the stimulation. Applying and inflating a blood pressure cuff to the patient's upper arm and having the patient hyperventilate are two methods of eliciting carpopedal spasm (Trousseau's sign). A positive Trousseau's sign also is indicative of hypocalcemia.

42 Correct answer—C

When assessing a patient for hypocalcemia, the nurse would observe for a prolonged QT interval on electrocardiogram (ECG), an indication of impaired cardiac contractility resulting from hypocalcemia. A prolonged QT interval predisposes the patient to a polymorphous ventricular tachycardia (torsades de pointes).

43 Correct answer—B

Oliguria is not one of the potential complications of hypocalcemia. Bleeding abnormalities occur in hypocalcemia because calcium assists in converting prothrombin to thrombin in the coagulation cascade. Bronchospasm can lead to laryngeal stridor and seizures as a result of neuromuscular irritability caused by reduced calcium levels.

44 Correct answer—A

A patient with myxedema coma typically suffers from hyponatremia, resulting from inappropriate secretion of antidiuretic hormone (ADH). A myxedematous state also may result from the interstitial accumulation of a mucopolysaccharide substance that attracts water and produces water retention. Therefore, the hyponatremia is caused by dilution from inappropriate ADH secretion as well as from water retention. Another common finding in myxedema coma is hypoglycemia, which results from the patient's hypometabolic state. Because the thyroid gland produces the calcium-lowering hormone calcitonin, calcium levels may rise in hypothyroidism.

45 Correct answer—A

The nurse would expect a patient with myxedema coma to have respiratory acidosis and CO_2 narcosis as a result of lowered thyroxine (T_4) and triiodothyronine (T_3) levels. These hormones increase metabolic functions, such as respiration. Thus, a decrease in T_3 and T_4 levels depresses respiratory function, thereby causing hypoventilation.

Metabolic acidosis also may develop as hypoxia increases serum lactate levels.

46 Correct answer — B

The nurse would expect to note oliguria and abdominal distention during the assessment of a patient with myxedema coma since this condition causes dilutional hyponatremia and a decreased cardiac output. Decreased cardiac output leads to a decreased renal perfusion and glomerular filtration rate (GFR), which results in oliguria. Dilutional hyponatremia may cause decreased intestinal peristalsis, resulting in abdominal distention and, possibly, paralytic ileus. The patient also may exhibit hypothermia, hypoventilation, seizures, hypoglycemia, and anemia.

47 Correct answer — C

Because myxedema coma is associated with dilutional hyponatremia, treatment usually consists of fluid restriction initially, followed by the administration of a hypertonic solution, such as dextrose 5% in normal saline (D_5NS). Since fluid therapy aims at correcting imbalances, an infusion of D_5NS would provide necessary calories, prevent hypoglycemia, and correct the underlying hyponatremia. Administering a hypotonic solution, such as D_5W or 0.3% sodium chloride, would worsen the patient's hyponatremic state. Although $D_{10}W$ would correct the hypoglycemia, it would be of no value in treating hyponatremia.

48 Correct answer — A

The nurse would anticipate the treatment of a patient with hyperkalemia to include of the administration of dextrose 50%, regular insulin, sodium bicarbonate, and calcium chloride, but not lactulose enemas; lactulose is used to treat hepatic failure. The dextrose converts to glucose, which drives potassium into the cells, as does the administration of I.V. insulin. Sodium bicarbonate corrects the accompanying metabolic acidosis, causing potassium to move out of the cell. I.V. calcium stimulates cardiac contractility, thereby counteracting the depressant effects of excess potassium on the heart.

49 Correct answer — B

During the initial stages of hyperkalemia, the nurse would expect to see peaked T waves on ECG. The impaired neuromuscular transmission that occurs in hyperkalemia produces intraventricular conduction disturbances, which manifest as repolarization changes (reflected as peaked T waves). As potassium levels increase, other

General Medical Emergencies Answers

changes occur, including prolongation of PR intervals, absence of P waves, and widening of QRS complexes.

50 Correct answer—B

During the physical assessment of a patient with hyperkalemia, the nurse would expect to note ascending muscle weakness and bradycardia. Ascending muscle weakness typically originates in the legs and travels to the trunk; because the diaphragm and intercostal muscles are usually spared, the respiratory function remains unimpaired. Because peristalsis is increased in a patient with hyperkalemia, diarrhea is common and hyperactive bowel sounds may be heard. Apathy is common to both hypokalemia and hyperkalemia. Polyuria is not a sign of hyperkalemia.

51 Correct answer—D

Hyperkalemia is commonly associated with metabolic acidosis. In an acidotic state, hydrogen shifts from the extracellular compartment into the cell to reduce the acidosis. As potassium is the major intracellular electrolyte, it shifts from the cell into the extracellular compartment in exchange. Thus, metabolic acidosis produces a relative increase in serum potassium levels.

52 Correct answer—B

In multiple myeloma, hypercalcemia results from the release of calcium from lesions into the extracellular compartment (plasma). Other causes of hypercalcemia unrelated to multiple myeloma include increased mobilization of calcium from the bone in primary hyperparathyroidism; altered renal tubular reabsorption of calcium; and increased intestinal reabsorption of calcium secondary to a large dietary intake or an excessive administration or intake of vitamin D.

53 Correct answer—A

Signs of hypercalcemia include flank or thigh pain, and polyuria, and constipation. Flank and thigh pain, which result from renal calculi, occur in approximately two-thirds of all hypercalcemic patients. Polyuria results from the inhibition of ADH by calcium in the distal tubules. Anuria or oliguria, diarrhea, and metabolic acidosis or alkalosis are not signs of hypercalcemia.

54 Correct answer—C

The increased extracellular levels of calcium predispose the patient to repolarization changes (as reflected in shortening of the ST segment) and ultimately cardiac arrest. If a patient is receiving digitalis therapy, hypercalcemia may cause an enhanced digitalis effect, which can contribute to arrhythmias or cardiac arrest.

55 Correct answer — A

Treatment for this patient would include the administration of normal saline solution and loop diuretics. Normal saline solution is administered to increase the patient's GFR and calcium excretion. Loop diuretics are used to prevent tubular reabsorption of calcium. Thiazide diuretics should be avoided, as they decrease calcium excretion. Other treatments for hypercalcemia include the administration of corticosteroids to decrease the GI absorption of calcium, plicamycin (mythramycin) to stimulate bone uptake of calcium, and oral phosphates to bind calcium. Sodium polystyrene sulfonate enemas, glucose, insulin, and hemodialysis are used to treat hyperkalemia.

56 Correct answer — C

The nurse would assess the patient for signs of hypokalemia. In hepatic failure, this occurs as a result of elevated aldosterone levels; aldosterone reabsorbs sodium and causes the kidneys to excrete potassium. Other signs of hepatic failure include decreased plasma protein level (hypoproteinemia), which results from hypoalbuminemia; decreased calcium levels (hypocalcemia), which results from inadequate storage of vitamin D; and free-water excess, as dilutional hyponatremia may result from increased ADH secretion.

57 Correct answer — A

Respiratory alkalosis results from increased ammonia levels, which act to stimulate the respiratory drive and lead to hyperventilation. Hypermagnesemia produces hypoventilation. Hypokalemia can result from metabolic alkalosis because, in this state, potassium shifts into the cell. Hypocalcemia usually is not associated with acid-base imbalances, except in the case of chronic renal failure, which produces metabolic acidosis.

58 Correct answer — B

Aldosterone causes the body to retain both sodium and water and to excrete potassium. Spironolactone is an aldosterone-blocking agent that is used to enhance sodium excretion and potassium retention; therefore, the nurse would assess for a decrease in serum sodium levels and an increase in serum potassium levels. It is important to prevent hypokalemia in the patient with liver dysfunction because decreased serum potassium levels can contribute to the development of hepatic encephalopathy. Magnesium levels should not be affected significantly by spironolactone.

59 Correct answer—A

The nurse would not expect the physician to order Kayexalate enemas in this situation, as they decrease potassium levels and the patient's levels are already decreased. Lactulose enemas are used to eliminate intestinal ammonia. Limiting the administration of hypotonic solutions restricts free-water intake, a necessary measure to prevent further dilution of intravascular sodium, as plasma hyponatremia is present in those with hepatic failure. Both dietary protein and sodium are restricted in patients with hepatic failure.

60 Correct answer—A

The goals of I.V. therapy for the patient in this situation would not be based on sex and medical history. Fluid replacement is a lifesaving step in the initial treatment of burns. Hemoconcentration (as determined by hemoglobin and hematocrit values), increased urine specific gravity, and oliguria are common sequelae in the early stages of burn injury. These result from intravascular depletion, as body fluids shift into the intracellular and interstitial compartments. Careful monitoring of urine specific gravity and urine output for signs of impending renal failure is necessary. The depth and percentage of burn injury (using the Rule of Nines) serve as the basis for determining the amount of fluid required.

61 Correct answer—B

During the initial treatment phase of a burn injury, one-half of the solution is given in the first 8 hours, during which time the patient undergoes generalized dehydration and decreased circulating volume peak, and the remaining fluid is administered over the next 16 hours. Nurses should keep in mind that this fluid replacement formula is only a guide; the patient's individual response to fluid therapy is the determining factor in replacement therapy. The patient's response is determined by hourly vital sign assessments, hourly urine output assessments, and monitoring of urine specific gravity every 8 hours.

62 Correct answer—B

During the initial stages of burn injury, the nurse would expect the patient to show signs of edema and hyperkalemia. At this time, the patient experiences a plasma-to-interstitial fluid shift, causing a leakage through the capillaries, resulting in tissue edema. Because of cellular trauma, potassium is released to the extracellular space, resulting in hyperkalemia. After the initial stage, usually after 36 hours, the body begins to mobilize burn edema; fluid shifts back into the intravascular space, thereby predisposing the patient to circulatory overload. Also at this time, potassium is excreted in large amounts in the urine because of an increase in intravascular volume. Aldosterone, which reabsorbs sodium and excretes potassium, is released in large quantities in response to the dilutional hyponatremia that develops as intracellular and interstitial fluid shifts back into the intravascular compartment.

63 Correct answer—A

During the later stages of a burn injury, the nurse would expect the patient to show signs of jugular venous distention and hypokalemia. At this time, the patient experiences an interstitial-to-plasma fluid shift into the intravascular compartment, resulting in circulatory overload (as evidenced by jugular venous distention) and dilutional hyponatremia. Aldosterone is released in response to hyponatremia, resulting in the reabsorption of sodium and excretion of potassium from the kidneys. Hypokalemia is further perpetuated as the expanding intravascular volume fosters an increase in urine output with resultant potassium loss.

64 Correct answer—A

The nurse would not expect to note jugular venous distention, a sign of fluid overload, in a patient with diabetic ketoacidosis (DKA). Instead, she would expect to note signs of severe intravascular dehydration, such as poor skin turgor. The nurse would also expect the patient to have hyperkalemia, an initial response to metabolic acidosis, as well as hyperventilation, as the body attempts to compensate for the metabolic acidosis by eliminating carbon dioxide.

65 Correct answer—D

The first priority in caring for *any* patient is to establish and maintain a patent airway. The patient with DKA typically displays Kussmaul's respirations (slow, deep, regular breathing) in response to the acidotic state. Frequent patient assessment and arterial blood gas (ABG) studies are vital. Administration of volume replacement fluids and I.V. insulin are secondary interventions in this situation.

66 Correct answer—A

Because a patient with DKA typically exhibits severe intravascular depletion and cellular dehydration, the nurse would expect the initial treatment to focus on stabilizing hemodynamic status by infusing isotonic saline solution to promote intravascular rehydration. If the circulatory system is stable but cellular dehydration is present, body fluid repletion can be achieved with a hypotonic solution, such as half normal saline solution. Because the circulatory system is unstable in DKA, hypotonic saline solution should be avoided. After fluid therapy and insulin administration have been initiated, careful monitoring of electrolyte and glucose levels is crucial. When the serum glucose level falls between 250 and 300 mg/dl, insulin is discontinued and fluid therapy is changed to a hypertonic solution containing glucose, such as $D_5\frac{1}{2}NS$, thereby preventing the development of hypoglycemia, hypokalemia, and cerebral edema.

67 Correct answer – A

During DKA therapy, the patient typically follows a pattern of initially elevated serum potassium levels followed by gradually decreasing levels. In DKA, serum potassium levels initially are elevated in response to the body's acidotic state, which causes shifting of cellular potassium into the intravascular space. However, in time, renal loss of potassium occurs from polyuria. Serum potassium is further depleted as potassium shifts into the intracellular compartment in response to insulin therapy and correction of acidosis.

68 Correct answer – C

Respiratory acidosis is an emergency in an asthmatic patient. During the early stages of an asthma attack, ABG measurements reveal respiratory alkalosis from hyperventilation. However, as airway obstruction progresses, respiratory acidosis results, as reflected in this patient's ABG measurements. The rationale for determining respiratory acidosis is that the PCO_2 is greater than 40 mm Hg (the respiratory component) and the pH is less than 7.35 (acidosis); the bicarbonate buffer remains unchanged.

69 Correct answer – D

Preparing for a possible tracheotomy is not a priority action in this situation. However, the nurse may need to prepare for oral intubation if initial therapy is unsuccessful. Initial management includes oxygen therapy, continuous cardiac monitoring, establishment of an I.V. line, and the delivery of inhaled bronchodilator therapy, as ordered.

70 Correct answer – A

If this patient is not treated, respiratory arrest will occur as a result of airway obstruction, acidosis, and hypoxemia.

71 Correct answer—B

Metabolic alkalosis is indicated by a pH greater than 7.45, an HCO_3^- level greater than 26 mEq/liter, and a normal PCO_2 (respiratory component). In this situation, the patient's metabolic alkalosis could only have been caused by overzealous administration of sodium bicarbonate. Respiratory arrest would have caused the patient to experience respiratory acidosis followed by metabolic acidosis. Hyperventilation would cause respiratory alkalosis. Excessive oxygen administration can cause O_2 toxicity and, in patients with obstructive lung disease, respiratory acidosis.

72 Correct answer—A

The correct treatment in this situation should have been limited to hyperventilation with a bag-valve-mask device. The patient's initial ABG measurements showed a respiratory acidosis secondary to ineffective ventilation. Hyperventilating this patient with a bag-valve-mask device would have blown off CO_2, thus correcting the acidosis. Sodium bicarbonate is unnecessary because the HCO_3^- level is normal. The patient's acid-base imbalance is unrelated to oxygen therapy. Epinephrine is not indicated because the patient did not lose pulse or blood pressure.

73 Correct answer—D

This patient is hyperventilating and, as a result, is in respiratory alkalosis. The pH is elevated above 7.45, and the PCO_2 (respiratory component) is low. The metabolic component of HCO_3^- is normal.

74 Correct answer—D

The goal of therapy for this patient is to increase CO_2 retention by helping the patient gain control of her respirations, which are presently uncontrolled because of hyperventilation. That can be accomplished by using a paper bag to induce rebreathing of exhaled air, which will lead to CO_2 retention, breaking the cycle and slowing the respiratory rate. The patient's oxygen and bicarbonate levels are already normal.

75 Correct answer—D

The patient does not require sodium bicarbonate administration, which is indicated for metabolic acidosis. The patient had an anxiety attack and took an overdose of medication; therefore, she requires either inpatient or outpatient follow-up.

General Medical Emergencies Answers

76 Correct answer—B

This patient is experiencing numbness and tingling because hypocapnia causes vasoconstriction and decreased calcium levels. Carbon dioxide is a potent vasoactive agent. Hypocapnia leads to vasoconstriction of cerebral and peripheral vessels, resulting in the paresthesias associated with hyperventilation. Alkalosis also decreases serum calcium levels, resulting in numbness, tingling, and paresthesias. Diazepam does not cause numbness or tingling.

77 Correct answer—A

The correct interpretation is metabolic acidosis. The pH is below 7.35, indicating acidosis; the respiratory component (PCO_2) is normal, but the metabolic component (HCO_3^-) is extremely low (normal is 22 to 26 mEq/liter), indicating an acid excess.

78 Correct answer—B

The bicarbonate deficit is the amount of bicarbonate anion that would theoretically be necessary to fully correct the acid-base imbalance. It can be calculated by subtracting the measured bicarbonate (10) from the desired bicarbonate (average, 24). Therefore, the bicarbonate deficit in this situation would be 14 mEq/liter.

79 Correct answer—D

A total of 245 mEq of sodium bicarbonate would be necessary to correct this acid-base imbalance. The patient may require a continuous infusion to receive this large amount of bicarbonate.
  The calculation to correct acidosis is as follows:
  bicarbonate deficit × weight (kg) × 0.25 (a conversion factor accounting for the bicarbonate space in the body) = dose of sodium bicarbonate (mEq).
  Therefore:
  14 × 70 × 0.25 = 245 mEq of sodium bicarbonate.

80 Correct answer—C

A lactate level and anion gap would provide essential information for the treatment of this patient because they give diagnostic clues to the source of the acid-base imbalance. An elevated lactate level (above 16 mg/dl) indicates lactic acidosis, usually a result of cardiogenic or septic shock or severe hypoxemia. An anion gap (normal is 12 mEq/liter) may be calculated by subtracting the total serum anions from the total serum cations. The calculation is as follows:
  anion gap = $(Na^+ + K^+) - (Cl^- + HCO_3^-)$.

A metabolic acidosis with a normal anion gap results from a loss of HCO_3^-, such as occurs in diarrhea or acute tubular necrosis or in chloride excess following the administration of calcium chloride or hydrochloric acid. A metabolic acidosis with an increased anion gap occurs in patients with lactic acidosis, DKA, or uremia.

Complete blood count (CBC) and electrolyte studies would also be performed to provide information about infection and electrolyte status. Creatine phosphokinase (CPK) isoenzyme levels are useful in diagnosing myocardial infarction. A reticulocyte count provides information about bone marrow function. Serum amylase levels aid in diagnosing pancreatitis, whereas acetone levels aid in diagnosing DKA.

81 Correct answer—D

In this situation, the patient has mixed metabolic and respiratory acidosis, a result of cardiopulmonary arrest. The pH is low; the respiratory component (PCO_2) is elevated, indicating CO_2 retention; and the metabolic component (HCO_3^-) is low, indicating excess systemic acids.

82 Correct answer—A

The initial therapy for this patient is to improve oxygenation and ventilation. If respiratory acidosis still exists after resuscitation measures have been instituted and the patient is intubated, some impediment to ventilation exits, such as pneumothorax, esophageal intubation, or pulmonary embolus. Improved oxygenation will prevent progression of metabolic acidosis. Sodium bicarbonate may then be required to reverse the metabolic acidosis. The patient's cardiac rhythm was not stated, so it is unclear whether defibrillation or epinephrine is indicated.

83 Correct answer—B

The two parameters that will cause a severe problem for this patient's myocardial function are acidosis and hypoxemia. Both depress contractility and reduce stroke volume. Myocardial contractility decreases dramatically as the pH falls below 7.25, a result of a dysfunction of calcium influx into the cell. Bicarbonate and carbon dioxide levels do not directly affect myocardial contractility.

84 Correct answer—C

Based on the presenting symptoms, the family probably is suffering from carbon monoxide poisoning. An O_2 saturation of 75% with a PO_2 of 97 mm Hg suggests that a molecule other than oxygen is occupying the hemoglobin molecule. Diagnosis is confirmed by a high arterial carboxyhemoglobin level (normal is 0% to 2% in nonsmokers, 2% to 5% in smokers).

85 Correct answer — B

The nurse would anticipate the initial treatment for a patient with carbon monoxide poisoning to be the administration of 100% O_2 via a nonrebreather mask. This should clear the blood of carbon monoxide in approximately 80 minutes. Breathing into a paper bag is the usual treatment for respiratory alkalosis induced by an anxiety attack. Administering acetylcysteine and bronchodilators is the treatment for an asthma attack. Acetylcysteine also is used to treat acetaminophen overdose.

86 Correct answer — A

Secondary treatment of carbon monoxide poisoning includes hyperbaric oxygen therapy. For carboxyhemoglobin levels above 20%, authorities recommend hyperbaric oxygen therapy. When carboxyhemoglobin levels approach 30%, permanent neurologic damage can occur if treatment is not begun.

87 Correct answer — D

An appropriate nursing diagnosis after treatment has been instituted and the family is stabilized would be *Knowledge deficit related to the medical diagnosis of carbon monoxide poisoning.* The nurse must instruct the family on the sources of carbon monoxide exposure, such as wood stoves, propane heaters, smoldering charcoal, and incomplete combustion of organic materials, as well as on the signs and symptoms of potential exposure, such as headache, dizziness, nausea, and vomiting. No information provided supports the formulation of the other nursing diagnoses listed.

88 Correct answer — A

When an ED patient is unconscious and the cause is unknown, the appropriate treatment is to administer one ampule of dextrose 50% and 0.8 to 2 mg of naloxone. Dextrose is administered in case the patient is in insulin shock, a condition more dangerous than DKA. Naloxone is administered to reverse respiratory depression, in case an overdose of narcotics caused the unconsciousness. Administering insulin to an unconscious patient before establishing the cause of unconsciousness could be harmful because it may result in furthering hypoglycemia. Not enough information is provided to determine the appropriateness of administering sodium bicarbonate, potassium, or activated charcoal.

89 Correct answer — B

Regular insulin and sodium bicarbonate should be administered to a patient whose serum glucose level is 592 mg/dl and pH is 7.03. Regular insulin is preferred over NPH insulin because of its rapid onset of action; sodium bicarbonate should be administered to a patient with DKA if the pH falls below 7.10. Naloxone, dextrose, and activated charcoal are not indicated in the treatment of DKA. Potassium therapy normally is instituted after correction of the acid-base imbalance.

90 Correct answer — B

The patient has tachycardia and hypotension, indicating intravascular volume depletion. Therefore, the most appropriate solution in this situation would be 0.9% (normal) saline solution. Usually, therapy involves the infusion of 1 liter of normal saline solution every hour for 2 to 3 hours, until the blood pressure returns to normal or urine output improves. Hypertonic solutions, such as dextrose 5% in 0.45% normal saline ($D_5\frac{1}{2}NS$) and dextrose 5% in normal saline, and hypotonic solutions, such as 0.45% saline, are inappropriate initially. Hypertonic solutions would cause further cellular depletion, and hypotonic solutions would cause further intravascular volume loss as fluid shifts into the cell.

91 Correct answer — B

The preferred initial insulin treatment would be an I.V. bolus of 20 units of regular insulin, followed by a continuous infusion of 4 to 8 units/hour. The insulin should be diluted in a glass bottle, because it will bind to plastic containers. The subcutaneous route should be avoided in hypotensive patients because absorption is variable. Continuous infusion maintains a steady blood insulin level. Use of NPH insulin should be avoided initially because of its delayed action.

92 Correct answer — D

Precipitating factors in the development of DKA include omission of or resistance to insulin in a patient with diabetes, surgery or trauma in a patient with diabetes, and pancreatitis, which interferes with insulin production and release. These conditions produce stress, thereby increasing glucocorticoid release, which results in elevated blood glucose levels.

93 Correct answer — A

Children at risk for DKA include those who have infections, who are under emotional stress, or who do not comply with insulin therapy.

General Medical Emergencies Answers

Younger children are more prone to infections, whereas adolescents tend to suffer more from emotional stress and to not comply with therapy. An increase in activity, such as participation in a gym class, may precipitate hypoglycemia by lowering insulin requirements. A child requiring two injections of insulin per day or who self-administers insulin is at no greater risk of developing DKA.

94 Correct answer—B

Signs and symptoms of DKA may also occur in a child with appendicitis or urinary tract infection; in fact, the symptoms are similar enough that misdiagnosis is possible. For example, the abdominal pain associated with DKA is so severe that it mimics an acute surgical abdomen or sickle-cell crisis; polyuria may cause DKA to be mistaken for a urinary tract infection.

95 Correct answer—D

During the initial stages of DKA, the nurse may note tall T waves on ECG. The appearance of tall T waves and wide QRS complexes, along with absence of P waves, signals hyperkalemia, a common initial finding in a patient with DKA. Hyperkalemia is caused by the shifting of potassium out of the cell as a result of metabolic acidosis. As the acidosis is reversed, potassium returns to the cell; this may result in hypokalemia caused by osmotic diuresis. ECG findings indicative of hypokalemia include ST-segment depression and the appearance of U waves. The patient with DKA typically experiences sinus tachycardia, not sinus bradycardia, from hypovolemia.

96 Correct answer—B

Hypophosphatemia, manifested by muscle weakness, may occur in DKA as a result of total body phosphate depletion resulting from diuresis and acidosis. Initial phosphate measurements may be normal or high, as seen with potassium measurements, but may drop after therapy. Both phosphate and potassium may be replaced by administration of potassium phosphate I.V. Hypomagnesemia, hyperchloremia, and hypercalcemia do not typically occur in DKA.

97 Correct answer—A

Slow respirations are not indicative of a patient with DKA. Clinical manifestations of this condition include altered level of consciousness, poor skin turgor, hypotension, and tachycardia, which are the result of dehydration. Hyperglycemia promotes osmotic diuresis, resulting in polyuria, polydipsia, and cellular and intravascular fluid depletion. The breakdown of body fats releases excessive ketones, resulting in metabolic acidosis and acetone breath odor. An increase in the rate and depth of respirations compensates for the acidosis by blowing off carbon dioxide; this is known as Kussmaul's respirations.

98 Correct answer—D

A decreased serum potassium level and decreased hematocrit would not support a diagnosis of DKA. Initial diagnostic studies typically reveal decreased arterial pH, HCO_3^-, and CO_2 levels caused by metabolic acidosis with respiratory compensation. The patient's blood urea nitrogen (BUN) and hematocrit levels and urine specific gravity increase as a result of dehydration. Potassium shifts from the cells into the intravascular fluid, with a corresponding hydrogen shift into cells. This compensatory mechanism is an attempt to buffer the acidosis, which produces an elevated potassium level.

99 Correct answer—D

Polyuria, the most obvious sign of DKA, initially results from the osmotic diuretic effect of hyperglycemia. Although the ketone-induced metabolic acidosis causes a shift of potassium into the serum, the resulting elevated serum potassium level is not so obvious. Metabolic acidosis decreases blood pH; Kussmaul's respirations compensate for this. A patient with DKA is typically hypotensive because of the associated fluid loss.

100 Correct answer—D

The priority nursing diagnostic category for a patient with DKA would be *Fluid volume deficit,* as an elevated serum glucose level results in intracellular dehydration and intravascular depletion. Hyperglycemia increases the serum osmolarity, thereby causing a shift of intracellular fluid into the intravascular space, producing intracellular dehydration. An increased serum osmolarity produces osmotic diuresis and polyuria (excessive urination).

Although a patient with DKA has altered nutrition, this is not a priority at this time. The other categories are inappropriate because the respiratory alkalosis that results from Kussmaul's respirations is a beneficial compensatory mechanism to combat metabolic acidosis.

101 Correct answer—C

Cerebral edema can result from overzealous fluid replacement and administration of sodium bicarbonate. Although a rare complication, it most commonly occurs in children and adolescents during the first day of treatment. Mannitol (Osmitrol), an osmotic diuretic, is the treatment of choice. Acute renal failure may occur if treatment is not instituted and dehydration continues. HNKS and respiratory acidosis are not treatment-related complications.

General Medical Emergencies Answers

102 Correct answer — D

After initiation of therapy, hypokalemia may result from the correction of acidosis or from insulin therapy. Once intravascular fluid depletion has been reversed, 20 to 40 mEq of potassium should be added to each liter of I.V. fluid.

103 Correct answer — A

A child is at highest risk for hypovolemic shock from DKA because, compared to an adolescent or adult, a child has less body fluid and therefore less to lose before becoming dehydrated. A child with DKA can lose up to 10% of his body weight through dehydration. Children and adolescents also have a higher risk of developing cerebral edema during fluid replacement. Elderly and cardiac patients are at increased risk of developing pulmonary edema.

104 Correct answer — C

Once the patient's serum glucose level has fallen between 250 and 300 mg/dl, the nurse would expect the physician to order $D_5\frac{1}{2}NS$ to prevent hypoglycemia and cerebral edema. The other solutions do not contain dextrose, which the patient now requires in small doses since his serum glucose level has fallen.

105 Correct answer — D

In the ED, the most effective parameter for determining a DKA patient's response to insulin therapy is taking bedside capillary measurements with a glucometer. This provides instantaneous results; sending serum specimens to the laboratory may take 1 to 2 hours for results. Urine measurements are inconsistent because urine glucose thresholds are variable, and glycosuria usually occurs when the serum glucose level is above 180 mg/dl.

106 Correct answer — A

Continuous administration of NPH insulin at 4 to 8 units/hour is inappropriate for a patient with DKA. NPH insulin is an intermediate-acting insulin and should never be administered I.V. Specific treatments for such a patient aim to restore fluid balance; restore normal carbohydrate, fat, and protein metabolism; and maintain electrolyte balance and function of related systems. During restoration of fluid balance, rapid administration of fluid (up to 1,000 ml/hour) may be ordered initially. When the patient's serum glucose level falls to 250 mg/dl, the initial infusions of 0.45% saline or normal saline solution should be changed to $D_5\frac{1}{2}NS$ with potassium to prevent hypoglycemia, hypokalemia, and cerebral edema. To restore normal carbohydrate, fat, and protein metabolism, rapid-acting insulin (regular) should be administered, preferably as a continuous infusion of 4 to 8 units/hour (alternatives include I.M. or I.V. loading doses) or as an I.V. bolus of 10 to 25 units/hour. During treatment, electrolyte levels, especially potassium, should be monitored.

107 Correct answer—A

Hyperglycemia results in an elevated plasma osmolarity (normal serum osmolarity is 275 to 295 mOsm/liter). This hyperosmolar state causes the brain cells to become dehydrated, thereby producing a change in level of consciousness. A BUN level of 50 mg/dl would not alter the patient's level of consciousness. A serum sodium level of 125 mEq/liter could cause a change in mental status, but serum sodium levels are typically elevated (not lowered) in HNKS. A nonketotic state would not cause a change in mental status.

108 Correct answer—C

Monitoring the patient's rectal temperature and notifying the physician if the temperature rises above 101° F (38.3° C) is not a priority nursing action during the initial management of HNKS. Although HNKS may be precipitated by prolonged total parenteral nutrition administration, pneumonia, burns, cerebrovascular accident, or recent surgery, and temperature assessment is an important component of managing these states, monitoring temperature is not a priority concern in the initial management. Initially, the patient should be rehydrated with a hypotonic solution, such as 0.45% saline solution if the blood pressure is stable, or normal saline solution if intravascular depletion occurs. Frequent neurologic assessments are necessary because cerebral intracellular dehydration results in mental status changes. The serum glucose level should be normalized by insulin administration.

109 Correct answer—B

The nurse would expect the patient with HNKS to require hypotonic fluid replacement and less insulin and potassium than that needed for a patient with DKA. Hypotonic (0.45% saline) solution is preferred to isotonic (0.9% saline) solution because of the marked hyperosmolarity associated with HNKS. Because of this severely dehydrated state, as much as 4 to 6 liters may be required in the first 10 hours. In the absence of acidosis, potassium loss in the urine is greatly decreased during the initial stages of glycosuria. Less insulin usually is required to reduce the hyperglycemia in a patient with HNKS as compared with a patient with DKA.

General Medical Emergencies Answers

110 Correct answer — D

Ineffective breathing pattern related to hyperventilation would be inappropriate because compensatory hyperventilation resulting from metabolic acidosis does not develop in HNKS. Appropriate nursing diagnoses for a patient with this condition would include *Fluid volume deficit related to osmotic diuresis,* which is induced by the hyperglycemic state; *Potential for injury related to altered level of consciousness* because of the possibility of confusion, obtundation, and seizures secondary to severe intracerebral dehydration; and *Altered peripheral tissue perfusion related to a decreased cardiac output,* which may result from fluid volume loss.

111 Correct answer — B

Based on the assessment findings, the nurse would suspect that the patient's change in level of consciousness resulted from syndrome of inappropriate antidiuretic hormone (SIADH) secretion. Dilutional hyponatremia and altered mental status are indications of this disorder; a mass in the right lung field may reflect oat-cell carcinomas, which produce antidiuretic hormone (ADH). Cerebral metastasis typically produces neurologic dysfunction of one area or one side of the body rather than a generalized state of confusion or stupor. Acute purulent meningitis could cause an altered mental status without such dysfunction, but the lack of a fever or an elevated white blood cell count makes meningitis a less likely diagnosis. A subarachnoid hemorrhage presents with a more abrupt onset of severe headache and photophobia.

112 Correct answer — B

Phenytoin has not been associated with SIADH; therefore, a 36-year-old patient receiving phenytoin sodium is not considered at risk for developing SIADH. Patients at risk include those with lung carcinomas, as oat-cell carcinoma accounts for 80% of all cases of SIADH and vasopressin is synthesized, stored, and released from the tumor tissue; those who have received prolonged positive-pressure ventilation, as a reduction in left atrial filling may stimulate central ADH release; and those with pneumonia, tuberculosis, lung abscesses, or empyema, as inflamed pulmonary tissue may lead to ADH secretion.

113 Correct answer — D

SIADH is caused by increased secretion of ADH by the posterior pituitary gland. Precipitating factors include tuberculous meningitis; extracranial malignant tumors, especially bronchogenic and pancreatic tumors; head traumas, such as skull fractures; medications, such as chlorpropamide, clofibrate, and thiazides; and viral respiratory infections.

114 Correct answer—A

A serum sodium level of 120 mEq/liter is characteristic of a patient with SIADH. An increase in ADH secretion promotes excessive water retention by the kidneys. This lowers the serum sodium level and produces a marked decrease in serum osmolarity (the normal range for serum osmolarity is between 275 and 295 mOsm/liter). Dilutional hypokalemia also results (normal potassium levels range from 3.5 to 5 mEq/liter). Urine output decreases as a result of increased reabsorption of water. The concentrated urine that is produced has high specific gravity and osmolarity (urine specific gravity ranges from 1.001 to 1.030, depending on its concentration).

115 Correct answer—D

Use of demeclocycline and other drugs that block the effect of ADH on the renal tubules are inappropriate for the acute treatment of SIADH but may be appropriate for long-term therapy. Hyponatremia and its resultant decreased osmolarity are responsible for the patient's seizures. The goal of initial treatment is to raise the serum sodium level to at least 125 mEq/liter to avoid neurologic symptoms. At this level, the patient's mental status should improve. Administering furosemide should produce diuresis; administering a 3% hypertonic saline solution and restricting fluids should raise the serum sodium level.

116 Correct answer—B

Preventing seizures is the primary goal of nursing care in a patient with SIADH. The clinical manifestations of SIADH result from excessive water retention, which leads to overhydration and water intoxication. Water intoxication dilutes serum sodium levels, producing hyponatremia, which results in neurologic changes. Signs and symptoms of hyponatremia and water intoxication vary from a mild headache to seizures, coma, and death. The patient is probably hypertensive because of the fluid overload. Tetany is a sign of hypocalcemia.

117 Correct answer—D

Diabetes insipidus may develop from various causes, one of which is head trauma, especially involving a basal skull fracture. It most commonly develops in neurosurgical patients. Other precipitating factors include inflammatory or degenerative conditions, such as tubercular meningitis, syphilis, sarcoidosis, Hodgkin's disease, and tumors. Severe pneumonia and therapy with thiazides and vasopressin predispose the patient to SIADH.

118 Correct answer — D

Laboratory findings for a patient with diabetes insipidus typically show a urine specific gravity betwen 1.001 and 1.005. Diabetes insipidus results from a defect in the release or synthesis of ADH within the pituitary or a defect in renal tubular response to ADH. In diabetes insipidus, the patient has impaired renal conservation of water; therefore, little water reabsorption occurs. As water is lost from the body, the serum sodium level rises, resulting in an increased serum osmolarity. As the kidneys fail to conserve water, the urine remains dilute, resulting in a decreased urine osmolarity and a specific gravity between 1.001 and 1.005.

119 Correct answer — A

Diabetes insipidus can be complicated by severe volume depletion and dehydration, resulting in hypovolemic shock. The appropriate nursing intervention would be to assess for signs and symptoms of rapidly developing hypovolemic shock. Meticulous recording of fluid intake and output, monitoring of vital signs, and daily weight monitoring are mandatory. Instituting seizure precautions and auscultating lung fields for crackles are appropriate interventions for a patient with SIADH. Although arrhythmias are possible in diabetes insipidus, they are uncommon and monitoring for them is not a priority.

120 Correct answer — C

The mainstay of management in diabetes insipidus is the administration of vasopressin tannate because the patient is deficient in ADH, or vasopressin. If Pitressin tannate is prescribed, the vial must be warmed under hot water for several minutes and vigorously shaken. In this situation, inadequate warming or agitation of the medication vial may have caused the patient's unresponsiveness to therapy. The other choices have no bearing on the effectiveness of vasopressin.

121 Correct answer — C

The nurse would question administering vasopressin to a patient with angina pectoris. Vasopressin must be used cautiously in patients with heart disease because its vasoconstrictive properties may precipitate myocardial ischemia. It increases water reabsorption by the renal tubules and constriction of the smooth muscle of the arterioles. Vasopressin may be safely administered in a patient with liver dysfunction, a brain tumor, or a transplanted kidney.

122 Correct answer — A

In this situation, the patient has symptoms of hypoglycemia that probably resulted from a neurologic response. During hypoglycemia, insulin-antagonist hormones, such as epinephrine, are released, causing the patient to experience the characteristic symptoms of neuroglycopenia (tachycardia, diaphoresis, tremors, and nervousness).

123 Correct answer — C

Emergency management of a patient in hypoglycemic coma includes the administration of 50 ml of dextrose 50% I.V. If there is any doubt about whether a comatose patient is hypoglycemic or hyperglycemic, the nurse should obtain a serum glucose measurement by finger stick. A fasting blood sugar level measurement is not feasible in this situation because the nurse would not know whether the patient had fasted before the measurement was obtained.

124 Correct answer — D

Myxedema occurs in patients with moderate to severe hypothyroidism. If the hypothyroidism is allowed to progress, the patient's condition will deteriorate and coma will eventually ensue. Myxedema coma is extremely advanced hypothyroidism; all persons who develop myxedema coma are in a hypothyroid state, but not all patients with hypothyroidism have myxedema coma.

125 Correct answer — A

The nurse would expect a patient with myxedema coma to have hyponatremia. Low sodium levels are caused by impaired water excretion, which is dilutational in nature. Potassium levels are typically normal in myxedema, unless the patient has another underlying condition.

126 Correct answer — B

Rewarming should take place gradually, using blankets or sheets only. The use of a hypothermia blanket is strongly contraindicated because rapid rewarming can precipitate vasodilation, which can cause cardiac arrhythmias, circulatory collapse, or death. Once thyroid replacement has begun, the body will begin to compensate and slowly return to a normal temperature. No benefit occurs from glycerin suppositories in this condition.

General Medical Emergencies
Answers

127 Correct answer — D

Diuretic therapy may result in sodium loss, thereby lowering sodium levels further; it is therefore contraindicated in patients with myxedema coma. Fluid restriction may be indicated in myxedema coma to correct hyponatremia. If the hyponatremia is severe (levels less than 115 mEq/liter), infusion of normal saline solution (electrolyte replacement) may be necessary to elevate the serum sodium level. Thyroid hormone replacement is essential to correct the decreased secretion of thyroid hormone.

128 Correct answer — D

The patient's CO_2 level is 64 mm Hg, indicating acute respiratory acidosis; therefore, the appropriate nursing intervention at this time would be to prepare for endotracheal intubation. Myxedema coma causes changes in the thoracic ventilatory capacity and respiratory center. The initial assessment indicated bilateral pulmonary congestion. The patient also may have pleural effusion and ascites. The nurse must assess the respiratory system carefully to determine the need for ventilatory assistance. Arterial blood gas measurements usually demonstrate respiratory acidosis with CO_2 narcosis.

129 Correct answer — D

The patient has a history of Addison's disease, which can be controlled by corticosteroids. However, because he had been fasting and did not take his medication, the blood level of corticosteroids decreased. Abrupt discontinuation of steroid therapy precipitated the adrenal crisis.

130 Correct answer — C

The most serious threat in adrenal crisis is peripheral vascular collapse. A patient may lose as much as 20% of extracellular fluid volume. Therefore, the first goal of emergency treatment is fluid replacement. Secondary interventions are aimed at achieving electrolyte balance and a normal glucose state. A patient with Addison's disease typically has hypoglycemia, hyperkalemia, and hyponatremia.

131 Correct answer — C

The most definitive diagnostic test for adrenal crisis is measurement of plasma cortisol levels. Abnormally low levels indicate adrenocortical insufficiency. Adrenocorticotropic hormone (ACTH) and 24-hour urine 17-hydroxycorticosteroid level measurements are used to help diagnose adrenal disorders; however, they are contraindicated for a patient with adrenal crisis because of the potentially life-threatening delay associated with the tests. Plasma carcinoembryonic antigen levels help diagnose cancer or abnormal cells in the body.

132 Correct answer – B

To combat the patient's fluid deficit, the nurse would expect to infuse 1 liter of dextrose 5% in normal saline. The infusion rate should be extremely rapid (1 to 2 hours), barring such complications as cardiac or renal disease. Fluid replacement should raise the blood pressure by volume expansion and contribute needed glucose and sodium. After the first liter, the patient may require additional fluids at a rate of 1 liter every 3 to 4 hours. A 0.45% saline solution, D_5W, and dextrose 5% in lactated Ringer's solution are inappropriate because they do not contain enough sodium, which is needed to correct the hyponatremia associated with adrenal crisis.

133 Correct answer – C

Hydrocortisone, a soluble cortisol replacement for lost glucocorticoids, is commonly used to treat adrenal crisis. The usual dosage is 100 to 200 mg I.V. immediately, then every 6 hours. Sodium levothyroxine is used to treat thyroid disease. Dexamethasone and fludrocortisone, mineralocorticoid replacements, may be used to treat adrenal crisis; however, they are not urgently required because saline solution and hydrocortisone adequately compensate for lost mineralocorticoids.

134 Correct answer – B

When adrenal crisis is complicated by hyperkalemia, the ECG will show peaked T waves, wide QRS complexes, and prolonged PR intervals. Hyperkalemia may cause bradycardia; it is not associated with bundle branch block or T-wave depression.

135 Correct answer – A

Adrenal crisis, or acute adrenocortisol insufficiency, is caused by decreased cortisol and aldosterone secretion by the adrenal cortex. ADH is secreted by the posterior pituitary and has no significance in adrenal crisis.

136 Correct answer – B

In this situation, the nurse would assess for signs and symptoms of hyperglycemia and hyponatremia. Excessive thyroid hormone levels appear to produce an increase in glycogenolysis and rapid intestinal glucose absorption. Also, increased adrenergic activity may cause insulin resistance and impair insulin secretion, resulting in hyperglycemia. Diaphoresis in a patient with a high fever who

General Medical Emergencies
Answers

consumes large quantities of water without adequate salt intake, may induce water toxicity or dilutional hyponatremia.

137 Correct answer—C

For patients who are iodine-sensitive, lithium carbonate is used to inhibit thyroid hormone release. Levothyroxine sodium is used for thyroid hormone replacement. ACTH is used mainly in treating adrenal diseases. Phenytoin is an antiepileptic agent.

138 Correct answer—A

Aspirin would be inappropriate in this situation because salicylates are thought to interfere with the binding of triiodothyronine (T_3) and thyroxine (T_4) to circulating thyroid-binding protein. The increase of free T_3 and T_4 may exacerbate the existing hyperthyroidism. Nonaspirin antipyretics should be used in thyroid storm. Administering muscle relaxants to control shivering, applying ice packs to the axillae and groin, and using a hypothermia blanket with a rectal probe are acceptable methods of treating fever.

139 Correct answer—D

Measurement of 24-hour urine 17-ketosteroids is used to assess adrenal, not thyroid, function. Serum protein-bound iodine, radioactive iodine uptake, and thyroid-stimulating hormone measurements help assess thyroid function.

140 Correct answer—D

In this situation, the patient's serum calcium level should be monitored because bone pain, muscle weakness, and hypotonic muscles are symptoms of hypercalcemia, which is caused by hypermetabolism of the bone. Hypercalcemia also causes thirst, lethargy, and drowsiness, which may progress to stupor and coma.

141 Correct answer—B

The patient's signs and symptoms are the classic manifestations of Cushing's syndrome and constitute the associated protein catabolic, glyconeogenic, mineralocorticoid, androgenic, and behavioral effects that are characteristic of this disorder.

142 Correct answer—C

Cushing's syndrome, the opposite of Addison's disease, presents with clinical manifestations of excessive rather than deficient adrenocortical activity. The syndrome may result from excessive administration of cortisone or ACTH or from hyperplasia of the adrenal cortex. Removal of the pituitary gland may cause vasopressin deficiency, resulting in diabetes insipidus.

143 Correct answer—D

A patient with Cushing's syndrome should be monitored for mineralocorticoid effects, including increased serum sodium levels (hypernatremia), decreased serum potassium levels (hypokalemia), hypertension, and edema. Increased blood glucose levels (hyperglycemia) are a glyconeogenic effect manifested by glucose intolerance.

144 Correct answer—B

Potential for infection related to altered metabolism best reflects the anti-inflammatory effects of excessive glucocorticoid levels seen in a patient with Cushing's syndrome. Such effects produce increased susceptibility to infection and mask infections that do occur. *Potential for injury related to decreased protein catabolism* is incorrect because the patient with Cushing's syndrome experiences excessive, not decreased, protein catabolism, resulting in muscle weakness and an increased risk for soft tissue injuries and fractures from progressive osteoporosis. *Altered body image related to physical appearance* and *Sleep pattern disturbance related to anxiety* may be relevant diagnoses; however, they are not associated with the anti-inflammatory effects of this disease.

145 Correct answer—A

The hypokalemia associated with Cushing's syndrome produces an increased heart rate, frequently with atrial premature complexes. Also, increased serum aldosterone levels result in an increased serum osmolarity and hypernatremia. Elevated calcitonin levels may be seen in hyperthyroidism. Chvostek's sign occurs in hypocalcemia.

CHAPTER 7

Genitourinary and Gynecologic Emergencies

1 The most appropriate nursing action for an uncircumcised male patient with a zipper injury would be to:

A. Delicately unzip the zipper after the physician administers a local anesthetic
B. Delicately unzip the zipper using no anesthesia
C. Cut the zipper around the injury, allowing the tracks to separate
D. Prepare the patient for circumcision to remove the injured foreskin

2 Which statement regarding urethral trauma is *true?*

A. Urethral trauma is most common in women
B. Urethral trauma commonly occurs when the bladder is full
C. Urethral trauma is diagnosed by intravenous pyelography (IVP)
D. The patient with urethral trauma should be instructed not to void

3 Which statement regarding the assessment or treatment of urethral trauma is *true?*

A. Urethral trauma is difficult to diagnose because it is painless
B. An indwelling urinary catheter should be inserted as soon as possible to maintain urethral patency
C. A suprapubic catheter may be inserted to divert urine
D. The patient typically suffers urinary incontinence as a result of sphincter damage

4 The nurse is assessing a patient with a hard scrotal mass that cannot be transilluminated. This finding most likely indicates:

A. Hydrocele
B. Spermatocele
C. Testicular tumor
D. Epididymitis

5 The nurse understands that IVP usually is not indicated for a patient with acute renal failure because:

A. It would be of no diagnostic value
B. It places the patient at increased risk for an allergic reaction to the contrast media
C. It may cause a fluid volume deficit because of the osmotic effect of the contrast media
D. The contrast media would have a nephrotoxic effect

6 Which finding differentiates decreased renal perfusion from acute tubular necrosis (ATN)?

A. Serum creatinine level of 4 mg/dl
B. Urine sodium level of 15 mEq/liter
C. Urine output of 350 ml/24 hours
D. Urine specific gravity of 1.010

7 Anuria is a common symptom of:

A. Urethral injury
B. Bladder injury
C. Postrenal acute renal failure ARF
D. All of the above

8 The nurse would expect a patient with ureteral trauma to be best managed by:

A. Surgical repair
B. Insertion of an indwelling urinary catheter
C. Insertion of a suprapubic catheter
D. Bed rest and monitoring of urine output

9 The nurse would anticipate a penile fracture to be treated by:

A. Insertion of a suprapubic catheter
B. Surgical repair
C. Splinting
D. Casting

10 Which common assessment finding is considered a nonspecific sign of genitourinary trauma?

A. Flank pain
B. Hypotension
C. Urine retention
D. Hematuria

11 Signs and symptoms of epididymitis may be confused with those of:

A. Testicular torsion
B. Priapism
C. Urinary tract infection (UTI)
D. Pyelonephritis

SITUATION

A 24-year-old man is brought to the emergency department (ED), after having sustained blunt trauma to the left kidney during a boxing match. He is awake and alert. His chief complaint is flank tenderness. Urinalysis reveals microscopic hematuria. All other laboratory data are within normal limits. Vital signs are blood pressure, 130/70 mm Hg; pulse rate, 76 beats/ minute; and respiratory rate, 20 breaths/minute. He is scheduled for transfer to the medical-surgical unit as soon as a bed is available.

Questions 12 to 19 relate to the above situation.

12 Which assessment findings indicate renal trauma?

A. Severe, colicky flank pain and diaphoresis
B. Hematuria and flank pain
C. Severe flank pain and urethral bleeding
D. Severe flank pain and no urine output

13 Which injury resulting from blunt renal trauma typically resolves without surgery?

A. Contusion
B. Rupture of a major renal artery
C. Renal pedicle injury
D. None of the above

14 The patient's assessment findings reveal ecchymoses around the left flank area. This would best be interpreted as:

A. Pulled muscles in the flank area
B. Fractured ilium
C. Retroperitoneal bleeding
D. All of the above

15 The physician determines that the patient has a renal contusion. Priority intervention would include:

A. Immediate surgery
B. Maintaining the patient on his affected side to apply pressure to the area
C. Percutaneous evacuation of blood from the abdominal cavity
D. No treatment other than observation for worsening of the injury

16 If the patient's pain increases, the nurse's main priority would be to:

A. Administer narcotics, as ordered
B. Monitor the patient's serum electrolyte studies, blood urea nitrogen (BUN) level, and glucose level
C. Monitor the patient's serum hematocrit
D. Measure the patient's blood pressure

17 The nurse should suspect renal trauma in any patient with:

A. A positive Chvostek's sign
B. Oliguria
C. Hematoma in the flank area
D. Dysuria

18 Which injury would lead the nurse to suspect kidney trauma?

A. Chest trauma
B. Fractured pelvis
C. Deceleration injury
D. All of the above

19 Which test would confirm a diagnosis of renal trauma most conclusively?

A. Kidney-ureter-bladder (KUB) urethrography
B. Abdominal computed tomography (CT) scan
C. IVP
D. Peritoneal tap

SITUATION

A 62-year-old man arrives at the ED after being unable to urinate for the past 2 days. He appears slightly confused and complains of nausea, vomiting, and swollen ankles. His history reveals no renal dysfunction but a history of benign prostatic hypertrophy. Laboratory findings indicate a serum BUN level of 38 mg/dl and a serum creatinine level of 4 mg/dl.

Questions 20 to 25 refer to the above situation.

20 The nurse suspects that this patient is exhibiting signs and symptoms of:

A. ARF
B. Congestive heart failure
C. Pyelonephritis
D. Chronic renal failure

21 Which symptom is considered the hallmark assessment finding in a patient with this condition?

A. Edema
B. Rising BUN and creatinine levels
C. Anuria
D. Confusion

22 Which test would the nurse expect the physician to order initially when diagnosing this patient's condition?

A. KUB urethrography
B. Abdominal CT scan
C. IVP
D. Peritoneal tap

23 After inserting an indwelling urinary catheter and draining 2,500 ml of urine from the patient's bladder, the nurse formulates a nursing diagnosis of:

A. Fluid volume excess related to kidney dysfunction
B. Fluid volume deficit related to restoration of urine flow
C. Potential for injury related to potassium excess
D. Potential for injury related to metabolic acidosis

24 The most important nursing intervention at this time would involve:

A. Clamping the catheter
B. Requesting an order for fluid replacement
C. Requesting an order for a diuretic
D. Preparing the patient for emergency surgery

25 After establishing an I.V. line, the nurse would expect to administer:

A. Dextrose 5% in water at a keep-vein-open rate
B. 3% saline solution at 20 ml/hour
C. Normal saline solution and potassium chloride at 30 ml/hour
D. Dextrose 5% in 0.45% saline solution and potassium chloride at 160 ml/hour

SITUATION

A 35-year-old woman arrives at the ED complaining of nausea, vomiting, malaise, and a decreased urine output. She recently completed a 2-week course of cephradine (Velosef) for a UTI. Urinalysis reveals a sodium level of 40 mEq/liter with a urine specific gravity of 1.0. Urine sediment includes casts, with few red blood cells (RBCs) or white blood cells (WBCs). Other laboratory findings include a serum BUN level of 40 mg/dl and a serum creatinine level of 4 mg/dl.

Questions 26 to 31 refer to the above situation.

26 Which condition is suggestive of the patient's assessment findings?

A. Recurrence of UTI
B. Dehydration from vomiting
C. Allergic drug reaction
D. ATN

27 Which assessment finding is the most accurate indicator of this patient's renal function?

A. Serum creatinine level
B. Serum BUN level
C. Urine sodium level
D. Urine specific gravity

28 Which laboratory finding is an indirect measurement of the patient's glomerular filtration rate (GFR)?

A. Creatinine clearance
B. BUN level
C. Urine sodium level
D. Urine specific gravity

29 The nurse would expect treatment for this patient to include:

A. Antibiotic therapy with penicillin or an aminoglycoside
B. Fluid restriction
C. Furosemide (Lasix) administration
D. Electrolyte replacement

30 The nurse should also assess this patient for:

A. Hypernatremia
B. Metabolic alkalosis
C. Hyperkalemia
D. Hypercalcemia

31 Which finding would indicate that the patient's treatment has been effective?

A. Serum BUN level of 54 mg/dl
B. Serum creatinine level of 7.2 mg/dl
C. Creatinine clearance of 125 ml/min
D. Urine sodium level of 50 mEq/liter

SITUATION

A male patient is admitted to the ED complaining of sudden onset of pain to the testicular area, especially upon elevation of the scrotum. The pain radiates to the flank area and is accompanied by nausea, vomiting, and testicular edema.

Questions 32 to 34 refer to the above situation.

32 The patient's signs and symptoms are characteristic of which condition?

A. Testicular tumor
B. Priapism
C. Acute epididymitis
D. Testicular torsion

33 This condition is most common among which age-group?

A. Children and adolescents
B. Young adults
C. Middle-age adults
D. Older adults

34 The nurse would expect treatment of this problem to include:

A. Antibiotic therapy
B. Application of ice packs and manual manipulation
C. Immediate orchiectomy
D. Sedation

SITUATION

A 52-year-old diabetic man with a 1-year history of chronic renal failure that is treated with continuous ambulatory peritoneal dialysis is unconscious when admitted to the ED. His blood pressure is 190/100 mm Hg; serum potassium level, 7.8 mEq/liter; serum BUN level, 200 mg/dl; and serum creatinine level, 10 mg/dl. Available medical records indicate that 2 years ago he had been receiving 28 units of NPH insulin daily.

Questions 35 to 41 refer to the above situation.

35 The nurse knows that end-stage renal disease (ESRD) develops when:

A. The serum creatinine level reaches 4 mg/dl
B. 90% of the nephrons are destroyed
C. The kidneys can no longer concentrate urine
D. The kidneys can no longer absorb sodium

36 The nurse anticipates that the patient's hyperkalemia will be treated with:

A. Ion-exchange resin
B. Sodium bicarbonate
C. Calcium chloride
D. All of the above

37 Which statement best describes how ESRD has most likely affected the patient's diabetes over the course of 2 years?

A. Insulin requirements have decreased
B. Insulin requirements have increased
C. Hyperglycemic episodes have occurred more frequently
D. Symptoms of diabetic neuropathy have increased

38 The patient has pulmonary edema, and peritoneal dialysis is indicated. Which percentage of glucose would the nurse expect to use in the dialysate solution?

A. 0.45%
B. 1.5%
C. 2.5%
D. 4.25%

39 When administering the dialysate solution, the nurse should assess for signs of:

A. Hypervolemia
B. Hyperkalemia
C. Hypercalcemia
D. Hyperglycemia

40 During peritoneal dialysis, the dialysate solution has difficulty draining from the abdomen. An appropriate nursing intervention to facilitate drainage would be to:

A. Aspirate drainage from the catheter using a syringe
B. Flush the catheter with a heparinized syringe
C. Instill another liter of dialysate
D. Reposition the patient from side to side

41 The nurse should also assess this patient for developing:

A. Coagulopathies
B. Heart block
C. Hypercalcemia
D. Metabolic alkalosis

SITUATION

A 58-year-old man arrives at the ED, diaphoretic and complaining of severe pain in the right side. He informs the nurse that he had been walking his dog when he suddenly felt a horrible pain. Assessment findings reveal that his blood pressure is 160/70 mm Hg; pulse, 124 beats/minute and regular; temperature, 98.6° F (37° C); and respiratory rate, 24 breaths/ minute. His abdomen, when palpated, reveals tenderness in the right flank. Urinalysis indicates RBCs in the urine. The patient has a history of hypertension and no known allergies. The physician diagnoses renal calculi and requests a consultation with the urologist.

Questions 42 to 47 relate to the above situation.

42 The nurse would expect the history of a patient with renal calculi to reveal a previous diagnosis of:

A. Prostatic hypertrophy
B. Hypothyroidism
C. Hyperparathyroidism
D. Chronic renal failure

43 Which question typically elicits the most valuable information from a patient complaining of flank pain?

A. "When did the pain start?"
B. "Is the pain steady, or does it increase and decrease in severity?"
C. "What helps to relieve your pain?"
D. "Does the pain radiate anywhere?"

44 Which action should be the nurse's priority when treating a patient with renal colic?

A. Straining the patient's urine
B. Encouraging the patient to drink fluids
C. Monitoring the patient's fluid intake and output
D. Relieving the patient's pain

45 Which procedure would most likely confirm a diagnosis of renal calculi?

A. IVP
B. Retrograde urography
C. KUB
D. Abdominal ultrasonography

46 If a kidney is partially obstructed by a calculus, the nurse would expect the patient's urine output to:

A. Increase
B. Decrease
C. Remain the same
D. Stop completely

47 Which medication should be avoided if renal calculi are suspected?

A. Atropine sulfate
B. Furosemide
C. Antacids
D. Antibiotics

SITUATION

A 26-year-old woman arrives at the ED complaining of dysuria, fever (101° F [38.3° C]), and urinary frequency. She has had these symptoms for 36 hours. Physical examination reveals suprapubic tenderness but no flank pain. No history of UTI or urologic instrumentation is evident. She informs the nurse that she had sexual intercourse 12 hours before the onset of symptoms. She has no significant medical history and takes no medications. Her complete blood count, serum electrolyte, BUN, and glucose levels are normal. A tentative diagnosis of UTI is made, and urine specimens for analysis and culture are sent to the laboratory.

Questions 48 to 53 refer to the above situation.

48 Which assessment data are characteristic of UTI?

   A. Dysuria, fever, many bacteria in the urine, urinary frequency
   B. Dysuria, low WBC count, acetone in the urine
   C. Dysuria, many platelets, and glucose in the urine
   D. Dysuria and acetone and protein in the urine

49 Which information about UTI should the nurse include in her discharge teaching for this patient?

   A. UTI is not a serious illness; therefore, the patient does not need to be anxious
   B. The patient must take the full course of antibiotic therapy ordered
   C. The patient should avoid sexual intercourse for the next 6 weeks to avoid contaminating her partner
   D. Now that the patient has a history of UTI, she should have a routine urinalysis every 3 months

50 Which diagnostic study would be necessary if the patient had hematuria?

   A. A count of RBCs in the urine
   B. A count of RBC casts in the urine
   C. A count of leukocytes in the urine
   D. A Gram stain of the urine

51 When taking the health history, the nurse should remember to ask the patient about:

   A. Previous surgeries or instrumentation of the genitourinary tract
   B. A previous diagnosis of hypoparathyroidism
   C. A history of sexually transmitted disease
   D. Which birth control methods the patient uses

52 Which organism is the most common cause of UTI?

A. *Staphylococcus saprophyticus*
B. *Klebsiella* species
C. *Proteus* species
D. *Escherichia coli*

53 Which nursing action is most appropriate in the treatment of UTI?

A. Avoiding catheterizing the patient to obtain a urine specimen so that the infection does not spread
B. Requesting an order for phenazopyridine hydrochloride (Pyridium) if the patient complains of bladder discomfort
C. Encouraging the patient to drink coffee or tea to aid in diuresis
D. Telling the patient that cranberry juice should be avoided because it is a bladder irritant.

SITUATION

A 35-year-old man arrives at the ED with pain in the right flank that began 2 hours ago, spontaneously abated, and then suddenly recurred. The pain is severe, sharp, and radiates to the groin. Physical examination reveals tenderness in the right costovertebral angle. The patient's pulse rate is 110 beats/minute; blood pressure, 150/94 mm Hg; temperature, 100° F (37.8° C); and respiratory rate, 24 breaths/minute. Laboratory results indicate a WBC count of 10,000/mm³; normal hemoglobin and hematocrit levels; and normal serum electrolyte, BUN, and glucose levels. Urinalysis reveals an RBC count greater than 100 cells via high-powered field. An indwelling urinary catheter is inserted, and 800 ml of urine is obtained. The patient is sent for an emergency IVP.

Questions 54 to 60 refer to the above situation.

54 The nurse knows that management of a patient with obstructive uropathy is directed primarily toward:

A. Preventing ARF
B. Correcting acidosis
C. Decompressing the urinary tract above the level of obstruction
D. Decompressing the urinary bladder to relieve pressure on the obstructed area

55 Which urinalysis finding is consistent with obstructive uropathy?

A. Normal urinalysis
B. Proteinuria of 3.5 g/day
C. Acetone 2+
D. Glycosuria 2%

56 The nurse notes that no urine has drained from the patient's catheter for 2 hours. Which is the most appropriate nursing action to take?

A. Change the patient's position
B. Check the catheter for patency
C. Reinsert a new catheter
D. Assume that the obstruction has worsened and call the physician

57 The IVP reveals 100% obstruction of the right ureter with severe hydronephrosis in the right kidney. The physician determines the need for percutaneous nephrostomy. Which is the *most* appropriate explanation the nurse can offer the patient about this procedure?

A. The nephrostomy will cure the patient's uropathy
B. Urine will temporarily drain through a tube in the patient's side
C. The procedure is necessary to prevent bilateral renal failure
D. All of the above

58 The initial goal in caring for this patient would be to:

A. Relieve the patient's pain
B. Reduce the patient's blood pressure
C. Prevent cardiac arrhythmias
D. Maintain normal fluid and electrolyte balance

59 Which test will provide the health care team with the most valuable diagnostic information in this situation?

A. Abdominal X-ray
B. Renal ultrasonography
C. Renal arteriography
D. IVP

60 Which nursing diagnosis would be appropriate for a patient who has undergone percutaneous nephrostomy?

A. Potential fluid volume deficit related to the creation of an additional source of urine flow
B. Potential for infection related to altered skin integrity
C. Potential for injury related to metabolic acidosis
D. Fluid volume excess related to decreased renal perfusion

SITUATION

A 56-year-old man is admitted to the ED because of shortness of breath. He has a history of congestive heart failure, myocardial infarction, and hypertension. Assessment findings reveal the following: blood pressure, 220/ 110 mm Hg; pulse rate, 100 beats/minute, full and bounding; and respiration rate, 34 breaths/minute, deep, fast, and labored. Auscultation reveals pericardial friction rub and crackles in both lung bases. ECG monitoring reveals normal sinus rhythm with tall, tented T waves. The nurse notes that the patient has distended jugular veins and edema of the hands, feet, periorbital areas, and sacrum. Indwelling urinary catheterization yields 20 ml of dark amber urine. Arterial blood gas studies show pH, 7.25; PO$_2$, 60 mm Hg; PCO$_2$, 36 mm Hg; and HCO$_3$$^-$, 14 mEq/liter. Laboratory results reveal a serum BUN level of 50 mg/dl and a serum creatinine level of 5.5 mg/dl. The physician diagnoses ARF.

Questions 61 to 64 refer to the above situation.

61 The nurse knows that prerenal azotemia results from all of the following *except:*

A. Shifting of fluid volume from the intravascular space to the interstitial space
B. Hemorrhage
C. Lodging of calcium oxalate calculi in a ureter
D. Hypotension

62 If a patient with ARF exhibits a pericardial friction rub, the nurse should immediately:

A. Notify the physician because the patient requires hemodialysis
B. Assess for pulsus paradoxus
C. Administer oxygen
D. Request an order for furosemide

63 The physician determines that hemodialysis is necessary for this patient. The nurse should explain to the patient that:

A. Because his kidneys no longer function, he is now in ARF and will need dialysis for the rest of his life
B. His kidneys do not function, but dialysis will repair them
C. His breathing will be easier once hemodialysis removes fluid and toxins that his kidneys cannot
D. Hemodialysis will not remove all toxins

64 The tall, tented T waves noted on the patient's ECG are indicative of:

A. Hypercalcemia
B. Hypochloremia
C. Hypophosphatemia
D. Hyperkalemia

SITUATION

A 24-year-old man who was involved in a head-on automobile accident is brought to the ED. Paramedics report that the dashboard and steering wheel were pinned against the patient's abdomen and legs for 1 hour before rescue workers were able to release him. The patient is conscious and in severe abdominal and pelvic pain. His vital signs are stable: blood pressure, 120/70 mm Hg; pulse rate, 86 beats/minute; and respiratory rate, 22 breaths/minute. The nurse notes that the patient's penis and testes are swollen and painful and that blood is oozing from his urethra. The physician diagnoses a pelvic fracture with genitourinary trauma, then calls the urologist.

Questions 65 to 69 relate to the above situation.

65 Which history finding would lead the nurse to suspect that the patient has a ruptured bladder?

A. The bladder was full when injury occurred
B. The patient is male
C. The patient suffered a straddle-type injury
D. The patient received injuries to the lower chest

66 A patient with a ruptured bladder should also be assessed for:

A. Ruptured spleen
B. Pancreatitis
C. Rectal injury
D. Spinal cord injury

67 The nurse would expect a patient with a ruptured bladder to exhibit which signs and symptoms?

A. Pyuria, fever, and distended bladder
B. Hematuria and fever
C. Pyuria and severe pelvic pain
D. Hematuria, pelvic discomfort, and difficulty voiding

68 Besides providing pain relief, which nursing action should be included in the plan of care for a patient who has sustained testicular trauma?

A. Application of ice packs and testicular elevation
B. Application of heat packs and testicular elevation
C. Application of heat packs and leaving the testes in their natural position to avoid further trauma
D. Application of ice packs and leaving the testes in their natural position to avoid further trauma

69 Which symptom is present when the urethra is completely transected?

A. Hematuria
B. Abdominal distention from urine extravasation
C. Urethral bleeding
D. Severe colicky pain

SITUATION

A 29-year-old woman is admitted to the ED with suspected pelvic inflammatory disease (PID). She is complaining of bilateral lower abdominal pain and a slight, whitish-yellow, odorless vaginal discharge. Her blood pressure is 100/70 mm Hg; pulse rate, 96 beats/minute; respiratory rate, 24 breaths/minute; and temperature, 100.6° F (38.1° C). The patient informs the nurse that she has had the discharge for 3 days and that the lower abdominal pain began 2 days ago and has become increasingly worse. Her fever has persisted since yesterday. She also mentions that she has an intrauterine device (IUD) in place. The physician orders a complete blood count, blood culture, and cervical culture as well as a urinalysis and ultrasound studies.

Questions 70 to 75 relate to the above situation.

70 Which organism causes PID?

A. *Neisseria gonorrhoeae*
B. *Mycobacterium tuberculosis*
C. *Chlamydia trachomatis*
D. All of the above

71 The nurse knows that the signs and symptoms of PID may be confused with those of:

A. Pregnancy
B. Gallbladder disease
C. Acute pancreatitis
D. Appendicitis

72 Which condition is a potential complication of PID?

A. Peritonitis
B. Ectopic pregnancy
C. Infertility
D. All of the above

73 Which history finding places a patient at increased risk for PID?

A. Abnormal menstrual cycles
B. Stress
C. IUD use
D. Continued use of antibiotics

74 Which statement indicates that a patient with PID who has been placed on continuing antibiotic therapy understands discharge instructions?

A. "I need to be on bed rest while taking the antibiotics"
B. "I need to take all of the medication"
C. "I can stop the medication when the discharge disappears"
D. "My partner does not need to be treated"

75 Discharge planning for a patient with PID should include:

A. Genetic counseling for future pregnancies
B. Education and treatment of sexual contacts
C. Education for stress reduction
D. Follow-up ultrasound studies every 6 months

SITUATION

A 27-year-old woman is admitted to the ED after losing consciousness at home. Now fully alert, she complains of achiness, nausea, vomiting, and fever, which began yesterday morning. The patient has no medical or gynecologic history. She is 3 days into her menstrual period. She informs the nurse that she uses super-absorbent tampons and, occasionally, contraceptive sponges. The patient's vital signs are blood pressure, 86/48 mm Hg; temperature, 103° F (39.4° C); pulse rate, 124 beats/minute; and respiratory rate, 28 breaths/minute.

Questions 76 to 82 refer to the above situation.

76 Based on the above symptoms, the nurse would suspect that the patient has:

A. Ectopic pregnancy
B. Vaginitis
C. Toxic shock syndrome
D. Ovarian cyst

77 What other symptoms would the nurse assess for in this patient?

A. Cutaneous petechiae over the trunk
B. Diffuse macular erythroderma
C. Mucous membrane lesions
D. Vesicular rash over the palms and soles

78 The nurse would suspect that the patient's condition is caused by:

A. *Staphylococcus aureus*
B. *Chlamydia trachomatis*
C. *Escherichia coli*
D. *Treponema pallidum*

79 Which factors place a patient at high risk for toxic shock syndrome?

A. Poor personal hygiene, deodorant tampon use, and IUD use
B. Prolonged use of super-absorbent tampons, contraceptive sponges, or a diaphragm
C. Prolonged use of tampons and frequent use of commercial douche preparations
D. Prolonged oral antibiotic therapy and alternating use of tampons and vaginal pads during menses

80 An appropriate nursing diagnosis for this patient would be:

A. Decreased cardiac output related to vasodilation and decreased myocardial contractility
B. Potential for infection related to fever and achiness
C. Fluid volume deficit related to vaginal hemorrhage and fever
D. Potential for injury related to seizures

81 Which nursing interventions would be the main priority in managing the patient's condition?

A. Rapidly infuse I.V. fluid, as ordered, and closely monitor the patient's vital signs and urine output
B. Administer antipyretic medications, as ordered, and administer tepid sponge bath to reduce fever
C. Draw blood for cultures, as ordered, and monitor the patient's vital signs
D. Prepare for a spinal tap and monitor the patient's temperature

82 The nurse should observe the patient for which condition associated with untreated toxic shock syndrome?

A. Adult respiratory distress syndrome
B. Disseminated intravascular coagulation
C. Severe metabolic acidosis
D. All of the above

SITUATION

A 24-year-old woman is admitted to the ED, complaining of a vaginal discharge and painful, frequent urination. An enzyme-linked immunosorbent assay of vaginal discharge reveals gonorrhea.

Questions 83 to 87 refer to the above situation.

83 The nurse knows that anyone infected with gonorrhea also should be tested for:

A. Chlamydia
B. Human immunodeficiency virus (HIV)
C. Syphilis
D. Herpes

84 Which question asked during the nursing history should elicit important information about the infection and possible treatment of this patient?

A. "When did you become sexually active?"
B. "Which birth control method do you use?"
C. "What kind of sexual practices do you engage in?"
D. "Have you ever had a sexually transmitted disease?"

85 The nurse explains that recurrence of sexually transmitted diseases places the patient at increased risk for all of the following conditions *except:*

A. Ectopic pregnancy
B. Renal disease
C. HIV
D. PID

86 The nurse initiates a discussion about sexually transmitted diseases and the use of contraceptives. The patient's decision to use which contraceptive method indicates the need for further teaching?

A. Oral contraceptives
B. Diaphragm
C. Condoms
D. Contraceptive sponges

87 The physician orders a single dose of amoxicillin (Amoxil) and probenecid (Benemid), followed by a week of tetracycline therapy. Which statement best reflects that the patient understands the reason for receiving probenecid?

A. "It enhances amoxicillin's effect"
B. "It relieves painful urination"
C. "It kills bacteria"
D. "It reduces fever"

SITUATION

A 20-year-old woman walks into the ED and states, "I was raped." Her clothes are torn and her face is severely bruised. Trembling and withdrawn, she avoids eye contact with immediate personnel and is escorted by the nurse to a private room.

Questions 88 to 92 refer to the above situation.

88 The receiving nurse knows that the most important message to convey initially to any victim of sexual assault is that:

A. All medical tests will be handled confidentially
B. The examination will be done quickly
C. The patient is now in a safe, secure environment
D. Medications are available to prevent pregnancy

89 When obtaining the nursing history, the nurse should determine whether the patient has done which activity since the assault?

A. Urinated or defecated
B. Changed clothes
C. Rinsed her mouth
D. All of the above

90 Which nursing action would be most appropriate when collecting this patient's clothing?

A. Have the victim place all of her clothing together in a plastic bag
B. Have the victim fold each piece of clothing inward and place each article in a separate paper bag
C. Shake each piece of clothing separately, then place all articles together in a paper bag
D. Not collect the clothing of the victim who had been totally undressed before the assault.

91 The patient should be instructed to return to her physician for a repeat serologic test for syphilis (Venereal Disease Research Laboratory test) within how many weeks?

A. 1 to 2
B. 3 to 4
C. 5 to 6
D. 7 to 8

92 Upon discharge, the nurse should provide the patient with:

A. Written discharge instructions
B. Suitable clothing, if the clothing has been retained for evidence
C. A list of referral telephone numbers
D. All of the above

Answer Sheet

	A B C D		A B C D		A B C D		A B C D
1	○ ○ ○ ○	31	○ ○ ○ ○	61	○ ○ ○ ○	91	○ ○ ○ ○
2	○ ○ ○ ○	32	○ ○ ○ ○	62	○ ○ ○ ○	92	○ ○ ○ ○
3	○ ○ ○ ○	33	○ ○ ○ ○	63	○ ○ ○ ○		
4	○ ○ ○ ○	34	○ ○ ○ ○	64	○ ○ ○ ○		
5	○ ○ ○ ○	35	○ ○ ○ ○	65	○ ○ ○ ○		
6	○ ○ ○ ○	36	○ ○ ○ ○	66	○ ○ ○ ○		
7	○ ○ ○ ○	37	○ ○ ○ ○	67	○ ○ ○ ○		
8	○ ○ ○ ○	38	○ ○ ○ ○	68	○ ○ ○ ○		
9	○ ○ ○ ○	39	○ ○ ○ ○	69	○ ○ ○ ○		
10	○ ○ ○ ○	40	○ ○ ○ ○	70	○ ○ ○ ○		
11	○ ○ ○ ○	41	○ ○ ○ ○	71	○ ○ ○ ○		
12	○ ○ ○ ○	42	○ ○ ○ ○	72	○ ○ ○ ○		
13	○ ○ ○ ○	43	○ ○ ○ ○	73	○ ○ ○ ○		
14	○ ○ ○ ○	44	○ ○ ○ ○	74	○ ○ ○ ○		
15	○ ○ ○ ○	45	○ ○ ○ ○	75	○ ○ ○ ○		
16	○ ○ ○ ○	46	○ ○ ○ ○	76	○ ○ ○ ○		
17	○ ○ ○ ○	47	○ ○ ○ ○	77	○ ○ ○ ○		
18	○ ○ ○ ○	48	○ ○ ○ ○	78	○ ○ ○ ○		
19	○ ○ ○ ○	49	○ ○ ○ ○	79	○ ○ ○ ○		
20	○ ○ ○ ○	50	○ ○ ○ ○	80	○ ○ ○ ○		
21	○ ○ ○ ○	51	○ ○ ○ ○	81	○ ○ ○ ○		
22	○ ○ ○ ○	52	○ ○ ○ ○	82	○ ○ ○ ○		
23	○ ○ ○ ○	53	○ ○ ○ ○	83	○ ○ ○ ○		
24	○ ○ ○ ○	54	○ ○ ○ ○	84	○ ○ ○ ○		
25	○ ○ ○ ○	55	○ ○ ○ ○	85	○ ○ ○ ○		
26	○ ○ ○ ○	56	○ ○ ○ ○	86	○ ○ ○ ○		
27	○ ○ ○ ○	57	○ ○ ○ ○	87	○ ○ ○ ○		
28	○ ○ ○ ○	58	○ ○ ○ ○	88	○ ○ ○ ○		
29	○ ○ ○ ○	59	○ ○ ○ ○	89	○ ○ ○ ○		
30	○ ○ ○ ○	60	○ ○ ○ ○	90	○ ○ ○ ○		

1 Correct answer—**C**

The most appropriate nursing action in this situation would be to cut the zipper around the injury, allowing the zipper tracks to separate. No further tissue trauma should ensue. Another effective method would be to delicately unzip the zipper, using petrolatum as a lubricant. Local anesthetics should be avoided because edema will result. Cutting the skin or performing a circumcision may cause extensive scarring or may damage the urethra if the patient has epispadias (a condition in which the urethra is located at the top of the glans) or hypospadias (a condition in which the urethra is located at the bottom of the glans).

2 Correct answer—**D**

A patient with urethral trauma should be instructed not to void because urine may extravasate into the peritoneum, causing pain and inflammation. Urethral injuries, which are more common in men, are associated with straddle-type injuries. This type of trauma can be diagnosed by kidney-ureter-bladder (KUB) or retrograde urethrography. Bladder injuries commonly occur when the bladder is full.

3 Correct answer—**C**

A suprapubic catheter may be inserted to divert urine in a patient with urethral trauma. The nurse should never catheterize a patient with this type of injury. The physician should request an emergency consultation with the urologist, who will insert either an indwelling urinary or a suprapubic catheter based on his own assessment. Urethral trauma is associated with localized dull or sharp acute pain in the suprapubic or perineal area. A patient with urethral trauma typically cannot void, although he may have the desire to do so, because sphincter damage may have occurred.

4 Correct answer—**C**

A hard scrotal mass that does not transilluminate most likely indicates a testicular tumor. In transillumination, a light beam is shone through the scrotum, resulting in a red glow emanating through the skin. This glow is not present in masses resulting from blood or tissue. Therefore, a mass filled with fluid, as in hydrocele or spermatocele, will not transilluminate. Epididymitis does not produce a mass, although the scrotum is edematous.

5 Correct answer—**D**

Intravenous pyelography (IVP) is contraindicated in acute renal failure (ARF) because the contrast media has an osmotic and nephrotoxic effect and can further compromise renal function. Contrast medium has a high osmolarity, which may cause further fluid overload in a patient with acute renal failure. A patient with iodine sensitivity may have an allergic reaction but may be premedicated with steroids or antihistamines to counteract it. IVP may help diagnose acute renal failure from obstructive causes.

6 Correct answer—**B**

A urine sodium level of 15 mEq/liter helps the nurse to differentiate decreased renal perfusion from acute tubular necrosis (ATN). In decreased renal perfusion, the kidneys reabsorb sodium and water in an effort to increase intravascular volume. This is reflected in a urine sodium level below 20 mEq/liter. The urine is concentrated, resulting in a urine specific gravity above 1.010. The serum creatinine level is typically normal. In ATN, the damaged kidney loses its ability to reabsorb sodium, as reflected by a urine sodium level greater than 40 mEq/liter. The urine is typically plasmalike, with a specific gravity of about 1.010. The serum creatinine level is typically elevated above 2 mg/dl. A low urine output, such as 350 ml/24 hours, is characteristic of both decreased renal perfusion and the early phase of ATN.

7 Correct answer—**D**

Anuria, the inability to void, is a common symptom of urethral injury, bladder injury, and postrenal ARF. Sphincter damage may have occurred from trauma to the urethra, resulting in urine retention. Extravasation of urine in the peritoneum typically occurs in bladder rupture and results in anuria. Urine outflow is obstructed in postrenal ARF, resulting in the patient's inability to void.

8 Correct answer—**A**

Ureteral trauma is best treated by surgical repair. In this type of injury, disruption of the structural integrity of the ureters occurs, usually as a result of penetrating abdominal trauma. Surgical anastomosis is required. Indwelling urinary and suprapubic catheterization are of no value because the urine cannot reach the bladder; hence, urine cannot be measured.

9 Correct answer—**C**

Penile fracture, which is commonly associated with straddle-type injuries or violent sexual intercourse, usually is treated by splinting and the application of ice packs. Surgical evacuation of a hematoma may be required if extravasation occurs. An indwelling urinary or suprapubic catheter may be inserted to divert urine if edema occurs;

however, catheterization does not aid in treating the fracture. Casting is inappropriate in this situation.

10 Correct answer — D

Hematuria, whether frank or microscopic, is a common, nonspecific sign of genitourinary trauma. However, it does not necessarily occur in all cases. Menstruation, anticoagulant overdose, and bleeding disorders must be ruled out before the bleeding can be attributed to genitourinary trauma. Flank pain may be indicative of renal hemorrhage or urinary calculi. Hypotension is not a sign of renal trauma except when massive hemorrhage occurs. Urine retention is common in bladder rupture and urethral trauma.

11 Correct answer — A

Epididymitis and testicular torsion are commonly mistaken for one another. Similar signs and symptoms include unilateral testicular pain, swelling, and fever. Differentiation occurs upon elevation of the scrotum, which relieves the pain of epididymitis but increases the pain of testicular torsion.

12 Correct answer — B

Hematuria and flank tenderness indicate renal trauma. Microscopic hematuria is associated with minor contusions, whereas gross blood in the urine is consistent with major renal damage. Flank pain may reflect hemorrhage or extravasation of urine. Colicky pain is associated with obstruction rather than trauma. Urethral bleeding is a manifestation of urethral trauma. Urine output does not initially change as a result of trauma but may become oliguric, if acute renal failure develops, or anuric, if complete obstruction occurs.

13 Correct answer — A

Contusion of the kidney, disruption of the fornix, and lacerations that do not extend beyond the renal cortex are considered minor renal injuries. These typically resolve without surgical intervention. Deep cortical lacerations and injuries involving the renal pedicle or renal pelvis are considered life-threatening and require surgery. Disruption of a major renal artery causes massive bleeding and also warrants surgery.

14 Correct answer — C

When trauma causes rupture of the renal vasculature, bleeding into the retroperitoneal space occurs. The amount of bleeding depends on the degree of injury. This condition may be so severe that the patient succumbs to shock, resulting from hemorrhage. Pulled muscles and a fractured ilium do not directly result in ecchymoses.

15 Correct answer – D

Renal contusions are minor injuries and require no immediate treatment other than observation for worsening of the injury.

16 Correct answer – D

The nurse's main priority in this situation would be to measure the patient's blood pressure. If the patient is hypotensive, bleeding should be suspected. Expansion of a hematoma in the kidney may cause increased pain or tenderness. The nurse may administer narcotics, as ordered, to control pain; however, this is not the primary intervention for bleeding. In some instances, narcotics are withheld to avoid masking symptoms, such as increased pain. Although monitoring the patient's serum hematocrit level is important, the initial action should be to assess vital signs. Monitoring serum electrolyte, blood urea nitrogen (BUN), and glucose levels is of no value in this situation.

17 Correct answer – C

Renal trauma should be suspected in any patient with a hematoma in the flank area. Other signs and symptoms of renal trauma include frank or microscopic hematuria, flank pain that increases with movement and possibly radiates to the groin, and abdominal rigidity. Hypotension and hypovolemic shock may result if significant blood loss occurs. Swelling or a mass in the flank area may be noted on palpation. Chvostek's sign, facial twitching that is elicited by tapping the facial nerve, indicates hypocalcemia. Oliguria is a common finding in acute prerenal and intrarenal failure. Dysuria, or painful urination, is a sign of urinary tract infection (UTI) and renal calculi.

18 Correct answer – D

Kidney trauma should be suspected in any patient with chest trauma, a fractured pelvis, or a deceleration injury. Chest trauma can cause kidney injuries, especially if the lower ribs have been fractured. Deceleration injuries, such as those caused by motor vehicle accidents and contact sports, are the most common cause of renal trauma. Although most kidney injuries are from blunt trauma, penetrating trauma, such as gunshot or stab wounds, may also result in renal trauma.

19 Correct answer — B

An abdominal computed tomography scan confirms renal trauma most conclusively because of its high accuracy, ease of performance, and ability to visualize all renal structures. KUB urethrography also may help determine renal injury; it is especially valuable in demonstrating the size, shape, and location of renal anatomy. IVP also may help to diagnose renal trauma that results in hematomas or lacerations; however, before this test, the patient should be checked for any allergy to contrast media or iodine. Hydrocortisone (Solu-Cortef) and diphenhydramine hydrochloride (Benadryl) should be available if the allergy history is unknown. Peritoneal tap is indicated if bowel trauma is suspected.

20 Correct answer — A

The patient has signs and symptoms consistent with postrenal ARF. Postrenal ARF occurs when urine flow becomes completely obstructed, most commonly from renal calculi, prostatic hypertrophy, or tumors of the bladder, pelvis, or prostate gland. Serum BUN and creatinine levels rise because metabolic waste products cannot be eliminated from the body. A patient with congestive heart failure typically has oliguria, not anuria. A patient with pyelonephritis has signs of infection and urine frequency. The fact that the patient has no history of renal dysfunction rules out chronic renal failure.

21 Correct answer — C

The hallmark symptom of postrenal ARF is anuria, the absence of urine output. Prerenal and intrarenal ARF are characterized by oliguria, a urine output of less than 400 ml/day. Polyuria typically develops later in intrarenal ARF. Other signs and symptoms of postrenal ARF — edema, shortness of breath, nausea, vomiting, and confusion — result from hypervolemia and uremia.

22 Correct answer — A

The physician will probably order KUB urethrography to help diagnose the patient's condition. This procedure should demonstrate enlargement of the structures distended with urine from the obstruction. Ultrasonography also may be used to diagnose postrenal obstruction.

23 Correct answer — B

In this situation, the nurse would formulate a diagnosis of *Fluid volume deficit related to restoration of urine flow.* After the restoration of urine flow, the patient with postrenal ARF is at risk for fluid volume deficit because the urine is characteristically dilute and rich in electrolytes. More fluid is drawn in the urine, therapy diluting the high osmolarity of electrolytes. The other nursing diagnoses would be appropriate before the urine flow is reestablished. Acute renal failure from postrenal obstruction causes a fluid volume overload, potassium excess, and metabolic acidosis. This occurs because of the inability to rid the body of urine, which results in a rise in electrolyte levels and metabolic waste products.

24 Correct answer—B

After the drainage of 2,500 ml of urine, the most important intervention would be to request an order for fluid replacement to restore fluid balance. Once the obstruction is removed, diuresis of dilute urine high in electrolytes results. If fluids are not replaced, dehydration and electrolyte imbalance may occur. The indwelling urinary catheter should be clamped after 800 ml of fluid drains. Emergency surgical consultation is not indicated because the obstruction has been temporarily relieved. Because the urine is already dilute, diuretics are not indicated.

25 Correct answer—D

The nurse would expect to administer dextrose 5% in 0.45% saline solution and potassium chloride at 160 ml/hour. The most appropriate solution for fluid replacement is dextrose 5% in 0.45% saline solution. Sodium and potassium must be replaced as per serum test results. A 0.45% saline solution is hypotonic and is used to replace total fluid volume (intravascular and intracellular). Standard fluid replacement calls for replacing two-thirds of lost urine over 24 hours, plus another 30 ml/hour for insensible water loss.

26 Correct answer—D

This patient has the signs and symptoms of ATN, a form of ARF resulting from drug-induced nephrotoxicity. When intrarenal damage occurs, the kidneys can no longer reabsorb sodium and concentrate urine. The urine sodium level is characteristically above 40 mEq/liter, and urine specific gravity is a plasmalike 0.01. Casts, or cellular debris, appear in the urine because the renal tubules have been damaged. BUN and creatinine levels rise as metabolic wastes accumulate, producing the symptoms of nausea, vomiting, and malaise. A recurrent UTI would produce more signs and symptoms of infection, such as fever and white blood cells in the urine. If the patient had been dehydrated only, the serum creatinine level would be normal. An allergic drug reaction typically occurs earlier in antibiotic therapy.

27 Correct answer – A

The serum creatinine level is the most accurate indicator of this patient's renal function. Creatinine, the end-product of muscle metabolism, is produced at a constant rate and excreted by the kidneys at a constant rate with no reabsorption. The normal serum creatinine level is 1 to 2 mg/dl. BUN, the end-product of protein metabolism, is a less accurate indicator than serum creatinine, because BUN is not produced at a constant rate and is excreted as well as reabsorbed. BUN levels are typically elevated in those who consume high-protein diets and in those are dehydrated or have blood in the GI tract. The normal serum BUN level is 10 to 20 mg/dl. Urine sodium levels provide information about the kidney's ability to reabsorb sodium. Urine specific gravity provides information about the kidney's ability to concentrate urine.

28 Correct answer – A

Creatinine clearance is an indirect measurement of the patient's glomerular filtration rate (GFR). GFR, the amount of water filtered out of the plasma through the glomerular capillary walls per minute, cannot be measured directly but only inferred from the creatine clearance because creatinine is produced and excreted at a constant rate. The creatinine clearance test involves the collection of a 24-hour urine specimen and a serum creatinine specimen. Normal GFR (and creatinine clearance) is 125 ml/minute.

29 Correct answer – B

The nurse would expect this patient's treatment to include fluid restriction to correct the hypervolemia and oliguria caused by impaired kidney function. Penicillin and aminoglycosides produce nephrotoxic effects and would not be indicated because the patient does not have signs of infection. Furosemide administration and electrolyte replacement are indicated in prerenal conditions; in this situation, such therapy could compound the patient's nephrotoxicity. Also, the patient is probably retaining electrolytes and would not require their replacement at this time.

30 Correct answer – C

A patient with ATN should also be monitored for hyperkalemia because of decreased renal excretion. Hyperkalemia occurs when the serum potassium level rises above 5 mEq/liter. It may be represented by tall T waves and cardiac arrhythmias on electrocardiogram. Symptoms of hyperkalemia include nausea, vomiting, and weakness. Other common electrolyte abnormalities associated with ATN include hyponatremia, which results from the kidney's inability to reabsorb sodium, and hypocalcemia and hyperphosphatemia (after 1 week) from decreased vitamin D utilization. Metabolic acidosis occurs because of the inability to excrete hydrogen ions.

31 Correct answer—C

A creatinine clearance of 125 ml/min is a normal finding and indicates that interventions have been successful in restoring normal kidney function. The other findings—elevated serum BUN and creatinine levels and a high urine sodium level—are still indicative of acute renal failure and the kidney's inability to reabsorb sodium.

32 Correct answer—D

This patient's signs and symptoms suggest testicular torsion, or twisting of the spermatic cord. If untreated for more than 4 hours, testicular ischemia may result. The pain is severe and increases upon elevation of the testes. Acute epididymitis, infection of the male reproductive system, can be confused with testicular torsion; however, pain from epididymitis is relieved by elevating the scrotum. Testicular tumor would be suspected if palpation reveals a hard, testicular mass; pain may or may not be present. Priapism, an involuntary, painful erection, is not associated with testicular torsion.

33 Correct answer—A

Testicular torsion is most common in children and adolescents, but it also may occur in young adults. It may be caused by a congenital abnormality of the spermatic cord.

34 Correct answer—B

Treatment of testicular torsion includes the application of ice packs to reduce edema and manual manipulation by a urologist to reduce the torsion. Surgery may be necessary if manipulation is unsuccessful. Antibiotic therapy is indicated for epididymitis. Testicular tumor requires orchiectomy. Analgesia, not sedation, is part of the therapy for testicular torsion.

35 Correct answer—B

End-stage renal disease (ESRD) develops when 90% of the nephrons are destroyed. Functional nephrons hypertrophy to maintain integrity of the renal system. The serum creatinine level is about 10 mg/dl when ESRD occurs. Inability to concentrate urine occurs during the recovery phase of acute tubular necrosis. Impaired sodium reabsorption occurs throughout all phases of acute and chronic renal failure.

36 Correct answer – D

Hyperkalemia can be treated with the administration of ion-exchange resins, sodium bicarbonate, calcium chloride, and insulin and dextrose 50% solution. Ion-exchange resins, such as sodium polystyrene sulfonate (Kayexalate), exchange sodium for potassium ions in the intestine. Sodium bicarbonate temporarily shifts potassium back into the cells by creating alkalosis. Although calcium chloride and calcium gluconate do not decrease the serum potassium level, these agents protect the heart from the adverse effects of hyperkalemia and enhance contraction. Insulin and dextrose 50% solution also decrease the serum potassium level by temporarily shifting potassium into the cell. Potassium enters the cell along with glucose; insulin helps glucose enter the cell.

37 Correct answer – A

This patient's insulin requirements most likely have decreased over the past 2 years; during the last year of ESRD, before dialysis is instituted, insulin requirements typically decrease by 40% to 50%. Peripheral tissues become resistant to insulin, resulting in an increased half-life. Institution of dialysis typically improves the use and excretion of insulin, thereby decreasing its half-life. As renal failure progresses, the catabolism of exogenous and endogenous insulin decreases, resulting in more frequent hypoglycemic, not hyperglycemic, episodes. Diabetic neuropathy is unaffected by ESRD.

38 Correct answer – D

A 4.25% glucose dialysate solution usually is indicated to treat pulmonary edema. In peritoneal dialysis, glucose creates a hyperosmolar condition in the peritoneal cavity, drawing fluid from the intravascular space. A 4.25% glucose dialysate has an osmolality of 486 mOsm/liter, compared with a normal serum osmolality of 285 to 295 mOsm/liter. Higher glucose concentrations draw more fluid, whereas lower concentrations draw too little fluid to be of benefit.

39 Correct answer – D

When administering the 4.25% dialysate solution, the nurse should assess for signs of hyperglycemia because of the solution's high glucose concentration. Careful monitoring is especially necessary in diabetic patients. If the glucose draws too much fluid, hypovolemia may occur. Dialysis may help correct hyperkalemia. A slight decrease in calcium levels may result from peritoneal dialysis because protein and calcium are drawn off.

40 Correct answer—D

Repositioning the patient from side to side may facilitate drainage of the dialysate from the abdomen. Disconnecting the catheter to aspirate drainage and flushing the catheter with a heparinized syringe are contraindicated because of the high risk of contamination and peritonitis. Instilling another liter of dialysate might impair ventilation by pushing on the diaphragm.

41 Correct answer—A

The nurse should also assess this patient with chronic renal failure for developing coagulopathies because of impaired platelet function and clotting mechanisms resulting from uremia. Capillary membranes become more fragile as a result of hypocalcemia. Anemia results from decreased erythropoiesis. All these problems place the patient at increased risk for hemorrhage. The patient with chronic renal failure also may have bradycardia and metabolic acidosis.

42 Correct answer—C

The nurse would expect a patient with renal calculi to have a history of hyperparathyroidism. Hyperparathyroidism is characterized by excess parathyroid hormone (parathormone) in the serum. Excess levels of this hormone pull calcium from the bone into the blood and increase renal tubular reabsorption of calcium. Excess calcium in the urine contributes to calculus formation. A patient with bone carcinoma is also at risk for renal calculus formation because bone lesions may release calcium into the blood. Prostatic hypertrophy, hypothyroidism, and chronic renal failure are not considered risk factors in the development of renal calculi.

43 Correct answer—B

The nurse must determine whether the patient's pain is colicky or noncolicky. To elicit this information, the nurse should ask whether the pain is steady or whether it increases or decreases in severity. Colicky pain is commonly associated with renal pelvis or ureter problems. Renal colic is characterized by severe, acute pain of a sudden onset. The patient typically experiences crescendo-decrescendo variations in the pain. Acute noncolicky pain is steady; its onset and severity vary from patient to patient. The other questions are helpful in understanding the patient's pain but are not helpful in establishing an association to renal calculi.

44 Correct answer—D

The priority nursing action would be to relieve the patient's pain. Straining the patient's urine, encouraging fluids, and monitoring fluid intake and output are important measures to include in the care plan for this patient; however, they are not the nurse's highest priority in this situation.

45 Correct answer—A

IVP is most helpful in identifying the location and size of renal calculi. If obstruction is present, this test is also helpful in identifying the extent of damage. Retrograde urography visualizes only the ureters and bladder, it may be performed after IVP if this test is inconclusive. KUB may be able to detect a stone and identify its general location. Abdominal ultrasonography would only be able to detect renal calculi that are located in the kidneys.

46 Correct answer—C

When a kidney is partially obstructed, urine output remains virtually the same. Because urine output and urine constituents are unchanged, the diagnosis may be delayed unless other symptoms are present.

47 Correct answer—A

Atropine sulfate causes urine retention and should be avoided if renal calculi are suspected. The patient with renal calculi probably is dehydrated from vomiting, fever, and diaphoresis. I.V. fluids are necessary to rehydrate the patient and to aid in the passage of calculi. Atropine would interfere with this process. Furosemide (Lasix), antacids, and antibiotics are not known to interfere with the passage of renal calculi.

48 Correct answer—A

Dysuria, fever, many bacteria in the urine, and urinary frequency are characteristic of UTI. Dysuria results from decreased bladder compliance and inflammation of the genitourinary mucosa. Normally, the bladder stretching reflex is stimulated at 350 to 400 ml, thereby producing the urge to urinate. Inflammation decreases bladder elasticity, producing pain with minimal distention. This decrease inbladder elasticity, along with irritation from inflamed tissues, produces urinary frequency. Fever is the body's normal response to infection. Urinalysis typically reveals many white blood cells (WBCs), which suggests bacteria in the urine, and must be followed up by a culture and sensitivity report.

49 Correct answer—B

Antibiotic therapy is the only treatment for UTI. The nurse must ensure that the patient understands the significance of the treatment and that she needs to continue the full course of medication even when symptoms are relieved. The nurse should stress that UTI is a serious illness that, if untreated, can ascend to the kidneys and cause severe complications. The patient should not be released from the ED without this information. The patient should avoid sexual intercourse during the course of antibiotic therapy to avoid reinfection. Routine urinalysis is not indicated.

50 Correct answer—B

When a patient with suspected UTI has hematuria, the physician should order a count of red blood cell (RBC) casts in the urine to help identify the source of bleeding and the appropriate treatment. Normally, no RBC casts are seen in UTI. The presence of casts indicates that the source of bleeding is glomerular. The presence of RBCs that are of normal contour indicates that the source of bleeding is the urinary tract. This differentiation is important, as the treatment plan differs significantly. A count of leukocytes in the urine and a Gram stain of urine would not help to identify the source of the patient's hematura.

51 Correct answer—A

History of surgery or instrumentation is associated with the development of UTI. A history of hypoparathyroidism, sexually transmitted disease, or birth control methods have no significance in UTI.

52 Correct answer—D

Escherichia coli, the most common causative agent of UTI, ascends the urinary tract after being transported to the urethra from the anal area. Although other microbes, such as *Staphylococcus saprophyticus* and certain *Klebsiella* and *Proteus* species may cause UTI, *E. coli* is by far the most common.

53 Correct answer—B

Requesting an order for an antispasmodic agent, such as phenazopyridine hydrochloride, if the patient complains of bladder discomfort is the most appropriate nursing action in this situation. If the patient is menstruating, catheterization may be necessary to obtain a true urine specimen. Encouraging the patient to drink coffee or tea to aid in diuresis is inappropriate because these substances are

bladder irritants and may increase bladder discomfort. The nurse
should instruct the patient to increase her fluid intake, especially that
of cranberry juice, which helps to acidify the urine and prevent
reinfection.

54 Correct answer—C

Decompressing the urinary tract above the level of the obstruction is
essential in a patient with obstructive uropathy, either through
percutaneous nephrostomy or cystostomy. This should allow urine to
flow out of the kidney, thereby relieving hydronephrosis, which results
from obstruction. An obstruction causes urine to flow back up to the
kidney, where it stagnates. The degree of damage depends on the
duration and completeness of the blockage and on the presence or
absence of infection. Treatment aims to drain the genitourinary tract
of urine above the level of obstruction to prevent kidney damage. The
type of procedure (cystostomy or nephrostomy) also depends on the
location of the obstruction. Cystostomy and nephrostomy are
temporary measures used to improve the general health of the patient
until more definitive procedures, such as surgery, can be performed. A
consequence of relieving hydronephrosis is the prevention of ARF.

The situation does not mention whether the patient is acidotic;
therefore, correcting acidosis is not applicable. Besides, acidosis would
not occur until ARF occurs. Decompressing the bladder would not
necessarily relieve pressure on the obstructed area and would be of no
value in restoring urine flow.

55 Correct answer—A

If only one kidney is obstructed, the urinalysis should remain normal
because an unobstructed kidney can function normally, releasing
urine of normal composition into the bladder. An obstructed kidney,
however, cannot release urine. Hematuria may be present because
trauma from the obstruction may cause some bleeding. Sediment is
not usually found in the urine. If the urinalysis is normal, the patient
should have no protein, acetone, or glucose in the urine.

56 Correct answer—B

The most appropriate action in this situation would be to check the
catheter for patency. Urine flow can stop when the catheter becomes
obstructed from blood clots or kinks. Changing the patient's position
would not be therapeutic. Reinserting a new catheter may be
necessary if the present catheter is dislodged; however, this should be
done only after the catheter's patency is checked. Assuming that the
patient's condition has worsened is premature; this should not be done
until after catheter placement is checked.

57 Correct answer—B

Percutaneous nephrostomy involves the insertion of a catheter tube above the level of obstruction to allow urine to flow from the kidney's collecting system, through the nephrostomy tube, and into a drainage bag. Obstructed urine flows backs into the kidney. Over time, this hydronephosis causes damage to the tubules, which allows greater reabsorption of tubular fluid, especially sodium and water. When the obstruction is chronic, tubular function diminishes until it becomes lost; the concentrating ability is the first to cease. The more severe and prolonged the obstruction, the worse the damage. Untreated chronic obstruction can lead to complete kidney failure, in this case, of the right kidney.

A nephrostomy rarely cures the patient's uropathy; rather, it temporarily alleviates such symptoms as pain or acidosis and promotes a better state of health before more permanent and definitive procedures, such as surgery, can be performed. A nephrostomy can help prevent further damage, but it cannot reverse damage already incurred.

58 Correct answer—A

The initial goal would be to relieve the patient's pain and distress, then decompress the urinary tract above the obstruction and improve the patient's condition to permit more definitive treatment. Pain relief measures will most probably help reduce the patient's blood pressure. Cardiac arrhythmias are not commonly associated with obstructive uropathy. Because this situation developed only recently, the patient's fluid and electrolyte status probably is still normal.

59 Correct answer—D

IVP, the best technique to delineate the urinary tract, would most clearly identify the exact location of obstruction and degree of hydronephrosis. An abdominal X-ray, the easiest and most readily available test, would show only calcifications or masses as well as the position of the kidneys. Renal ultrasonography would not provide information about the patient's renal function; however, it would yield information about the size, shape, and location of the kidneys and the presence or absence of hydronephrosis. It is typically used to help guide the physician during percutaneous nephrostomy. Renal arteriography shows the condition and distribution of the renal vasculature, which is not the primary problem in obstruction.

60 Correct answer—B

Since a percutaneous nephrostomy drains urine from the kidney through the abdominal wall and into a drainage bag, the patient is at risk for infection. Therefore, *Potential for infection related to altered skin integrity* would be an appropriate nursing diagnosis. The patient is not at risk for fluid volume deficit from an additional source of urine flow because the kidney will continue to produce the same amount of urine. The patient also would not be at risk for metabolic acidosis or fluid volume excess because urine flow has been reestablished.

61 Correct answer—C

Prerenal azotemia does not result from the lodging of calcium oxalate calculi in a ureter. It results from any condition that reduces perfusion of the kidneys, such as fluid shifting from the intravascular space to the interstitial space, hemorrhage, or hypotension. When the blood supply is reduced, the efferent arteriole will constrict in an attempt to maintain filtration. The filtate will then remain in the glomerulus for a longer period. This allows for a backflow of urea into the blood, accounting for a disproportionate rise in BUN levels compared to creatinine levels. As poor oxygenation to the kidneys persists, ischemic changes occur and cellular debris obstructs the flow of filtrate into the tubules. If perfusion is restored, renal blood flow and oxygenation will improve, thereby restoring kidney function. If the cause is not corrected, ischemic changes persist, the patient remains oliguric, and recovery from ARF can take months. Obstruction in a ureter from calculi can cause postrenal failure.

62 Correct answer—B

The nurse should immediately assess for pulsus paradoxus, an exaggerated decline in the pulse or blood pressure during inspiration. Pericardial friction rub is a manifestation of pericarditis that results from the accumulation of uremic toxins and fluid in the pericardial sac. Although pericarditis can be reversed by hemodialysis, the nurse's primary responsibility in this situation would be to assess for a pulsus paradoxus, which would indicate the extent of fluid accumulation in the pericardial sac. When the pericarditis progresses to pericardial effusion, a friction rub can no longer be heard. Although oxygen may be necessary, the nurse would not necessarily assume that it should be administered, as oxygen needs are determined on an individual basis. Furosemide (Lasix) is of no value in treating pericarditis.

63 Correct answer—C

The nurse must remember that the patient is extremely ill and short of breath. Offering the simplest explanation that is truthful and that offers hope and support would be most appropriate in this situation. Therefore, the nurse should tell the patient that he will be able to breathe easier once hemodialysis removes fluid and toxins that the kidneys cannot. Hemodialysis does not repair kidney function but effectively removes metabolic waste products. The nurse in this situation would not know whether the patient requires only a short course of hemodialysis or ongoing therapy for the rest of his life.

64 Correct answer—D

Tall, tented T waves and prolonged PR intervals are indicative of hyperkalemia, a common complication of ARF. As hyperkalemia progresses, wide QRS complexes develop; if hyperkalemia is not treated promptly, asystole ensues. Chronic renal failure results in hypocalcemia and hyperphosphatemia. Calcium and phosphorus imbalances usually do not occur in ARF.

65 Correct answer—A

A ruptured bladder is most likely to occur when the bladder is full. It occurs equally in both sexes and is commonly associated with blunt adominal (not chest) trauma and fracture of the pelvis. The nurse would suspect urethral trauma in a patient with a straddle-type injury.

66 Correct answer—C

A patient with a ruptured bladder should also be assessed for rectal injury, which significantly increases morbidity and mortality. Damage to the iliac vesels also may occur. Ruptured spleen, pancreatitis, and spinal cord injury usually are not associated with bladder ruptures.

67 Correct answer—D

Signs and symptoms of bladder rupture include hematuria, pelvic discomfort, and difficulty voiding. Hematuria and pelvic discomfort result from tissue trauma. The degree to which the patient experiences these symptoms depends on the extent of damage and the presence of other injuries. Difficulty voiding occurs because the muscles responsible for urination are unable to function. Pyuria and fever indicate infection. A ruptured bladder would not be capable of distention.

68 Correct answer—A

Besides pain relief measures, the plan of care should include the application of ice packs and testicular elevation. Because the patient is in severe pain, pain relief is a priority for this patient. Applying ice packs will help to reduce swelling and pain. Trauma may cause bleeding into the penis and scrotal sac. The collection of extravasated blood typically produces pain. Immobilizing and elevating the testes

will help minimize further bleeding, thereby minimizing the pain.
Applying heat packs will contribute to further bleeding.

69 Correct answer — C

Urethral bleeding is present when trauma to the urethra occurs. This
must be distinguished from hematuria, which occurs from injury to
other parts of the genitourinary system. Hematuria does not occur
with urethral trauma because urine cannot travel down the transected
urethra. When the posterior urethra is completely transected, urine
extravasation typically does not occur because the bladder neck
remains competent. Because an incomplete transection can become
completely transected, catheterization is not recommended. The patient
with urethral trauma may have acute dull or sharp pain; colicky pain
is associated with renal calculi.

70 Correct answer — D

Pelvic inflammatory disease (PID), an inflammation of the female
reproductive organs, can result from various causes but most
commonly from a sexually transmitted bacterial infection. Pathogens
carrying sexually transmitted disease, such as *Neisseria gonorrhoeae*
and *Chlamydia trachomatis*, enter the body from the outside via the
cervical canal and travel to the uterus and pelvis via the lymphatic
channels, uterine veins, or fallopian tubes. *Mycobacterium tuberculosis*
enters through the lungs and is transported via the bloodstream.

71 Correct answer — D

Signs and symptoms, such as lower abdominal pain, fever, chills,
nausea, and vomiting, may be confused with those of appendicitis or
ectopic pregnancy. Ultrasound studies and cultures help in making the
correct diagnosis.

72 Correct answer — D

As with any infection in the lower abdominal region, peritonitis can be
a potential complication if appropriate treatment is not prescribed and
maintained. Because of the inflammatory process affecting the
reproductive organs, patients with PID are at a higher risk for tubal
ectopic pregnancies and subsequent infertility problems.

73 Correct answer — C

The risk of acquiring PID is four to eight times greater in women who
use an intrauterine device (IUD). During an episode of PID, many
physicians recommend removal of the IUD once antibiotic therapy has

been initiated. Abnormal menstrual cycles, stress, and continued use of antibiotics are not considered risk factors for PID.

74 Correct answer – **B**

"I need to take all of the medication" indicates that the patient understands the discharge instructions involving continuing antibiotic therapy – that the patient must finish taking all of the medication, even when the signs and symptoms, including vaginal discharge, have disappeared or she is feeling better. The patient does not need to be on bed rest or reduce her activity level during antibiotic therapy. The patient's sexual partner should also be treated to prevent the recurrence of infection.

75 Correct answer – **B**

Depending on the infecting organism, the discharge instructions for this patient should include the education and treatment of all sexual contacts to prevent reinfection. Genetic counseling and education for stress reduction are not necessary in this situation. Follow-up urine and cervical cultures, not ultrasound studies, may be necessary.

76 Correct answer – **C**

Characteristically, toxic shock syndrome has a rapid onset of nausea and vomiting followed by profuse diarrhea. Severe abdominal pain or rebound tenderness may occur. Fever in excess of 102° F (38.9° C) is an early sign and nearly always present. Volume loss with postural dizziness and hypotension develops quickly. Disorientation or altered consciousness without focal neurologic signs is sometimes prominent. Other symptoms may include photophobia, headache, diffuse muscle aches, joint stiffness, and sore throat. Toxic shock syndrome primarily affects previously healthy young women during their menstrual periods, although it may occur in nonmenstruating women and in children.

The nurse would not suspect ectopic pregnancy because the patient is menstruating. She also would not suspect vaginitis because the symptoms are too severe. Although the symptoms are similar to those of an ovarian cyst, the history of tampon use leads the nurse to suspect toxic shock syndrome over a cyst.

77 Correct answer – **B**

The symptoms of toxic shock syndrome are accompanied by diffuse macular erythroderma that desquamates and progresses to marked peeling of the palms and soles about 10 days after onset.

78 Correct answer—A

The toxin that causes toxic shock syndrome—enterotoxin F—is
secreted by *Staphylococcus aureus,* group I.

79 Correct answer—B

The vagina is a favorable environment for the growth of *S. aureus* and
its toxins, and it is believed that insertion of a tampon, contraceptive
sponge, or diaphragm may traumatize the vaginal mucosa, thereby
facilitating infection and absorption of the toxin. Extra-absorbent
tampons seem to cause increased incidence because of increased
absorbency and fewer tampon changes. The extra absorbency may
cause occlusion of the menstrual flow and less frequent changes,
permitting a contaminated environment for a longer time. Such
contamination also may occur with contraceptive sponges and a
diaphragm that is left in the vagina for 6 to 24 hours. The use of
IUDs, douches, and oral antibiotics is not associated with toxic shock
syndrome.

80 Correct answer—A

An appropriate nursing diagnosis for this patient would be *Decreased
cardiac output related to vasodilation and decreased myocardial
contractility* because the endotoxins released from bacteria produce
vasodilation, which impairs myocardial contractility. The other
diagnoses would be inappropriate because the patient already has an
infection, not a potential for one, and because vaginal hemorrhage and
seizures are not associated with toxic shock syndrome.

81 Correct answer—A

The hypotension of toxic shock syndrome is frequently difficult to
control, and immediate supportive care for shock should be initiated.
Immediate volume replacement is imperative, or refractory hypotension
with resulting vascular, cardiac, and renal abnormalities may result.
Systolic pressure should be maintained at 90 mm Hg. Treating fever
and drawing blood for cultures are secondary nursing interventions to
be performed after the patient has been stablizied. A spinal tap is not
indicated for a patient with toxic shock syndrome.

82 Correct answer—D

Adult respiratory distress syndrome, severe metabolic acidosis, and
disseminated intravascular coagulation have developed in patients
with toxic shock syndrome in response to vascular depletion, which
causes decreased peripheral perfusion.

83 Correct answer — A

About 40% of those with gonorrhea also are infected with chlamydia, which is commonly asymptomatic in women. Tetracycline (Tetracyn) is effective against chlamydia.

84 Correct answer — C

Asking the patient what kind of sexual practices she engages in, such as oral or anal sex, may elicit information about infection in other areas of the body, which may be asymptomatic and treated differently. Although the other questions may be useful in eliciting information about the patient's sexual history, allowing the nurse to concentrate on specific areas for patient teaching, they are not useful in determining the course of treatment for this infection.

85 Correct answer — B

Recurrence of sexually transmitted diseases does not place the patient at increased risk for renal disease. However, such a patient would be at increased risk for PID, which may result in infertility or ectopic pregnancy. High-risk sexual practices also place the patient at increased risk for contracting HIV.

86 Correct answer — A

The patient's decision to use oral contraceptives would indicate the need for further patient teaching in this situation. Sexually active women with a history of sexually transmitted disease are recommended to use a barrier type of contraception, such as a condom, contraceptive sponge, or diaphragm, which may decrease the risk of recurrence. Oral contraceptives do not offer this kind of protection.

87 Correct answer — A

The patient's acknowledgment that probenecid enhances amoxicillin's effect best reflects her understanding of the reason for receiving probenecid. Probenecid, an anti-gout medicine, increases the effectiveness of penicillin-type drugs; it does not relieve painful urination, kill bacteria, or reduce fever.

88 Correct answer — C

The first message that must be conveyed is that the victim is in a safe, secure environment. Most sexual assaults occur in places known to the victim and, because the victim may know the attacker, even familiar surroundings may be perceived as threatening. The fact that

sexual attacks commonly occur without warning contributes even
more to the victim's fear and sense of loss of control. Telling the
victim that all medical tests will be handled confidentially, that the
examination will be done quickly, and that medications are available
to prevent pregnancy may be conveyed after the patient's safety needs
are met.

89 Correct answer—D

Asking the victim whether she urinated or defecated, changed her
clothes, or rinsed her mouth since the assault is an important part of
the nursing history. Semen can be detected in urine and in a rectal
swab specimen. In cases of oral assault, semen is likely to be found in
oral secretions around the gum line. Such evidence as hair, blood,
semen, and grass may be retained in clothing. The ultimate goal is to
collect and maintain all evidence to ensure its admission into court.

90 Correct answer—B

Having the victim fold each piece of clothing inward and place each
article in a separate paper bag is the correct procedure. Folding
rather than shaking the clothing will retain evidence and prevent
contamination by staff members. Plastic bags should not be used
because they may retain moisture and alter the evidence. If the victim
consents, all clothing and other belongings should be retained for
evidence, even if they had been removed during the assault. Minute
pieces of hair, clothing, semen, blood, leaves, and dirt provide concrete
evidence that should be identified by a qualified laboratory.

91 Correct answer—C

The patient should return to her physician within 5 to 6 weeks
because syphilis takes from 4 to 6 weeks to be detected serologically.

92 Correct answer—D

The victim's basic needs of food, shelter, and clothing must be met to
allow her to begin reestablishing control. Clear, concise, written
instructions are necessary because the victim is unlikely to remember
oral instructions. A list of referral telephone numbers is critical and
should include at least one 24-hour resource.

CHAPTER 8

Neurologic Emergencies

1 Which physiologic event precipitates most neurologic emergencies?

A. Head trauma
B. Cerebrovascular accident
C. Intracerebral hemorrhage
D. Increased intracranial pressure

2 The nurse understands that consciousness is determined by the:

A. Reticular activating system
B. Spinothalamic tract
C. Extrapyramidal tracts
D. Hypothalamus

3 Which method is the best way of determining a patient's level of consciousness in the emergency department (ED)?

A. Assessing pupillary reaction
B. Assessing vital signs
C. Assessing muscle strength in the extremities
D. Using the Glasgow Coma Scale

4 The nurse typically begins to assess level of consciousness by using:

A. Auditory stimulation
B. Tactile stimulation
C. Light pain
D. Deep pain

5 Which of the following is the most reliable index of a patient's neurologic condition?

A. Level of consciousness
B. Pupillary response
C. Vital signs
D. Motor function

6 Which symptom is least likely to be exhibited by a patient who sustains a cerebral concussion?

A. Dizziness
B. Loss of memory
C. Headache
D. Bizarre behavior

7 When planning discharge instructions for a patient with a cerebral concussion, the nurse should anticipate telling the patient that he can expect all neurologic symptoms to subside within:

A. 2 to 4 hours
B. 4 to 8 hours
C. 8 to 12 hours
D. 24 to 48 hours

8 Which condition would the nurse expect to note in a patient who has sustained a head injury and damage to the sixth cranial nerve?

A. Absent gag reflex
B. Fixed and dilated pupils
C. Nystagmus
D. Inward deviation of the eyes

9 A man is brought to the ED by ambulance after hitting his head when he dove into a 4'-deep swimming pool. Which procedure would hold the highest priority after the patient's level of consciousness and vital signs have been checked?

A. Computed tomography (CT) scan of the head
B. X-ray of the cervical spine
C. Arterial blood gas measurements
D. Routine laboratory workup

10 The nurse assesses a comatose patient who is exhibiting decerebrate posturing. Which brain areas are likely to have been injured in this patient?

A. Cerebrum and cerebellum
B. Cerebrum and brain stem
C. Hypothalamus and brain stem
D. Cerebellum and hypothalamus

11 The nurse would anticipate a patient with a lesion at the lower midbrain level to demonstrate which breathing pattern?

A. Hyperventilation
B. Hypoventilation
C. Apneustic breathing
D. Cluster breathing

12 A 23-year-old man is brought to the ED after suddenly feeling ill while exercising with weights at a local health spa. While in the ED, he complains of a sudden, explosive headache. The nurse suspects:

A. Subarachnoid hemorrhage
B. Epidural hematoma
C. Basal skull fracture
D. Brain stem contusion

13 A man arrives at the ED via ambulance after sustaining a hemisection of the spinal cord from a stab wound to the right side of the back. He experiences loss of movement on the right side and loss of pain and temperature sensations on the left. The nurse knows that this syndrome is called:

A. Brown-Séquard syndrome
B. Anterior cord syndrome
C. Partial cord syndrome
D. Central cord syndrome

SITUATION

A 45-year-old man with a history of seizure arrives at the ED via an ambulance. His family informs the nurse that the patient suffered a seizure 30 minutes ago and that he takes phenytoin (Dilantin) and phenobarbital (Luminal) daily. Vital signs are blood pressure, 120/60 mm Hg; pulse rate, 110 beats/minute; and respiratory rate, 12 breaths/minute. His pupils are equal and reactive to light. The nurse notes that he grimaces only in response to tactile stimuli.

Questions 14 to 20 refer to the above situation.

14 Which statement accurately describes the mechanism of a generalized seizure?

A. The abnormal excessive firing of brain cells causes the clinical signs and symptoms of a seizure
B. The entire brain is involved in a seizure
C. The metabolism of the involved cells is greatly decreased during a seizure
D. The abnormal firing of neurons, once initiated, is perpetuated indefinitely until therapy is instituted

15 The nurse's highest priority when caring for a patient in a postictal state is to:

A. Obtain a complete family history
B. Begin an infusion of normal saline solution
C. Place the patient on his side
D. Call the physician

16 Which of the following is least likely to precipitate a seizure?

A. Head trauma
B. Heavy-metal ingestion
C. The patient's discontinuation of anticonvulsant therapy
D. Cerebral edema

17 Which nursing diagnostic category reflects the clinical problems associated with this patient's seizures?

A. Ineffective airway clearance
B. Altered tissue perfusion
C. Potential for injury
D. All of the above

18 When administering phenytoin intravenously, the nurse must:

A. Institute cardiac monitoring
B. Obtain a serum phenytoin level immediately after administration
C. Administer the drug in a dextrose solution
D. Administer the drug at a rate no faster than 500 mg/minute

19 Which life-threatening situation would the nurse expect to occur if phenytoin is administered by rapid I.V. bolus?

A. Ventricular tachycardia
B. Supraventricular tachycardia
C. Third-degree heart block
D. Electromechanical dissociation

20 Which information regarding phenytoin should the nurse include in her discharge teaching for this patient?

A. Alcohol may cause phenytoin toxicity
B. Phenytoin must be taken even in the absence of seizures
C. Missed doses should not be made up
D. Aspirin, rather than acetaminophen, should be taken for headaches

SITUATION

A 21-year-old woman is admitted to the ED in a coma. She is accompanied by her husband, who states that she had a seizure. The patient is 1 week postpartum. Her vital signs are blood pressure, 180/128 mm Hg; pulse rate, 120 beats/minute; and respiratory rate, 12 breaths/minute. The physician diagnoses eclampsia.

Questions 21 and 22 refer to the above situation.

21 Which statement about eclampsia is *true?*

A. Signs and symptoms typically occur during the third trimester but can occur up to 2 months postpartum
B. Signs and symptoms include hypertension, proteinuria, oliguria, and seizures
C. Eclampsia most commonly occurs in multigravida women
D. Eclampsia is idiopathic and not associated with any preexisting disease

22 After the initial management of this patient, the nurse would expect the physician to order which medication?

A. Phenobarbital
B. Diazepam (Valium)
C. Magnesium sulfate
D. Phenytoin

SITUATION

A middle-aged man who was found unconscious on the street is brought to the ED by paramedics. No identification or further information is available. Vital signs are blood pressure, 160/90 mm Hg; pulse rate, 120 beats/minute; and respiratory rate, 16 breaths/minute. Upon arrival, the patient begins experiencing sustained grand mal seizures and requires intubation. The nurse establishes an I.V. line.

Questions 23 to 25 relate to the above situation.

23 Which drug treatment is usually preferred to control status epilepticus?

A. 18 mg/kg of phenytoin I.V.
B. Diazepam 5 mg/minute I.V. every 5 to 10 minutes
C. 10 to 20 mg/kg of phenobarbital I.V.
D. 4 mg of lorazepam (Ativan) I.V. over 2 minutes

24 After the patient's seizure is controlled, the nurse would expect to administer all of the following *except:*

A. 50 ml of dextrose 50%
B. 10 to 20 mg/kg of phenobarbital I.V.
C. 100 mg of thiamine I.V.
D. 2 mg of naloxone (Narcan) I.V.

25 Which drug is the treatment of choice to prevent seizures from traumatic head injury?

A. Diazepam
B. Dexamethasone (Decadron)
C. Phenytoin
D. Phenobarbital

SITUATION

A 60-year-old man with a history of seizures is brought to the ED because of recurrent seizure activity. While in the ED, he develops tonic-clonic movements of the right arm and leg.

Questions 26 and 27 refer to the above situation.

26 The nurse correctly determines that this patient is exhibiting a:

A. Grand mal seizure
B. Petit mal seizure
C. Jacksonian seizure
D. Psychomotor seizure

27 Which postictal manifestation should the nurse anticipate and adjust for in the patient's plan of care?

A. Paralysis of the right side
B. Loss of consciousness
C. Incontinence
D. Seizure activity of the left side

SITUATION

A 25-year-old man, disoriented to time and place, is admitted to the ED. His co-worker states that the patient was hit on the head with a beam 2 hours ago and that the incident caused momentary unconsciousness. The patient was fine until 30 minutes ago, when he became tired and confused. Physical examination reveals a dilated nonreactive left pupil. Vital signs are blood pressure, 160/80 mm Hg; pulse rate, 80 beats/minute; and respiratory rate, 16 breaths/minute.

Questions 28 to 41 refer to the above situation.

28 Which diagnostic test would the nurse anticipate the physician to order initially?

A. Lumbar puncture
B. CT scan
C. Cervical spine X-ray
D. Cerebral angiography

29 Diagnostic studies reveal a temporal fracture with a pineal shift. The nurse would interpret this finding to indicate:

A. Subdural hematoma
B. Epidural hematoma
C. Subarachnoid hemorrhage
D. Intracerebral bleeding

30 The ED nurse would anticipate the medical treatment for this patient to include:

A. Direct intracranial pressure (ICP) monitoring in the intensive care unit (ICU)
B. Pharmacologic management
C. Lumbar puncture
D. Surgical evacuation of the clot

31 The primary objective in the plan of care for a patient with a traumatic head injury typically involves:

A. Decreasing the patient's ICP
B. Maintaining the patient's oxygenation
C. Maintaining the patient's body alignment
D. Hyperventilating the patient

32 Which independent nursing intervention best relieves increased ICP?

A. Elevating the head of the bed 30 degrees
B. Administering oxygen
C. Administering diuretics
D. Hyperventilating the patient

33 Which sign is typically the first indication of increased ICP?

A. Elevated systolic blood pressure
B. Elevated body temperature
C. Altered respiratory pattern
D. Altered level of consciousness

34 While caring for a patient with a head trauma, the nurse would assess for signs of uncal herniation. Which sign is an early indication of this condition?

A. Absent doll's eye reflex
B. Ipsilateral pupil dilation
C. Ataxic breathing
D. Impaired motor function

35 The nurse is aware that signs of increased ICP include:

A. Narrowing pulse pressure, rising systolic blood pressure, and bradycardia
B. Narrowing pulse pressure, rising systolic blood pressure, and tachycardia
C. Widening pulse pressure, rising diastolic blood pressure, and bradycardia
D. Widening pulse pressure, rising systolic blood pressure, and bradycardia

36 Although several nursing diagnostic categories would be applicable for a patient with increased ICP, which category is most appropriate for this patient?

A. Altered cerebral tissue perfusion
B. Increased cerebral perfusion pressure
C. Potential for brain injury
D. Increased intracranial adaptive capacity

37 The nurse knows that all of the following statements about epidural and subdural hematomas are false *except:*

   A. Epidural bleeding occurs below the dura mater and above the arachnoid layer

   B. Signs and symptoms of epidural bleeding develop more slowly than do those of subdural bleeding

   C. Epidural hematomas usually are caused by arterial bleeding, and subdural hematomas usually are caused by injury to a vein

   D. Temporal bone fractures are associated with subdural hematomas

38 When planning the care of a patient with increased ICP, the nurse includes appropriate interventions to prevent further worsening of the patient's condition. The nurse realizes that the patient's condition may worsen with the development of:

   A. Hypoxemia, hypercapnia, and respiratory alkalosis

   B. Hypoxemia, hypercapnia, and respiratory acidosis

   C. Hypoxemia, hypocapnia, and respiratory alkalosis

   D. Hypoxemia, hypocapnia, and respiratory acidosis

39 Which rationale best supports the use of mannitol in treating increased ICP?

   A. It induces diuresis by raising the osmotic pressure of glomerular filtrate

   B. It increases the rate of electrolyte excretion, particularly of sodium, chloride, and potassium

   C. It increases plasma osmolality, thereby inducing diffusion of water from cerebrospinal fluid back into the plasma and intravascular space

   D. It results in a shifting of intracellular fluid into the interstitial space, thus decreasing cellular edema

40 The nurse should include avoidance of which activity in the care plan of a patient with increased ICP?

   A. Valsalva's maneuver

   B. Coughing or sneezing

   C. Isometric muscle contraction or hip flexion

   D. All of the above

Neurologic Emergencies
Questions

41 Which method of determining ICP is considered unsafe in a patient with a head injury?

A. Lumbar puncture
B. Epidural monitoring
C. Intraventricular catheterization
D. Subarachnoid screw insertion

SITUATION

A patient admitted to the ED after a motor vehicle accident is found to have a basal skull fracture with middle meningeal artery damage.

Questions 42 to 47 refer to the above situation.

42 The nurse would expect a patient who sustained damage to the middle meningeal artery to develop:

A. A subdural hematoma
B. A subarachnoid hemorrhage
C. An epidural hematoma
D. An aneurysm

43 The nurse assesses this patient for Battle's sign, which is best described as:

A. A postconcussion syndrome
B. An ecchymosis over the mastoid bone
C. Black-and-blue discoloration around the eyes
D. A superficial hematoma on the skull

44 This patient is also at risk for injury to the:

A. Oculomotor nerve
B. Olfactory nerve
C. Optic nerve
D. Ophthalmic nerve

45 The nurse would anticipate further assessment of a patient with a basal skull fracture to possibly reveal:

A. Otorrhea
B. Meningism
C. Facial paresis
D. Hemianopia

46 Which nursing measure will benefit a patient with a basal skull fracture?

A. Instructing the patient to blow his nose gently
B. Instructing the patient to avoid Valsalva's maneuver
C. Encouraging the patient to cough and breathe deeply
D. Carefully inserting a nasogastric tube

47 The nurse understands that raccoon's eyes usually indicate:

A. Meningitis
B. Intracerebral hemorrhage
C. Epidural hematoma
D. Anterior fossa fracture

SITUATION

A man is brought to the ED by emergency medical service after involvement in a motor vehicle accident. He is suspected of having a spinal cord injury.

Questions 48 to 56 refer to the above situation.

48 Spinal X-rays confirm a lesion at the C5 to C6 level. The nurse anticipates that the patient has:

A. Quadriplegia with intact triceps and biceps and intercostal breathing
B. Quadriplegia with gross arm movements and diaphragmatic breathing
C. Paraplegia with diaphragmatic breathing
D. Diaphragmatic and intercostal breathing with loss of intrinsic hand muscle power

49 Which nursing diagnosis would be the highest priority for a patient with a cervical spinal cord injury?

A. Impaired gas exchange related to pulmonary embolism
B. Dysfunctional grieving related to paralysis
C. Ineffective breathing pattern related to weakened respiratory muscles
D. Potential for multisystem dysfunction related to spinal shock

50 While in the ED, the patient develops spinal shock. This condition is defined as a state of:

A. Spastic paralysis caused by a lesion of the upper motor neuron
B. Inhibition of parasympathetic outflow
C. Sudden initiation of the facilitory influences from higher brain centers
D. Transient reflex depression below the level of the lesion

51 Nursing assessment of the patient reveals all of the following *except:*

A. Urinary incontinence
B. Bradycardia
C. Poikilothermy
D. Hypotension

52 One of the nurse's major concerns in caring for a patient with a spinal cord injury is to maintain optimal respiratory function. Which development would *not* lead to hypoventilation in this patient?

A. An injury below C4 resulting in diaphragmatic breathing and decreased tidal volume
B. A cervical lesion at C8 resulting in spinal shock
C. Paralysis of abdominal and intercostal muscles leading to ineffective cough and retention of secretions
D. Abdominal distension from gastric dilation, possibly restricting diaphragmatic excursion

53 When assessing the patient's motor function, the nurse determines spinothalamic tract function by:

A. Applying a tuning fork to a bony prominence and asking the patient to identify the vibration
B. Asking the patient to close both eyes and to touch his nose with his finger
C. Asking the patient to identify areas stimulated by pinprick
D. Testing the patient's position sense

54 Which assessment finding would indicate deterioration of this patient's respiratory status?

A. Arterial blood gas (ABG) measurements of pH, 7.28; PCO_2, 36 mm Hg; HCO_3^-, 18 mEq; and PO_2, 86 mm Hg
B. Inspiratory force of -20 cm
C. Tidal volume of 500 ml
D. Bronchial breath sounds over the lung lobes

55 At which level does the phrenic nerve innervate the diaphragm?

A. C2 to C3
B. C3 to C4
C. T1 to T3
D. T3 to T4

56 In the patient with a spinal cord injury, early hypoventilation is best manifested by:

A. Poor respiratory exchange
B. Cyanosis
C. Shortness of breath while talking
D. ABG changes

57 A patient is admitted to the ED with possible spinal cord injury between T4 and T12. Which clinical finding would the nurse *not* expect to note?

A. Bladder and bowel incontinence
B. Paraplegia of the lower part of the body
C. Complete loss of motor function in the legs
D. Loss of feeling below the truncal dermatome level, corresponding with the site of cord damage

58 If a cervical spinal cord injury is suspected, the best way to open the patient's airway would be to:

A. Tilt the head forward, supporting the neck
B. Use a modified jaw-thrust maneuver
C. Log-roll the patient on his side and pull down the chin
D. Perform a tracheotomy

59 The nurse knows that loss of motor function in the right arm and leg may indicate a lesion in the:

A. Pyramidal tract of the left hemisphere
B. Spinocerebellar tract
C. Motor nerve fibers in the anterior horn of the spinal cord
D. Spinal cord at C7

60 The most reliable technique for testing the motor strength of a patient's arm is to:

A. Observe for spontaneous movement
B. Test the patient's muscle reflexes
C. Ask the patient to squeeze the nurse's hands
D. Ask the patient to close his eyes and to raise his arms straight in front of him

61 A patient admitted to the ED with an injury to the left cerebral hemisphere may exhibit:

A. Left hemiparesis
B. Left homonymous hemianopia
C. Deviation of the eyes to the left
D. Left-sided hemiplegia

62 The nurse understands that pinpoint pupils usually are indicative of a lesion in the:

A. Pons
B. Optic nerve
C. Medulla
D. Midbrain

63 An unconscious patient with pinpoint pupils is most likely to exhibit which breathing pattern?

A. Apneustic breathing
B. Biot's respirations
C. Ataxic breathing
D. Cheyne-Stokes respirations

64 Which patient assessment technique is the best way to check for meningeal irritation?

A. Flex the patient's leg at the hip and knee, then straighten the knee and watch for pain and resistance
B. Stroke the lateral aspect of the patient's sole and watch for dorsiflexion of the great toe
C. Check the patient's temperature; a reading above 102° F (38.9° C) indicates meningeal irritation
D. Check for papilledema

65 Which nursing action would be inappropriate for a patient who has just been diagnosed as having viral meningitis?

A. Institute seizure precautions
B. Institute isolation precautions
C. Monitor the patient's temperature frequently
D. Institute measures to control increased ICP

66 Which of the following findings is a common sign of meningococcal meningitis?

A. Petechiae
B. Hypothermia
C. Nystagmus
D. Hypertensive crisis

Neurologic Emergencies
Questions

Answer Sheet

	A	B	C	D		A	B	C	D		A	B	C	D
1	○	○	○	○	31	○	○	○	○	61	○	○	○	○
2	○	○	○	○	32	○	○	○	○	62	○	○	○	○
3	○	○	○	○	33	○	○	○	○	63	○	○	○	○
4	○	○	○	○	34	○	○	○	○	64	○	○	○	○
5	○	○	○	○	35	○	○	○	○	65	○	○	○	○
6	○	○	○	○	36	○	○	○	○	66	○	○	○	○
7	○	○	○	○	37	○	○	○	○					
8	○	○	○	○	38	○	○	○	○					
9	○	○	○	○	39	○	○	○	○					
10	○	○	○	○	40	○	○	○	○					
11	○	○	○	○	41	○	○	○	○					
12	○	○	○	○	42	○	○	○	○					
13	○	○	○	○	43	○	○	○	○					
14	○	○	○	○	44	○	○	○	○					
15	○	○	○	○	45	○	○	○	○					
16	○	○	○	○	46	○	○	○	○					
17	○	○	○	○	47	○	○	○	○					
18	○	○	○	○	48	○	○	○	○					
19	○	○	○	○	49	○	○	○	○					
20	○	○	○	○	50	○	○	○	○					
21	○	○	○	○	51	○	○	○	○					
22	○	○	○	○	52	○	○	○	○					
23	○	○	○	○	53	○	○	○	○					
24	○	○	○	○	54	○	○	○	○					
25	○	○	○	○	55	○	○	○	○					
26	○	○	○	○	56	○	○	○	○					
27	○	○	○	○	57	○	○	○	○					
28	○	○	○	○	58	○	○	○	○					
29	○	○	○	○	59	○	○	○	○					
30	○	○	○	○	60	○	○	○	○					

1 Correct answer—**D**

Increased intracranial pressure (ICP) commonly precedes most neurologic emergencies, such as head trauma, cerebrovascular accident, and intracranial hemorrhage. An ICP less than 10 mm Hg is considered normal; any measurement above 15 mm Hg is considered abnormal. Increased ICP can be caused by conditions that increase brain volume, such as hematomas, tumors, and cerebral edema; those that increase blood volume, such as hypercapnia; and those that increase cerebrospinal fluid, such as hydrocephalus.

2 Correct answer—**A**

The reticular activating system is responsible for maintaining consciousness by coordinating sensory input and responding, in proportion, to incoming stimuli. The spinothalamic tract is responsible for transmitting pain and temperature sensations to the brain. The extrapyramidal tracts regulate and control voluntary motor activity. The hypothalamus is responsible for temperature regulation, behavior, autonomic responses, and control of the pituitary gland.

3 Correct answer—**D**

The Glasgow Coma Scale is the standard means of assessing a patient's level of consciousness in the emergency department (ED). The nurse uses the scale to assign a numeric value to the patient's ability to open his eyes, respond verbally, and demonstrate motor response to different stimuli. The totaled scores, ranging from 1 to 15, indicate the level of consciousness (alert, lethargic, obtunded, stuporous, semicomatose, or comatose); a total of 7 or less indicates a comatose state. Using the Glasgow Coma Scale allows the nurse to quickly determine any deterioration in the patient's neurologic status.

4 Correct answer—**A**

The nurse typically begins to assess consciousness by using auditory stimulation and observing for a response. Because it is always best to start with the minimum amount of stimulation necessary to evoke a response, speaking to the patient is commonly the first step.

5 Correct answer—**A**

Level of consciousness, the most important and reliable index of a patient's neurologic condition, is the earliest and most sensitive indicator of a change in neurologic status. Altered consciousness is the hallmark of cerebral injury.

Neurologic Emergencies
Answers

6 Correct answer—**D**

Bizarre behavior is characteristic of a patient with a cerebral contusion, not a cerebral concussion. A patient with a cerebral concussion may experience dizziness, loss of memory, and headaches. A cerebral concussion is a shock to the brain's soft tissues; a contusion involves bruising and laceration of brain tissue.

7 Correct answer—**D**

All symptoms of a concussion should subside within 24 to 48 hours. Any problems lasting longer than that time indicate a more serious injury and require reevaluation by a physician.

8 Correct answer—**D**

The nurse would expect to note inward deviation of the eyes because the sixth cranial (abducens) nerve controls this movement. The gag reflex is controlled by the ninth and tenth (glossopharyngeal and vagus, respectively) cranial nerves. Pupillary constriction and dilation is controlled by the third cranial (oculomotor) nerve. Nystagmus is caused by an interruption of cerebellar function.

9 Correct answer—**B**

An X-ray of the cervical spine with a view of C7 is vitally important to determine whether the patient has a compression injury to the spinal cord and the level at which it has occurred. The patient should not be moved to obtain the X-rays; a cross-table lateral view should be obtained.

10 Correct answer—**B**

Decerebrate posturing is indicative of a patient with damage to the brain stem and cerebrum, because both areas control motor function. The cerebellum coordinates muscle tone with movement and maintains equilibrium. The hypothalamus does not regulate motor function.

11 Correct answer—**A**

Altered breathing patterns are directly related to specific levels of brain dysfunction. Central neurogenic hyperventilation, which is characterized by rapid, regular respirations (in excess of 24 breaths/minute) with an increase in depth of respiration, is typical of a patient with a lesion at the lower midbrain level. Apneustic breathing, which is characterized by prolonged inspiration with a 2- to 3-second pause at the end of inspiration, typically occurs in a patient with a lesion at the pons level. Cluster breathing, which is characterized by irregular breathing with periods of apnea at irregular intervals, is associated with medullary damage. Hypoventilation typically occurs in a patient with metabolic or drug-induced coma, respiratory depression, or increased ICP.

12 Correct answer—**A**

The patient is probably experiencing a subarachnoid hemorrhage caused by an arteriovenous malformation and brought on by strenuous activity. Epidural hematoma, basal skull fracture, and brain stem contusion typically occur as a result of traumatic injury.

13 Correct answer—**A**

In Brown-Séquard syndrome, the damage is located on one side of the spinal cord. As a result, complete motor paralysis occurs on the same side (ipsilateral motor loss), with nearly complete loss of pain and temperature sensation on the opposite side below the level of the lesion (contralateral loss of pain and temperature sensation). In anterior cord syndrome, which may be caused by a forward dislocation or compression injury, the damage is mainly concentrated in the anterior aspect of the cord. Complete motor paralysis usually occurs below the level of the lesion, with complete loss of pain and temperature sensations. In central cord syndrome, the mechanism of injury usually is hyperextension of the cervical spine with compression, resulting in greater motor loss of upper extremities than of lower ones. No type of spinal cord damage is known as partial cord syndrome.

14 Correct answer—**A**

The abnormal excessive firing of brain cells causes the clinical signs and symptoms of a seizure. Either a portion of or the entire brain may be involved. The metabolism of the involved cells is greatly increased during seizure activity. The abnormal firing of neurons may terminate as abruptly as it begins.

15 Correct answer—**C**

Maintaining a patent airway is the primary nursing goal in this situation; placing the patient in a side-lying position with the head and body aligned ensures airway patency and helps prevent aspiration. An airway should be placed in the patient's mouth before a tonic phase begins. To prevent injury, objects should never be forced into the mouth during a seizure. The nurse should stay with the patient during the seizure and summon assistance if further equipment is needed. The nurse may need to establish an I.V. line to administer

Neurologic Emergencies Answers

anticonvulsants. Once the patient is stabilized, the nurse may obtain a complete family history.

16 Correct answer—B

Heavy-metal ingestion is least likely to precipitate a seizure. Common precipitating events include the discontinuation of anticonvulsant therapy, which typically occurs as a result of the patient's forgetting to take the medication or not complying with the drug regimen; craniocerebral trauma; infections, particularly of the central nervous system; cerebral tumors; or metabolic brain disorders.

17 Correct answer—D

All of these nursing diagnostic categories reflect the clinical problems associated with this patient's seizures, including ineffective airway clearance, altered tissue perfusion, and potential for injury. Appropriate nursing interventions would include inserting an artificial airway, providing supplemental oxygen, turning the patient to his side, initiating an I.V. line, administering prescribed drugs to stop the seizure activity, maintaining upright bed side rails, measuring the patient's temperature by the rectal route only, and protecting the patient's head during seizures.

18 Correct answer—A

When administering phenytoin intravenously, the nurse should institute cardiac monitoring and observe the patient carefully. Therapeutic blood phenytoin levels of 10 to 20 mcg/ml can be achieved quickly by I.V. administration; however, rapid administration depresses the myocardium and can cause cardiac arrest. Because this patient had been taking this medication at home, the nurse would obtain a level before administration to provide a baseline level and prevent possible toxicity. Nystagmus with lateral gaze is the first sign of toxicity; ataxia, slurred speech, diplopia, lethargy, and coordination disturbances may result from acute overdose. I.V. phenytoin must be administered slowly at a rate no faster than 50 mg/minute in a saline solution. If given in a dextrose solution, the drug will precipitate into crystals.

19 Correct answer—C

Phenytoin is a myocardial depressant. Administering this drug by rapid I.V. bolus or in excessive doses may induce third-degree heart block and cardiac arrest.

20 Correct answer—B

Phenytoin must be taken as ordered, even in the absence of seizures, because the drug is effective only when therapeutic blood levels are maintained. The patient should know the signs and symptoms of toxicity, such as slurred speech, confusion, diplopia, nausea, gingival hyperplasia, and fever. Because phenytoin is absorbed slowly from the GI tract, daily doses can be adjusted to the patient's convenience, and missed doses can be made up safely. The patient should be encouraged to wear a medical alert identification bracelet or necklace. The patient should be advised against using drugs that potentiate or inhibit phenytoin's action. Phenytoin's action may be potentiated by the concurrent use of aspirin, estrogen, disulfiram (Antabuse), chlordiazepoxide (Librium), or anticoagulants (especially dicumarol). Drugs that inhibit phenytoin's action include alcohol, antihistamines, barbiturates, hypnotics, and sedatives.

21 Correct answer—B

Signs and symptoms of eclampsia include hypertension, proteinuria, oliguria, and seizures. These manifestations typically occur during the third trimester but also can occur up to 2 weeks postpartum. Eclampsia, which is most common in primagravida patients, is associated with diabetes, hypertension, and renal disease.

22 Correct answer—C

The nurse would expect the physician to order magnesium sulfate, the anticonvulsant of choice in treating eclampsia. Hydralazine (Apresoline) or nitroprusside sodium (Nipride) also may be ordered to control the patient's hypertension. Diazepam and other sedatives should be used judiciously in this condition.

23 Correct answer—B

The drug of choice to manage status epilepticus is diazepam, a rapid-acting anticonvulsant with less tendency to produce hypotension. Phenytoin and phenobarbital would be indicated to prevent further seizures. Lorazepam is typically used to treat anxiety.

24 Correct answer—B

In this situation, the nurse would expect to administer all of the drugs except phenobarbital. After the patient's seizure is controlled, secondary management should focus on finding the underlying cause of the seizure. If no one provides the ED team with this information, dextrose 50%, naloxone, and thiamine should be administered. Dextrose is administered to reverse possible hypoglycemia; naloxone,

Neurologic Emergencies Answers

to reverse potential drug intoxication. Thiamine is commonly administered to alcoholic patients and those with a potential vitamin deficiency. All of these conditions can result in seizure activity.

25 Correct answer — C

Phenytoin is the drug used to treat seizures resulting from head trauma because a therapeutic blood level is rapidly established. Phenytoin works by stabilizing the seizure threshold, thereby reducing seizure activity. Diazepam and phenobarbital should be avoided in the patient with head trauma because they cause sedation and will inhibit an accurate assessment of level of consciousness. Dexamethasone is used to decrease cerebral edema; however, its action is decreased when used concurrently with phenytoin.

26 Correct answer — C

Jacksonian seizures are characterized by tonic-clonic movement limited to one side of the body. Grand mal seizures produce tonic-clonic movement of the entire body and loss of consciousness, followed by a postictal state of drowsiness. Petit mal seizures produce transient loss of consciousness with no postictal state. Psychomotor seizures, which are more common in children, are characterized by bizarre behavior with no loss of consciousness and by postictal drowsiness and amnesia about the seizure episode.

27 Correct answer — A

A patient with jacksonian seizures typically develops Todd's paralysis, transient postictal paralysis of the affected side. Unconsciousness and incontinence are associated with grand mal seizures.

28 Correct answer — C

Once the patient's vital signs are stabilized, the nurse would expect the physician to order cervical spine X-rays to rule out spinal injuries. This usually is done before further diagnostic procedures or treatments, such as a computed tomography scan (to pinpoint the area of damage), are begun.

29 Correct answer — B

An epidural hematoma is commonly associated with a temporal fracture. The development of such a hematoma causes a contralateral pineal shift. These findings, along with a nonreactive left pupil and a deteriorating level of consciousness, are indicative of an epidural hematoma.

30 Correct answer – D

The nurse would anticipate the medical treatment for this patient to include surgical evacuation of the hematoma and ligation of the damaged vessel. Early diagnosis and immediate surgical treatment are directly related to a good prognosis.

31 Correct answer – B

Although all these measures are important, the primary objective in caring for a patient with a traumatic head injury involves maintaining oxygen supply to the brain, as hypoxia and carbon dioxide retention cause cerebral vasodilation and increase ICP.

32 Correct answer – A

All of these interventions decrease ICP. However, elevating the head of the bed 30 degrees to allow for venous drainage by gravity is the only independent nursing intervention listed. The other interventions require a physician's order.

33 Correct answer – D

Altered level of consciousness is typically the first sign of increased ICP. It results from decreased blood supply to the cortex. Changes in vital signs and temperature are late indicators because the brain stem is not compressed until later stages of this condition.

34 Correct answer – B

Ipsilateral pupil dilation is the earliest sign of uncal herniation. An expanding lesion of the lateral middle fossa, most commonly of the temporal lobe, causes shifting of the inner basal temporal lobe. This area contains the uncus, which is forced through the tentorium as pressure builds. The third cranial nerve and the posterior cerebral artery on the same side of the expanding temporal lobe lesion are frequently caught between the uncus and the tentorium. Ataxic or irregular respirations are seen in the later stages of herniation. An absent doll's eye reflex indicates brain stem dysfunction and is a late sign of herniation. Impaired motor function is a common sign in various neurologic and neuromuscular diseases, such as cerebrovascular accident, multiple sclerosis, and myasthenia gravis.

35 Correct answer – D

The classic signs of increased ICP involving the brain stem include widening pulse pressure, rising systolic blood pressure, and bradycardia. These three signs, known as Cushing's response, are a compensatory mechanism for maintaining blood pressure and cerebral blood flow when ICP increases. Vital signs, such as blood pressure and pulse rate, are controlled in the vital centers of the brain stem. Hypertension stimulates the baroreceptors in the carotid and aortic bodies, stimulating the vagus nerve and producing bradycardia.

36 Correct answer — A

Altered cerebral tissue perfusion is an appropriate nursing diagnostic category for this patient with increased ICP. Nursing interventions should focus on assisting with medical decompression of the cranial vault, ensuring adequate cerebral perfusion pressure, continuously monitoring the patient's neurologic status, preparing for surgical decompression, and instituting appropriate measures to prevent complications.

37 Correct answer — C

Epidural hematomas usually are caused by arterial bleeding, and subdural hematomas usually are caused by injury to a vein. Epidural hematomas occur between the skull and the dura mater; subdural hematomas, between the dura mater and arachnoid layer. Signs and symptoms develop more rapidly in epidural bleeding than in subdural bleeding because epidural bleeding is usually associated with arterial bleeding, whereas subdural bleeding results from venous bleeding. Approximately 85% of patients in whom epidural hematomas develop have sustained a skull fracture, with the most common site being the temporal bone. The middle meningeal artery, located under the temporal bone, is usually the affected artery.

38 Correct answer — B

Hypoxemia, hypercapnia, and respiratory acidosis are potent vasodilating factors in the body's attempt to increase oxygen supply to the brain. Cerebral vasodilation causes an increase in blood volume in the brain and a subsequent increase in ICP.

39 Correct answer — C

Mannitol is used to treat increased ICP because it increases plasma osmolality, thereby inducing diffusion of water from cerebrospinal fluid (CSF) back into the plasma and intravascular space. Although mannitol induces diuresis by raising the osmotic pressure of the glomerular filtrate and increasing the rate of electrolyte excretion, neither of these actions decreases ICP. Shifting intracellular fluid to the interstitial space will not decrease edema.

40 Correct answer – D

Valsalva's maneuver, an exertion against a closed epiglottis, increases intrathoracic pressure, impedes venous return from the brain, and increases ICP. Isometric muscle contractions, those that do not lengthen the muscle, cause a rise in systemic blood pressure, thereby elevating ICP. Coughing and sneezing elevate intra-abdominal and intrathoracic pressures. An increase in these pressures is transmitted to the spinal and intracranial subarachnoid spaces through the veins that communicate with the dural venous sinuses and intracranial subarachnoid space. The venous return from the cranial vault is impeded, resulting in an increase in ICP. Positions that obstruct venous return from the brain and increase ICP include extreme flexion of the hips, Trendelenburg's position, and angulation of the neck.

41 Correct answer – A

Although a lumbar puncture is a means of measuring ICP, it is considered unsafe and therefore contraindicated in a patient with an expanding cerebral mass. A lumbar puncture will give accurate pressure readings only if CSF is flowing freely within the subarachnoid space. An expanding lesion, as well as adhesions and constrictions, will alter the flow of CSF and result in an inaccurate pressure reading. Also, with increased ICP, lumbar puncture may cause brain stem herniation by reducing spinal pressure. Epidural monitoring, intraventricular catheterization, and subarachnoid screw insertion are the three commonly used methods to measure ICP.

42 Correct answer – C

The nurse would expect a patient who sustained damage to the middle meningeal artery to develop an epidural hematoma, which commonly results from arterial bleeding. A subdural hematoma commonly results from venous bleeding. A subarachnoid hemorrhage is commonly caused by a ruptured cerebral aneurysm, which involves the weakening of a vessel wall.

43 Correct answer – B

Battle's sign, which is commonly associated with basal skull fractures involving the middle fossa, is best described as bleeding with resultant ecchymosis over the mastoid bone. Because this sign takes 24 hours to develop, it may be undetectable to the ED nurse. A basal skull fracture may involve the anterior, middle, or posterior fossa at the base of the skull.

44 Correct answer—B

The patient with a basal skull fracture is also at risk for injury to the cranial nerves. Injury to the first cranial (olfactory) nerve is common and typically causes anosmia, or loss of the sense of smell. Other common cranial nerve injuries include those to the seventh (facial) nerve, which causes ipsilateral facial paralysis, and the eighth (acoustic) nerve, which may lead to disturbances in hearing or equilibrium.

45 Correct answer—A

Further assessment of the patient with a basal skull fracture may reveal cerebrospinal otorrhea or rhinorrhea. Cerebrospinal otorrhea occurs if the dura mater is torn and the tympanic membrane is ruptured; cerebrospinal rhinorrhea results if the tympanic membrane is intact. Drainage samples from either site test positive for glucose.

46 Correct answer—B

The patient with a basal skull fracture will benefit from any nursing measure that aims to avert further tearing of the dura by preventing transient increases in ICP; therefore, the nurse should instruct the patient to avoid coughing and performing Valsalva's maneuver. The nurse should instruct the patient to avoid blowing his nose and to allow the fluid to drain freely. If rhinorrhea is significant, a small, loose dressing may be applied. Nothing should be put into the patient's nose or ears, including suction catheters or nasogastric tubes.

47 Correct answer—D

Raccoon's eyes, bilateral ecchymoses from bleeding into the sinuses, usually indicates a basal skull fracture involving the anterior fossa. Anterior fossa fractures may also result in cerebrospinal rhinorrhea if the dura mater is torn.

48 Correct answer—B

The nurse would expect a patient with a lesion at the C5 to C6 level to have quadriplegia with gross arm movements and diaphragmatic breathing. Such an injury would result in complete loss of motor power in the trunk and legs (quadriplegia), along with bladder and bowel retention. Although paralysis of intercostal respiration also occurs, diaphragmatic respiration would continue without abdominal muscle action because the diaphragm is innervated at the C2 to C4 level.

49 Correct answer—C

The priority nursing diagnosis for a patient with a cervical spinal cord injury would be *Ineffective breathing pattern related to weakened respiratory muscles,* because the nurse's immediate concern in such cases is always maintaining effective breathing.

50 Correct answer—D

Spinal shock is a state of transient reflex depression below the level of the lesion. Although the pathophysiology of spinal shock is incompletely understood, the shock results, in part, from sudden withdrawal of facilitory influences from higher brain centers. A loss of sympathetic outflow occurs in lesions higher than T5. Flaccidity typically occurs during shock caused by a lesion of the upper motor neuron; spasticity returns after the shock subsides.

51 Correct answer—A

Urine retention, rather than incontinence, is seen in spinal shock because of bladder atony. Spinal shock may result in such life-threatening symptoms as hypotension and bradycardia from sympathetic blockade. Poikilothermy results from the interruption of sympathetic pathways to the temperature-regulating centers in the hypothalamus.

52 Correct answer—B

A cervical lesion at C8 accompanied by spinal shock would not lead to hypoventilation because spinal shock results in a transient reflex depression below this area; respiratory musculature should not be affected by this type of injury. A lesion at C8 typically results in hand weakness and paraplegia.

53 Correct answer—C

To assess spinothalamic tract function, the nurse should ask the patient to close both eyes and then identify areas stimulated by pinprick. The lateral spinothalamic tract conveys pain and temperature sensation, whereas the anterior spinothalamic tract conveys light touch, pressure, pain, and temperature sensation. Identifying vibrations and position assesses proprioreceptive sensation. Point-to-point testing assesses coordination.

54 Correct answer—D

Bronchial breath sounds over the patient's lung lobes indicate the development of pneumonia, probably the result of immobility, an ineffective cough, and a decreased vital capacity. The arterial blood gas (ABG) results indicate metabolic acidosis, which is not an indicator of the patient's respiratory status. An inspiratory force of −20 cm and a tidal volume of 500 ml are normal values.

55 Correct answer—B

The phrenic nerve innervates the diaphragm at the C3 to C4 level. Respiratory paralysis is seen with complete lesions at C2 or above, caused by the loss of innervation to the diaphragm and the intercostal and abdominal muscles. A lesion at C3 or C4 results in a weakened diaphragm with absent intercostal muscle power. Diaphragmatic breathing is seen with lesions below C4.

56 Correct answer—D

In spinal cord injury, early hypoventilation is manifested by ABG level changes. Poor values indicate inadequate oxygenation and ventilation. Cyanosis, a late sign of hypoventilation, may not be an accurate indicator because it may never develop in an anemic patient and is difficult to assess in a black patient.

57 Correct answer—A

The nurse would not expect the patient with a possible spinal cord injury between T4 and T12 to have bladder and bowel incontinence. An injury to this area typically results in paraplegia of the lower part of the body, including complete loss of motor function in the legs. However, the patient can perform all activities of daily living, achieve mobility with a wheelchair, and transfer easily. The T11 to L2 level is a particularly important area of the cord; sympathetic motor fibers exiting the spinal cord at this level innervate the trigone muscle of the bladder. Thus, injury at this level produces loss of voluntary bowel and bladder control, resulting in retention.

58 Correct answer—B

If a cervical spinal cord injury is suspected, the patient's airway should be opened by a modified jaw-thrust maneuver. This is the safest approach to opening the airway of a patient with a suspected neck injury. The modified jaw-thrust maneuver is accomplished by grasping one of the angles of the patient's lower jaw in each hand and lifting both hands, thus displacing the mandible forward. If the lips close, the lower lip can be retracted with the thumb. The head of the bed should not be tilted because paralysis may ensue. Pulling down the chin alone will not open the airway. A tracheotomy would not be indicated at this time.

59 Correct answer—A

Loss of motor function in the right arm and leg may indicate a lesion in the pyramidal tract of the left hemisphere. The lateral corticospinal (pyramidal) tract is the most important upper motor neuron tract. Damage to this area results in contralateral motor loss. Middle cerebral artery syndrome is by far the most common of all cerebral occlusions. If the main stem of the middle cerebral artery is occluded, a massive infarction of most of the hemisphere results.

60 Correct answer—D

The most reliable technique for testing upper extremity motor strength is for the nurse to ask the patient to close his eyes and raise his arms straight in front of him, palms up. The nurse should watch how well this position is maintained. By asking the patient to squeeze her hands, the nurse can assess equality of strength in hand grasps, but this is less accurate than that of arm extension. Observing for spontaneous movement does not assess strength. Testing reflexes assesses the intactness of the reflex arcs.

61 Correct answer—C

A patient admitted with an injury to the left cerebral hemisphere would exhibit contralateral findings, such as right-sided hemiparesis and hemiplegia, and right homonymous hemianopia (loss of vision in the right half of both visual fields). In an injury to the left cerebral hemisphere accompanied by right-sided visual loss, the eyes deviate to the left to permit better visualization.

62 Correct answer—A

Pinpoint pupils usually are indicative of a lesion in the pons. Small, bilateral, nonreactive pupils may result from the loss of sympathetic innervation. Parasympathetic innervation remains, causing pupillary constriction. A lesion in the midbrain may result in midposition, nonreactive pupils. Bilateral fixed and dilated pupils are seen in severe cerebral anoxia.

63 Correct answer—A

Apneustic breathing and pinpoint pupils occur in the patient with an injury, or lesion, of the pons. In apneustic breathing, the patient experiences a prolonged inspiration with a pause at the end of the inspiratory and expiratory cycle.

Neurologic Emergencies Answers

64 Correct answer—**A**

One of the best techniques for assessing meningeal irritation is to elicit Kernig's sign by flexing the patient's leg at the hip and knee, then straightening the knee and watching for pain and resistance. In a patient with meningitis, pain and spasm of the hamstrings occur when any attempt is made to extend the knee. Eliciting Brudzinski's sign is another effective technique to assess meningeal irritation. A positive sign is indicated by the flexing of both legs at the hips and knees in response to passive flexion of the neck and head onto the chest. A stiff neck (nuchal rigidity) and photophobia are other symptoms of meningeal irritation.

65 Correct answer—**B**

Instituting isolation precautions is unnecessary and therefore inappropriate for a patient who has just been diagnosed as having viral meningitis. Appropriate interventions would include monitoring the patient's temperature frequently, because fever increases ICP, and instituting seizure precautions, because seizure activity is common in patients with central nervous system infection. A major responsibility in caring for a patient with viral meningitis involves monitoring and managing increased ICP.

66 Correct answer—**A**

A common sign of meningococcal meningitis is petechiae. Petechiae, rash, purpuric lesions, or ecchymoses develop in 50% of patients with this condition. Patients with bacterial meningitis may also have fever, headache, lethargy, confusion, irritability, and neck stiffness.

CHAPTER 9

Obstetric Emergencies

1 Which finding would the nurse expect to note when assessing a patient who is bleeding from abruptio placentae?

A. Premature labor
B. Severe abdominal pain
C. Nontender uterus
D. Boggy uterus

2 Any third-trimester vaginal bleeding calls for close fetal monitoring. Which fetal heart rate pattern would alert the nurse to a deterioration in the client's condition?

A. Late decelerations below the normal baseline level
B. Accelerations, to 160 beats/minute, lasting 15 seconds
C. Stable heart rate of 120 beats/minute
D. All of the above

3 If impending shock is suspected in a pregnant patient with vaginal bleeding, the initial nursing action would be to stay with the patient and alert the other staff. The next action would be to:

A. Start an infusion of dextrose 5% in water
B. Monitor the fetal heart rate
C. Position the patient on her right side
D. Massage the fundus

4 During the nursing assessment of an antepartal patient, which blood pressure change would signal the onset of mild preeclampsia?

A. An increase in systolic pressure of 30 mm Hg or greater
B. A blood pressure reading of 140/90 mm Hg or greater
C. Any increase in diastolic pressure above 90 mm Hg
D. A minimum of three consecutive blood pressure measurements above the patient's baseline

SITUATION

A woman in the 38th week of pregnancy arrives at the emergency department (ED) complaining of painless vaginal bleeding that occurred, without warning, upon arising this morning. Her abdomen is soft, and her uterus is nontender. The fetal heart rate is assessed at the umbilical level at 120 beats/minute.

Questions 5 to 7 refer to the above situation.

5 Based on the patient history and physical findings, the nurse would suspect that the patient has:

A. Abruptio placentae
B. Disseminated intravascular coagulation
C. Spontaneous abortion
D. Placenta previa

6 An appropriate nursing diagnosis for this patient would be:

A. Fluid volume deficit related to uterine rupture
B. Fluid volume deficit related to uterine hemorrhage
C. Altered peripheral tissue perfusion related to abnormal coagulation
D. Spiritual distress related to neonatal death

7 The nurse's highest priority in caring for this patient involves:

A. Preparing for a potential cesarean section
B. Maintaining the patient on strict bed rest and observing for further bleeding
C. Assessing for signs of shock caused by blood loss
D. Avoiding pelvic examinations or the insertion of any foreign objects into the vagina

SITUATION

A woman is brought to the ED while in labor. Her membranes had ruptured earlier. Uterine contractions are now occurring every 2 to 3 minutes, lasting approximately 60 to 90 seconds. With the next contraction, the patient experiences the urge to bear down. Pelvic examination indicates the cervix is fully dilated and 100% effaced, the fetal station is +2, and the presenting part is the head.

Questions 8 to 12 refer to the above situation.

8 Which equipment should be available for the delivery?

A. Sterile gloves and scissors, two sterile Kelly clamps, warm blankets, a bulb syringe, and a bag-valve-mask device
B. Sterile gloves and a basin, a sterile Kelly clamp, and a DeLee suction apparatus
C. Sterile gloves and scissors, a sterile Kelly clamp, and 1% lidocaine solution
D. Sterile gloves and scissors and two sterile Kelly clamps

Obstetric Emergencies
Questions

9 Which sign indicates imminent delivery?

A. Bulging of the perineum
B. Crowning of the fetal head
C. Receding of the fetal head between contractions
D. Involuntary bowel movements

10 The nurse instructs the patient to pant or breathe through contractions during the delivery. The primary rationale for this intervention is to:

A. Help the patient to cope with the pain of contractions
B. Avoid fetal hypoxia or distress
C. Avoid a too-rapid or uncontrolled delivery ,
D. Assist the physician in a more efficient and safe delivery

11 The patient gives birth to a girl. The physician performs an initial neonatal assessment and assigns an Apgar score of 8. Which statement about the Apgar scoring system is *true?*

A. Scores are assigned immediately after delivery and 10 minutes later
B. Scores are based on assessment of the neonate's heart rate, respiratory effort, muscle tone, reflex irritability, and skin color
C. A score of 1 to 3 is considered excellent
D. All of the above

12 The nurse would expect the first sign of placental separation to be:

A. Lengthening of the umbilical cord
B. A gush of blood from the vagina
C. Rising of the fundus as it contracts and separates from the placenta
D. Shakes and chills

SITUATION

A woman in the 36th week of pregnancy arrives at the ED complaining of a persistent headache and a feeling of indigestion. Her blood pressure is 150/100 mm Hg. Her ankles show 2+ pitting edema. Urinalysis reveals 3+ proteinuria. She is placed in a quiet, private ED evaluating room, and the physician is notified.

Questions 13 to 17 refer to the above situation.

13 While waiting for the physician, the nurse assesses the patient for the possible development of eclampsia. Which finding would the nurse expect to note in a patient with this condition?

A. Blood pressure of 150/100 mm Hg
B. Generalized edema
C. Seizures
D. 3+ proteinuria

14 Which intervention would be the nurse's highest priority when caring for an eclamptic patient?

A. Turn the patient on her right side to prevent aspiration
B. Insert an I.V. line for medication administration
C. Monitor the patient's vital signs continuously
D. Maintain a patent airway and administer supplemental oxygen

15 The priority nursing diagnosis for this patient at this time would be:

A. Altered renal tissue perfusion related to hypertension
B. Fluid volume excess related to hypertension and edema
C. Fluid volume deficit related to uterine hemorrhage
D. Potential for injury related to seizures

16 The primary rationale for placing this patient in a quiet, private room is to:

A. Prevent onset of early labor
B. Reduce external stimuli
C. Protect the patient from becoming emotionally upset by seeing other patients
D. Protect her from infection

17 The physician orders magnesium sulfate at 1 g/hour via a continuous infusion. During the infusion, the nurse should monitor for and immediately report:

A. A blood pressure of 120/80 mm Hg
B. A urine output of 50 ml/hour
C. A respiratory rate less than 12 breaths/minute
D. Increased serum calcium levels

SITUATION

A woman is brought to the ED via an ambulance after having given birth at home, 1 hour ago, to a normal, healthy girl. Since arriving in the ED, the patient has completely saturated five perineal pads. Her blood pressure is 100/70 mm Hg; pulse rate, 82 beats/minute and regular; and respiratory rate, 18 breaths/minute. She has no sign of syncope or light-headedness and has not lost consciousness. Blood specimens are sent to the laboratory for a complete blood count (CBC) with differential, electrolyte levels, and type and cross match. Two units of packed red blood cells are available, if necessary.

Questions 18 to 22 refer to the above situation.

18 The nurse palpates the fundus and determines that it is soft. Which nursing intervention would be most appropriate at this time?

A. Recheck the patient's vital signs
B. Massage the fundus gently until firm
C. Request an order for oxytocin (Pitocin)
D. Assess the amount of bleeding

19 The nurse knows that a slow rate of continuous postpartum vaginal bleeding usually indicates:

A. Cervical laceration
B. Clots in the uterus
C. Retained placental fragments
D. Too-vigorous uterine massage

20 The physician orders ergonovine maleate (Ergotrate Maleate), 0.2 mg I.M. stat and every 4 hours for two doses. After the first dose, the nurse evaluates the effectiveness of therapy. The nurse should withhold the next dose of this medication and notify the physician if assessment reveals:

A. Tachycardia of 102 beats/minute
B. Positioning of the fundus at the umbilical level
C. Ataxia
D. Blood pressure greater than 130/90 mm Hg

21 Two hours later, the bleeding decreases but continues to be heavier than normal. The fundus is soft and located above and to the right of the umbilicus. The most appropriate initial nursing intervention would be to:

A. Notify the physician and prepare the patient for a dilation and curettage
B. Record the findings on the patient's chart
C. Encourage voiding and assist the patient in using a bedpan
D. Assist the patient in getting out of bed and encourage her to ambulate

22 The patient now has a blood pressure of 90/60 mm Hg; pulse rate, 92 beats/minute; and respiratory rate, 16 breaths/minute. She complains of light-headedness and appears restless. The fundus is firm with a moderate amount of lochia rubra. The appropriate nursing action would be to stay with the patient, alert other staff, and:

A. Place the patient in modified Trendelenburg's position
B. Increase I.V. fluids to 150 ml/hour
C. Obtain a specimen for a second CBC with differential
D. Massage the fundus to remove clots

SITUATION

A 26-year-old woman is admitted to the ED with complaints of severe right lower quadrant abdominal pain and moderate, bright-red vaginal bleeding that began as spotting this morning. The patient has not menstruated for 2 months. She has had five or six episodes of nausea without vomiting in the morning. She states she has swollen breasts and occasionally feels fatigue. She thinks she is pregnant but has not yet had a pregnancy test. Her medical history reveals an episode of pelvic inflammatory disease (PID) 3 years ago, which was treated with a course of antibiotic therapy. Vital signs, which are taken every 15 minutes, remain stable: blood pressure is 110/70 mm Hg; pulse rate, 100 beats/minute; respiratory rate, 24 breaths/minute; and temperature, 100.6° F (38.1° C). She is pale, but alert and responsive. The physician orders a CBC, type and cross match for 2 units of blood, a radioimmunoassay, and a pelvic ultrasound. The nurse begins an infusion of 1,000 ml of lactated Ringer's solution, as ordered. Within 2 hours, the laboratory and ultrasound data confirm an ectopic pregnancy.

Questions 23 to 26 refer to the above situation.

Obstetric Emergencies
Questions

23 Over 90% of all ectopic pregnancies are located at which site?

A. Fallopian tube
B. Cervix
C. Abdominal cavity
D. Retroperitoneal area

24 Which finding indicates the potential for development of an ectopic pregnancy?

A. Amenorrhea for 8 weeks
B. Nausea without vomiting
C. History of PID
D. Positive radioimmunoassay of human chorionic gonadotropin

25 Which clinical sign of ectopic pregnancy would the nurse expect to note in this patient upon further assessment?

A. Back pain
B. Shoulder and neck pain
C. Leg cramping
D. Intestinal cramping

26 Which nursing action is essential to performing a pelvic ultrasound?

A. Monitoring the patient's vital signs every 15 minutes
B. Increasing the patient's fluid intake before the test
C. Obtaining informed consent
D. Placing the patient on her right side

SITUATION

A 33-year-old woman, para 6006, is admitted to the ED on a stretcher. She arrived by ambulance approximately 1 hour after an extramural delivery of a healthy, 6-lb, 5-oz (2.9-kg) girl at home. While assisting with transferring the patient from the ambulance stretcher to the ED stretcher, the ED nurse notes that the sheets under the patient are saturated with bright-red blood. The patient is pale and restless. Her blood pressure is 90/60 mm Hg; pulse rate, 108 beats/minute; respiratory rate, 28 breaths/minute; and temperature, 99.6° F (37.5° C). The fundus is firm at the umbilical level. The patient's perineal pad is completely saturated with lochia rubra. Blood loss is estimated at greater than 500 ml. After examining the patient, the physician diagnoses postpartum hemorrhage caused by a vaginal laceration.

Questions 27 to 30 refer to the above situation.

27 Which assessment finding indicates that the patient is at risk for postpartum hemorrhage?

A. Blood pressure
B. Home birth
C. High parity
D. Neonatal birth weight

28 Which finding suggests postpartum hemorrhage related to a vaginal laceration?

A. Extramural delivery of an infant weighing 6 lb, 5 oz (2.9 kg)
B. Vital signs, restlessness, and pallor
C. Blood loss of greater than 500 ml
D. Bright-red bleeding and a firm fundus

29 The priority nursing action at this time would be to assess the patient's:

A. Vital signs
B. Need for oxytocin therapy
C. Response to fundal massage
D. Response to verbal stimuli

30 The patient is to be admitted to the medical-surgical unit for further observation. The nurse explains to the patient the reason for the admission. Which of the following best indicates that the patient has understood the explanation?

A. The patient seems to have understood the nurse's explanation
B. The patient verbalizes an understanding of the reason for the admission
C. The patient is resting quietly while awaiting admission
D. The patient's blood pressure stabilizes at 110/70 mm Hg

Answer Sheet

	A	B	C	D
1	○	○	○	○
2	○	○	○	○
3	○	○	○	○
4	○	○	○	○
5	○	○	○	○
6	○	○	○	○
7	○	○	○	○
8	○	○	○	○
9	○	○	○	○
10	○	○	○	○
11	○	○	○	○
12	○	○	○	○
13	○	○	○	○
14	○	○	○	○
15	○	○	○	○
16	○	○	○	○
17	○	○	○	○
18	○	○	○	○
19	○	○	○	○
20	○	○	○	○
21	○	○	○	○
22	○	○	○	○
23	○	○	○	○
24	○	○	○	○
25	○	○	○	○
26	○	○	○	○
27	○	○	○	○
28	○	○	○	○
29	○	○	○	○
30	○	○	○	○

Obstetric Emergencies
Answer Sheet

1 Correct answer—**B**

The bleeding in abruptio placentae is typically accompanied by severe abdominal pain related to changes in the uterus as the placenta separates from the myometrium. This is described as uteroplacental apoplexy, or Couvelaire uterus; a boardlike abdomen accompanies the pain. An extremely tense and painful abdomen indicates placental bleeding into the myometrium; an enlarging uterus may indicate blood accumulating behind the placenta.

2 Correct answer—**A**

Any significant changes in the baseline fetal heart rate, which is normally 120 to 160 beats/minute, are significant, particularly late decelerations of any degree. Periodic late decelerations are indicative of fetal hypoxia or anoxia. Accelerations to 160 beats/minute, lasting 15 seconds, and a stable fetal heart rate of 120 beats/minute are considered normal. Periodic baseline accelerations are indicative of an adequate fetal-placental circulation. Any situation that disturbs maternal hemodynamics or the uteroplacental blood flow will eventually affect fetal well-being. Continuous or frequent monitoring with a Doppler ultrasound stethoscope or bell stethoscope is necessary.

3 Correct answer—**B**

In this situation, the priority action would be to monitor the fetal heart rate for significant changes from the normal baseline rate and for late decelerations that may indicate dysfunction in uteroplacental blood flow. Positioning the patient on her left side while monitoring the fetal heart rate minimizes compression of the ascending vena cava by the gravid uterus. Such compression can impede blood return to the right atrium, resulting in a drop in cardiac output and hypotension. An alternative would be to place the patient in a supine position with the right hip elevated. Supplemental oxygen should be provided. An I.V. infusion of isotonic fluid, such as normal saline or lactated Ringer's solution, should be started to administer fluids and to allow for medication administration. Massaging or stimulating the fundus is always contraindicated to avoid putting pressure on the presenting part, particularly if it is the placenta.

4 Correct answer—**A**

Mild preeclampsia is indicated by an increase in systolic pressure of 30 mm Hg or more and an increase in diastolic pressure of 15 mm Hg or more on two occasions, at least 6 hours apart. The patient should be maintained on bed rest in the left lateral position during these 6 hours. A prepregnancy or first-trimester blood pressure reading is necessary as a baseline level to assess any blood pressure changes in the second or third trimester. Blood pressure normally decreases in the second trimester as a result of blood volume expansion.

5 Correct answer — D

Based on the patient's history and physical findings, the nurse would suspect that this patient has placenta previa. Painless vaginal bleeding is the hallmark of placenta previa in women who carry until midterm or later. The degree of placental placement over the internal cervical os determines the bleeding's severity and the onset of the initial episode. Bleeding associated with spontaneous abortion occurs earlier in a pregnancy, usually before the 20th week. Abruptio placentae is usually associated with pain. Disseminated intravascular coagulation most commonly occurs postpartally.

6 Correct answer — B

An appropriate nursing diagnosis for this patient would be *Fluid volume deficit related to uterine hemorrhage* because the patient has suffered blood loss caused by premature separation of the placenta from the uterine wall. The other diagnoses are inappropriate because neither uterine rupture nor abnormal coagulation has occurred. Although the fetus is certainly compromised, the situation does not indicate that neonatal death has occurred.

7 Correct answer — C

The highest priority would be to assess for signs of shock caused by blood loss. This is best accomplished by monitoring the patient's vital signs and obtaining a blood specimen for a complete blood count (CBC) and type and cross match. Two units of blood should be available in case the patient's hemoglobin and hematocrit values decrease significantly. I.V. fluids, such as lactated Ringer's or normal saline solution, should be started to replace lost fluids and to prepare an access site for blood transfusion if this becomes necessary.

When stabilized, the patient should be restricted to complete bed rest. Perineal pads should be counted to assess further blood loss. A cesarean section may be unnecessary if bleeding is not severe and fetal well-being is maintained. If no emergency exists, the physician should assess maturity of the fetus before delivery is performed. Pelvic examinations are contraindicated in the emergency department because manipulating the cervix without knowing the cause of the problem may result in placental tearing. Any pelvic examination of a patient with suspected placenta previa should be performed in the labor and delivery suite under a "double set-up"; that is, the patient is prepared and draped for a cesarean section and all personnel are ready to operate should hemorrhage occur.

8 Correct answer—**A**

The nurse's priorities in an imminent or emergency delivery include establishing effective respirations in the neonate, maintaining asepsis, and preventing hypothermia. Sterile gloves and scissors and two sterile Kelly clamps are preferable to maintain asepsis and to clamp and cut the umbilical cord. Warm, dry blankets are used to dry the neonate's face, nose, and mouth and to wrap the neonate's head and body for warmth. If the fetal head is delivered slowly while the thorax is being squeezed in the birth canal, seepage of fluid into the neonate's nose and mouth can occur. A bulb syringe is used to suction the mouth, then the nose. Suctioning the nose first may elicit a reflex inhalation of amniotic fluids into the respiratory tract before the mouth has been cleared. If no respirations are noted, a bag-valve-mask device is used for resuscitation.

9 Correct answer—**B**

Crowning, the process by which the vaginal opening completely encircles the neonate's head, is a sign of imminent delivery, especially in a multiparous patient. In a nulliparous patient, delivery may occur up to 30 minutes after crowning occurs. If the amniotic sac is still intact at this point, the nurse will tear it to prevent the neonate from aspirating amniotic fluid with his first respiration. Bulging of the perineum may occur during contractions as the fetus moves down the birth canal; this may not be an indication of imminent delivery. If the fetal head recedes between contractions, the fetus still needs to move further down the vagina before delivery. Although feces may be excreted during contractions, this does not signify immediate delivery.

10 Correct answer—**C**

The patient usually is instructed to continue to pant or breathe through contractions and to bear down only when asked to do so, to avoid a too-rapid or uncontrolled delivery, which consequently prevents fetal hypoxia or distress and assists the physician in a more efficient and safe delivery. The nurse typically uses one hand to apply gentle pressure on the advancing head to control the delivery and prevent a precipitous birth; she uses the other hand to support the patient's perineum and receive the neonate's head as it emerges. Depending on the patient, one or more contractions may be necessary to distend maternal tissues and allow passage of the head through the introitus. The nurse should be sure to maintain a supportive and calm attitude at this time. Usually, the head is delivered between contractions. Breathing through contractions may help the patient to maintain control over the situation and help her to cope with the pain of contractions.

11 Correct answer—B

The Apgar scoring system, a means of measuring neonatal transition to extrauterine life, is based on assessment of the neonate's heart rate, respiratory effort, muscle tone, reflex irritability, and skin color. Typically, two assessments are performed—one immediately after delivery and another in 5 minutes. At each assessment, the individual categories are rated 0 (poor) to 2 (excellent), then added to reveal the total Apgar score. A score of 0 to 3 indicates that the neonate is in poor condition; 4 to 6, fair condition; and 7 to 10, excellent condition. The heart rate, the most important parameter of a neonate's condition, is typically 150 to 180 beats/minute during the first few minutes after delivery, then quickly subsides to 130 to 140 beats/minute. A rate below 100 beats/minute indicates neonatal asphyxia, for which resuscitative measures may be necessary. Respiratory effort should be assessed with the heart rate; crying is a good indicator of a normal condition. Muscle tone, the degree of flexion and muscle resistance, may be assessed with normal handling after delivery. A normal neonate should not appear flaccid or floppy. Reflex irritability may be assessed by eliciting a cough or gag reflex with the first suctioning effort or by eliciting a startle reflex by tickling the neonate's feet. Most neonates do not appear pink immediately after delivery. Commonly, the extremities are blue and the torso, pink (acrocyanosis). This condition is typically reversed by providing warmth to the neonate.

12 Correct answer—B

The first sign of placental separation is typically a gush of blood from the vagina. This is followed by lengthening of the umbilical cord and rising of the fundus as the uterus contracts and separates from the placenta. Pushing on the fundus or pulling on the umbilical cord is contraindicated before delivery of the placenta. A patient may feel an uncomfortable contraction as the placenta passes through the cervix. After the placenta is delivered, it must be examined for completeness and the presence of all cotyledons. Shaking and chills are benign phenomena that may occur during the transitional stage of labor or postpartally; they are not associated with placental separation.

13 Correct answer—C

The nurse would expect to note seizures in an eclamptic patient. Such seizures occur as a result of the hyperreflexivity associated with preeclampsia. The patient in this situation is exhibiting signs of severe preeclampsia (headache, hypertension, edema, hyperreflexia, proteinuria, and sudden weight gain); however, the severity of symptoms is not always indicative of the potential for seizures. Although seizures are not necessarily life-threatening to the patient, they may result in fetal hypoxia. Efforts toward delivering the fetus should be made after a seizure occurs.

14 Correct answer—D

The priority action in managing an eclamptic patient is to establish a patent airway and provide supplemental oxygen. The patient should also be positioned on her left side to reduce compression of the inferior vena cava by the enlarged uterus, thereby increasing the blood supply to the fetus. After a patent airway has been established, the nurse should insert an I.V. line for medication administration and monitor the patient's vital signs, especially the blood pressure, continuously.

15 Correct answer—D

Because this patient is at greatest risk for seizures from the hyperreflexivity associated with preeclampsia, the priority nursing diagnosis would be *Potential for injury related to seizures.* The other diagnoses are inappropriate because altered renal perfusion and fluid volume excess have not been indicated and uterine hemorrhage is not associated with preeclampsia.

16 Correct answer—B

The primary rationale for placing the patient in a quiet, private room is to reduce external stimuli, because the reduction of environmental stimuli plays an important role in limiting central nervous system (CNS) stimulation and preventing seizures.

17 Correct answer—C

The nurse should monitor for and immediately report a respiratory rate of less than 12 breaths/minute, because respiratory depression may indicate that the patient is receiving too much of the medication. Magnesium sulfate, a CNS depressant, reduces synaptic activity at the neuromuscular junction and helps prevent convulsions. Assessment parameters include respirations, deep tendon reflexes, and urine output. An absent or sluggish patellar reflex also suggests overdose. Serum magnesium levels should be checked every 4 to 6 hours to maintain therapeutic levels of 4 to 7 mg/dl; levels above 20 mg/dl can result in cardiac arrest. Usual dosage is 4 to 6 g I.V., given over 10 minutes, followed by a continuous infusion of 1 to 2 g/hour; or 4 g I.M. every 4 hours. Calcium gluconate should be available at the bedside to reverse the effects of magnesium sulfate, if necessary. A blood pressure of 120/80 mm Hg and a urine output of 50 ml/hour are normal. Use of magnesium sulfate may result in hypocalcemia.

18 Correct answer — **B**

The most appropriate nursing intervention at this time would be to massage the fundus until it is firm. Bleeding soon after delivery usually is caused by uterine atony. Massaging the fundus stimulates the myometrium to contract, promoting hemostasis and clot expulsion. The nurse should always use two hands to massage the fundus: one hand to anchor the lower uterine segment just above the symphysis pubis, and the other hand to gently massage the fundus. Anchoring the lower segment of the uterus provides support because the uterus may be relaxed after delivery. Using gentle massage helps prevent partial or complete uterine prolapse. If massage is ineffective, oxytocin may be ordered; overmassage may cause muscle fatigue and relaxation. Some physicians routinely use I.M. or I.V. oxytocin after delivery to aid in uterine contraction. Nipple stimulation from breast-feeding also helps to promote uterine tone and hemostasis. Rechecking vital signs and the amount of bleeding are considered additional secondary interventions.

19 Correct answer — **A**

A slow rate of continuous postpartum vaginal bleeding usually indicates a cervical laceration. Lacerations of the vagina, perineum, and labia also can occur. Continued bleeding is typically observed despite efficient postpartum uterine contractions. This requires immediate vaginal inspection because continuous bleeding can lead to hemorrhagic shock. In this situation, the potential for lacerations is increased because the delivery was spontaneous and unattended at home. Retained placental fragments usually result in vaginal bleeding at a fast rate, as may overmassaging the uterus. Clots in the uterus may slow or stop bleeding until they are passed.

20 Correct answer — **D**

The nurse should withhold the next dose and notify the physician if the patient has a blood pressure greater than 130/90 mm Hg. Ergonovine maleate is commonly administered after delivery of the placenta to produce firm uterine contractions and decrease uterine bleeding. Because this drug may cause increased blood pressure, it should not be administered to a patient with an already elevated pressure. Other potential adverse effects include nausea and vomiting, dizziness, headache, cramps, dyspnea, and chest pain. Positioning of the fundus at the umbilical level is a normal finding in an immediate postpartum patient. Ataxia and tachycardia are not among the side effects of ergonovine maleate.

21 Correct answer—C

The most appropriate initial action in this situation would be to encourage voiding and assist the patient in using a bedpan. Positioning of the uterus to the right of the umbilicus is a sign of bladder distension, which increases uterine pressure and, in some cases, vaginal bleeding. If the patient cannot urinate on the bedpan, catheterization may be necessary to empty the bladder and control bleeding. Afterward, the nurse should record the amount of urine obtained, the status of the uterus, the presence of bleeding, and the patient's comfort level on the patient's chart.

22 Correct answer—A

The appropriate nursing action in this situation would be to place the patient in modified Trendelenburg's position because the patient is showing signs of a fluid volume deficit. In this position, the patient's legs would be higher than her head, which would increase circulation back to the heart. Increasing I.V. fluids, as ordered, and obtaining a new specimen for a CBC and differential are appropriate subsequent interventions. The nurse should keep in mind, however, that this CBC may not be indicative of the immediate blood loss because it may take several hours for the hemoglobin and hematocrit to drop. Massaging the fundus at this time would be unnecessary because it is already firm.

23 Correct answer—A

Although ectopic pregnancies can also develop at the cervix, ovary, retroperitoneal area, and abdominal cavity, approximately 90% develop in the fallopian tubes. A tubal ectopic pregnancy may result from any condition that causes narrowing or constriction within the fallopian tube. Under such circumstances, the lumen of the fallopian tube is large enough to permit spermatozoa to ascend but not large enough to permit the fertilized ovum to pass downward.

24 Correct answer—C

A patient with a history of pelvic inflammatory disease (PID), such as the one in this situation, is at increased risk for ectopic pregnancy. Kinking of the fallopian tube, segmental narrowing of the tube, and partial agglutination of the opposing surfaces of the tube can be caused by endometriosis, developmental defects, or inflammatory disorders, such as PID. A positive radioimmunoassay of human chorionic gonadotropin and nausea (with or without vomiting) are signs of pregnancy.

Obstetric Emergencies Answer Sheet

25 Correct answer—B

The nurse would expect to note shoulder and neck pain that may radiate into sharp lower abdominal pain. Such pain is commonly precipitated by activities that increase abdominal pressure, such as defecation.

26 Correct answer—B

Increasing the patient's fluid intake before the test is essential for a pelvic ultrasound, because filling the bladder lifts the uterus and allows for better visualization of the uterus and other structures. Monitoring vital signs is unnecessary. An informed consent is not required. Usually, the patient is placed in a supine position for this procedure.

27 Correct answer—C

High parity is considered a predictive assessment factor associated with potential postpartum bleeding; other factors include rapid labor, an overdistended uterus, and a high neonatal birth weight. Any relaxation of the uterine muscle fibers, as occurs in a high-parity patient, gives rise to a continuous oozing of blood, one of the forms of postpartum hemorrhage. Assessing the patient before delivery helps determine the patient's risk of postpartum hemorrhage. In the obstetric designation para 6006, the first number indicates the number of pregnancies; the second, the number of induced or spontaneous abortions; the third, the number of premature deliveries; and the fourth, the number of full-term deliveries. Blood pressure and home birth are not associated with postpartum hemorrhage.

28 Correct answer—D

Vaginal lacerations are particularly likely to cause serious bleeding. Bright-red arterial blood and a firm fundus suggest postpartum hemorrhage related to a vaginal laceration; however, a vaginal inspection is necessary to confirm the diagnosis. A firm fundus indicates that the uterine muscle is contracted and an unlikely source of bleeding.

29 Correct answer—A

The priority nursing action in this situation would be to assess the patient's vital signs for onset of shock. When hemorrhaging occurs, the body activates certain compensatory mechanisms, such as tachycardia and vasoconstriction, to delay the onset of shock. The patient's condition and size determine the amount of blood loss that can be tolerated. However, when hemorrhaging is profuse, compensatory mechanisms can fail and shock ensues. As shock deepens, restlessness, diaphoresis, cool and clammy skin, tachypnea, unconsciousness, and death may follow. Assessing for response to verbal stimuli would be appropriate if the patient were unconscious or losing consciousness. Oxytocin administration and fundal massage would be inappropriate in this situation because they do not stop bleeding from a vaginal laceration.

30 Correct answer—**B**

The best indication that the patient has understood the nurse's explanation is a verbalization of her understanding of the reason for admission. Explaining to the patient the reason for treatment and care and ensuring that the patient understands the reason are part of the nurse's responsibilities. Because the nurse is the health professional who typically spends the most time with the patient and can best evaluate the patient's comprehension, the nurse is liable for the patient's understanding. The nurse must document that the patient can verbalize an understanding of what is taught or, if it is a specific skill, demonstrate what has been taught. Noting that the patient *seems* to understand the explanation is based on the nurse's perception, not the patient's acknowledgment that she understands. Objective data, such as a blood pressure measurement or observing that the patient is resting quietly, do not reflect that learning has occurred.

CHAPTER 10

Organ Donation

1 In terms of organ donation, the word *tissue* commonly refers to:

A. All organs
B. Organs, eyes, and bone
C. Skin only
D. Eyes, bone, skin, and heart valves

2 The emergency department nurse knows that the responsibilities of an organ procurement coordinator include:

A. Managing the organ donor
B. Communicating with the donor's family
C. Coordinating organ retrieval
D. All of the above

3 Which statement about brain death is *true?*

A. It is defined as the irreversible cessation of entire brain function, including brain stem function
B. A patient in a deep coma is considered brain-dead
C. A patient in a persistent vegetative state is considered brain-dead
D. Brain death is not a necessary criterion for organ retrieval

4 Brain death should be declared:

A. Before retrieving organs and discontinuing ventilator support
B. After retrieving organs but before discontinuing ventilator support
C. After retrieving organs and discontinuing ventilator support
D. None of the above

5 Legally, the time of death is when:

A. The second brain-death note is placed on the donor's chart
B. The ventilator is turned off in the operating room
C. The first brain-death note is placed on the donor's chart
D. The donor's heart is removed during organ retrieval

6 The nurse is aware that most organ donors die from:

A. Severe head injuries
B. Cardiopulmonary arrest
C. Myocardial infarction
D. Respiratory arrest

7 Consent for organ donation must be given by:

A. The potential donor before his death
B. The legal next of kin
C. Any member of the potential donor's family
D. The physician

8 The nurse understands that kidney donations usually are accepted from persons:

A. Aged 2 to 60
B. Aged 15 to 50
C. Under age 50
D. Of any age

9 For solid-organ retrieval to be effective, the donor must have:

A. An intact heartbeat
B. Adequate blood pressure
C. Mechanical ventilator support
D. All of the above

10 A urine output greater than the I.V. fluid intake in a potential organ donor is indicative of which condition?

A. Fluid overload
B. Diabetes insipidus
C. Polyuric phase of renal failure
D. Adequate renal function

11 Which condition does not initially contribute to hypotension in an organ donor?

A. Brain stem herniation
B. Collapse of peripheral vascular resistance
C. Therapeutic dehydration
D. Disseminated intravascular coagulation

12 Which situation would *not* fall under the jurisdiction of the medical examiner?

A. Death by homicide
B. Death by suicide
C. Death by accidental traumatic injury
D. Death by a witnessed cardiac arrest in a person known to have cardiovascular disease

13 Which rationale best describes the reason for administering 1 g of methylprednisolone sodium succinate (Solu-Medrol) I.V. to a potential organ donor?

A. To decrease the body's inflammatory response
B. To stabilize the kidney membrane during organ retrieval
C. To help prevent infection
D. To prevent tissue rejection

14 The nurse knows that evaluation of a potential organ recipient is based on all of the following criteria *except:*

A. Urgency of need
B. ABO blood-group compatibility
C. Sex
D. Tissue typing

15 The nurse is aware that most people over age 65 are ineligible for heart transplantation because:

A. They are not within the age limit for organ recipients
B. They typically have little or no health insurance
C. They typically have poor health
D. Their life expectancy will not increase substantially to warrant transplantation

16 Who may be considered for tissue donation?

A. Any patient who dies in a hospital
B. An individual referred within 6 to 12 hours after a cardiac-related death
C. Deceased patients of any age
D. All of the above

17 Which age-group is the established parameter for lung donation?

A. Newborn to age 40
B. Ages 2 to 50
C. Ages 4 to 60
D. Ages 10 to 50

18 Which age-group is the established parameter for bone donation?

A. Ages 2 to 50
B. Ages 15 to 65
C. Ages 20 to 50
D. All ages

19 Which age-group is the established parameter for eye donation?

A. Newborn to age 65
B. Ages 6 to 55
C. Ages 10 to 90
D. All ages

20 When caring for a potential organ donor, the nurse should keep in mind that norepinephrine (Levophed) and epinephrine should not be used as vasopressors because they:

A. Are extremely potent vasoconstrictors and may cause kidney and liver damage
B. Cannot be metabolized by a dying patient
C. Are ineffective in a brain-dead patient
D. Cause donor reactions

21 The nurse knows that the cost of organ retrieval is paid by the:

A. Donor's family
B. Donating hospital
C. Transplant center
D. Federal government

22 Which conditions are *not* considered contraindications for organ donation?

A. Urinary tract infection and intracranial cancer
B. Sepsis and I.V. drug abuse
C. Metastatic cancer
D. Human immunodeficiency virus infection and heroin addiction

23 The goals of donor maintenance include ensuring:

A. Adequate ventilation
B. Hemodynamic stability
C. Asepsis
D. All of the above

24 When discussing organ donation with a potential donor's family, the nurse should focus on:

A. Details about the intended recipient
B. Details relating to the surgical procedure
C. The monetary value of the organs to be transplanted
D. The positive aspects of transplantation

25 Which organ is commonly associated with the term *living related donor?*

A. Liver
B. Heart
C. Kidney
D. Pancreas

26 Which nursing intervention is most appropriate for kidney donor maintenance?

A. Maintaining a systolic blood pressure of 100 to 110 mm Hg
B. Maintaining a urine output greater than 100 ml/hour
C. Maintaining adequate ventilation
D. All of the above

27 When should the organ procurement agency be notified about a potential donor?

A. After consent is obtained
B. When the operating room is ready
C. As soon as a potential donor is identified
D. When the physician orders

28 The nurse would expect all of the following patients to be considered potential organ donors *except:*

A. A 35-year-old man with acquired immunodeficiency syndrome and a self-inflicted gunshot wound to the head
B. A 2-year-old near-drowning victim with hypoxic encephalopathy
C. A 56-year-old man with a massive intraventricular hemorrhage
D. A 14-year-old boy with massive head injuries and chest trauma

29 The nurse is aware that a thorough medical history can prove invaluable because:

A. It can help predict future organ functioning in the recipient
B. It can give important information to the recipient about the donor
C. It can help determine the existence of a disorder that may preclude organ donation
D. It is necessary for accurate record keeping

30 The nurse knows that a potential organ donor under age 5 may require extended observation because:

A. A young child has increased resistance to brain damage and may recover

B. Federal law mandates it

C. This type of observation is comforting to the parents

D. Test results of a young child typically are difficult to interpret

Answer Sheet

	A	B	C	D
1	○	○	○	○
2	○	○	○	○
3	○	○	○	○
4	○	○	○	○
5	○	○	○	○
6	○	○	○	○
7	○	○	○	○
8	○	○	○	○
9	○	○	○	○
10	○	○	○	○
11	○	○	○	○
12	○	○	○	○
13	○	○	○	○
14	○	○	○	○
15	○	○	○	○
16	○	○	○	○
17	○	○	○	○
18	○	○	○	○
19	○	○	○	○
20	○	○	○	○
21	○	○	○	○
22	○	○	○	○
23	○	○	○	○
24	○	○	○	○
25	○	○	○	○
26	○	○	○	○
27	○	○	○	○
28	○	○	○	○
29	○	○	○	○
30	○	○	○	○

1 Correct answer—**D**

In terms of organ donation, *tissue* typically refers to eyes, bone, skin, and heart valves. Tissue transplantation does not require a heartbeating donor, whereas organ transplantation does.

2 Correct answer—**D**

An organ procurement coordinator is responsible for managing the organ donor, coordinating organ retrieval, and communicating with the deceased donor's family. Other responsibilities include public and professional education and the development of organ donation programs in hospitals.

3 Correct answer—**A**

Brain death is the irreversible cessation of entire brain function, including brain stem function. Clinical criteria for establishing brain death include the absence of all cortical brain stem function, including cerebral responses to light, noise, motion, and pain; reflexes or muscle activity; spontaneous respirations; and cranial nerve reflexes and responses. Neither a comatose patient nor a patient in a persistent vegetative state is considered brain-dead because brain stem function still exists. A patient in a persistent vegetative state typically has severe, irreversible damage to the higher brain centers; however, the brain stem remains intact.

4 Correct answer—**A**

Brain death should be declared before retrieving organs and discontinuing ventilator support. Two attending physicians are necessary to declare a patient brain-dead. Brain death is a necessary criterion for organ retrieval.

5 Correct answer—**A**

Legally, the time of death is when the second brain-death note is placed on the patient's chart. No notation or pronouncement of death should be made in the operative note. The potential donor must be declared brain-dead before entering the operating room.

6 Correct answer—**A**

Most organ donors die from severe head injuries. Patients who die from cardiopulmonary reasons are excluded from organ donation but may donate tissue.

7 Correct answer — **B**

Consent for organ donation must be given by the legal next of kin, including (in order of priority) the patient's spouse, an adult brother or sister, the patient's legal guardian at the time of death, and a representative appointed by a court of competent jurisdiction who has ascertained that no person of higher priority exists who objects to organ donation.

8 Correct answer — **A**

Kidney donations usually are accepted from persons aged 2 to 60. Because the kidneys of children under age 2 are immature, they usually are unacceptable for donation; this policy, however, may vary, depending on the procurement center. The kidneys of those over age 60 are at increased risk for kidney disease and therefore are unacceptable for donation.

9 Correct answer — **D**

For solid-organ (heart, kidney, lung, or liver) retrieval to be effective, the organ donor must have an intact heartbeat, adequate blood pressure, and effective mechanical ventilator support. These criteria are necessary to maintain the proper organ function and adequate tissue oxygenation and perfusion required for effective organ procurement.

10 Correct answer — **B**

A urine output greater than the I.V. fluid intake in a potential organ donor indicates diabetes insipidus. This endocrine disorder, commonly seen in those who have sustained a severe head injury, typically results from the impaired ability of the hypothalamus to produce antidiuretic hormone (ADH) or the posterior pituitary gland to secrete ADH because of increased intracranial pressure. Decreased or absent ADH levels prevent the kidneys from reabsorbing water back into systemic circulation. This causes an increase in urine output, which is typically greater than the patient's fluid intake.

11 Correct answer — **D**

Disseminated intravascular coagulation (DIC) does not contribute to the development of hypotension in an organ donor; this disorder commonly results from prolonged hypotension but does not cause it. Hypotension, the most common complication during postmortem organ donor management, may result from brain stem herniation, collapse of peripheral vascular resistance, and therapeutic dehydration. In an organ donor, brain stem herniation may impair the medulla's vasomotor center, resulting in decreased blood vessel tone and eventual collapse of peripheral vascular resistance. Hypotension typically results from therapeutic dehydration caused by such intravascular depletion. Prolonged hypotension in an organ donor may cause cardiac death, acute tubular necrosis in transplanted kidneys, or DIC.

12 Correct answer — **D**

A witnessed cardiac arrest in a person known to have cardiovascular disease would not normally fall under the jurisdiction of the medical examiner. The medical examiner would be responsible for investigating any death resulting from an unknown cause, a suspected homicide, a suicide, or an accidental traumatic injury. The medical examiner typically gives consent for organ retrieval except when removal of a particular organ may inhibit the investigation.

13 Correct answer — **B**

Methylprednisolone sodium succinate is commonly administered I.V. to a potential organ donor because it stabilizes the kidney membrane during the retrieval process. This medication should be given immediately before retrieving the organ in the operating room.

14 Correct answer — **C**

Sex is not one of the criteria used when evaluating a potential organ recipient, because it has no bearing on the selection process. The most important criterion governing recipient selection is urgency of need, followed by ABO blood-group compatibility and tissue typing.

Blood-group compatibility is the most important physiologic criterion involved in the selection process. Age usually is the second factor considered. Body size also is a necessary criterion for matching heart and liver recipients. Body size and tissue typing are necessary criteria for kidney transplants.

15 Correct answer — **C**

With few exceptions, those over age 65 are ineligible for heart transplantation because they typically have poor health. Because of the tremendous shortage of organ donors, transplant candidates must be chosen carefully, with special consideration given to the potential recipient's overall health status. The ability to comply with changes in diet, drug regimens, and life-style also must be evaluated when considering a potential candidate.

16 Correct answer — D

A patient of any age who dies in a hospital or a person who is referred within 6 to 12 hours after a cardiac death may be considered for tissue donation. If the tissue is not used for transplantation, it may be used for research.

17 Correct answer — D

The age parameters for lung donation are ages 10 to 50. This range provides for lung maturity as well as optimal lung health.

18 Correct answer — B

The age parameters for bone donation are ages 15 to 65. Before age 15, bone growth typically is incomplete. After age 65, bone strength tends to deteriorate, particularly in women, from osteoporosis.

19 Correct answer — D

No age limit exists for eye donation. Eye tissue not used for corneal transplantation may be used for research.

20 Correct answer — A

Norepinephrine and epinephrine should not be used as vasopressors in a potential organ donor because they are extremely potent vasoconstrictors and may cause kidney and liver damage. In case of severe hypotension, however, they may be used as a last resort. The extreme vasopressor action of these medications produces marked vasoconstriction, resulting in acute tubular necrosis of the kidneys, and severely decreases blood flow to the liver, causing irreversible organ engorgement.

21 Correct answer — C

The cost of organ retrieval is paid by the receiving transplant center. The donor's family, the donating hospital, and the federal government do not pay for organ donation retrieval.

22 Correct answer — A

Urinary tract infection and intracranial cancer are not considered contraindications for organ donation. If a potential organ donor has evidence of a urinary tract infection, the ureters can be cultured during the retrieval process; the recipient can then be treated with appropriate antibiotics. A patient with intracranial cancer can donate organs as long as the cancer is confined intracranially. Although

Organ Donation
Answers

pneumonia is a contraindication for lung donation, it does not affect other types of donation. Such conditions as sepsis, I.V. drug abuse, human immunodeficiency virus (HIV) infection, and metastatic cancer are contraindications for all types of organ donation.

23 Correct answer—**D**

The goals of donor maintenance include ensuring adequate ventilation, hemodynamic stability, and asepsis. Adequate ventilation and hemodynamic stability are necessary for proper tissue perfusion and oxygenation. Asepsis is necessary because the organ recipient is immunosuppressed and likely to become further suppressed once antirejection drugs have been started; the introduction of microorganisms to his already-compromised system may be detrimental.

24 Correct answer—**D**

When discussing organ donation with a potential donor's family, the nurse should limit the discussion to the positive aspects of transplantation as well as to answering their questions about brain death. Details about the potential organ recipient are strictly confidential. The family should not be concerned with surgical techniques or the monetary value of organs. They should understand that organ donation involves no cost or monetary compensation. Primary nursing concerns include offering the family clear, concise, and nontechnical explanations as well as supportive measures, such as a quiet, private room; pastoral support; and time alone with the donor.

25 Correct answer—**C**

Living related donor is the term used to describe a person who donates one kidney to a blood relative, typically a son, daughter, mother, father, sister, or brother.

26 Correct answer—**D**

Nursing interventions related to kidney donor maintenance include maintaining a systolic blood pressure of 100 to 110 mm Hg, a urine output greater than 100 ml/hour, and adequate ventilation. All these interventions are necessary to ensure proper kidney perfusion and function and tissue oxygenation.

27 Correct answer—**C**

The organ procurement agency should be notified as soon as a potential donor is identified. The procurement coordinator is specially trained to assess the person and to approach the family tactfully.

28 Correct answer — **A**

A 35-year-old man with acquired immunodeficiency syndrome (AIDS) and a self-inflicted gunshot wound to the head would not be an acceptable candidate for organ donation because AIDS, which is caused by HIV, is a contraindication for all types of organ donation. All of the other patients in this situation are likely candidates for organ donation.

29 Correct answer — **C**

A thorough medical history of a potential organ donor can prove invaluable because it can help determine the existence of a disorder that may preclude organ donation. A good medical history can give evidence of chronic renal impairment, previous myocardial injury, or alcohol abuse, which could exclude the patient as a kidney, heart, or liver donor.

30 Correct answer — **A**

A child's brain is typically more resilient to brain damage than an older child's or adult's and may recover even after brain function appears lost. Electroencephalograms and cerebral arteriography may be necessary.

CHAPTER 11

Orthopedic Emergencies

1 Which early complication should the nurse assess for in a patient with a femoral shaft fracture?

A. Delayed union
B. Nonunion
C. Fat embolism
D. Infection

2 The nurse knows that the most serious complication of a femoral shaft fracture to assess for in a child would be:

A. Post-traumatic avascular necrosis
B. Volkmann's ischemia of nerves and muscles
C. Nonunion
D. Progressive coxa vara

3 Which primary treatment would the nurse expect a child between ages 2 and 9 with an uncomplicated femoral shaft fracture to receive?

A. Bryant's skin traction
B. Fixed skeletal traction
C. A double-hip spica cast
D. Intramedullary nailing

4 Which pelvic fracture is considered stable (minor)?

A. Straddle fracture
B. Malgaigne's hemipelvis fracture-dislocation
C. Combined hemipelvis fracture
D. Fracture of the ipsilateral rami

5 The nurse would prepare all of the following patients with a pelvic fracture for surgery *except* for the patient with:

A. A bilateral pelvic fracture
B. An open pelvic fracture
C. A major vessel injury
D. Hypovolemic shock

6 The nurse would expect which patient to be at highest risk for a pelvic fracture?

A. A 16-year-old boy who sustained a football-related injury
B. An 80-year-old woman who fell while walking in a nursing home
C. A 30-year-old man who was involved in a motorcycle accident
D. A 30-year-old man who fell from a window, landing on his feet

Orthopedic Emergencies
Questions

7 Which complication is considered most severe in a patient with a fractured pelvis?

A. Pneumothorax
B. Ruptured bladder
C. Intestinal perforation
D. Bleeding from iliac vessels

8 Which technique would be inappropriate for stabilizing a severely displaced pelvic fracture in the early resuscitative period?

A. External fixation
B. Internal fixation
C. Medical antishock trousers (MAST, or a pneumatic antishock garment) application
D. Skeletal traction

9 The nurse notes blood at the urethral meatus while assessing a male patient with a pelvic fracture. This indicates that:

A. Indwelling urinary catheterization is necessary
B. Indwelling urinary catheterization is contraindicated
C. The bladder has been traumatized
D. The patient has a retroperitoneal hematoma

10 The principle clinical effects of MAST for a patient with multiple injuries, including a pelvic fracture, include all of the following *except:*

A. Hemostasis (tamponade)
B. Autotransfusion
C. Decreased venous return
D. Increased peripheral vascular resistance

11 The nurse begins to deflate the MAST used to immobilize a patient who was admitted to the emergency department (ED) with multiple injuries and a pelvic fracture. The nurse knows that further deflation is contraindicated when the patient experiences a:

A. 5-mm Hg decrease in systolic blood pressure
B. 10-mm Hg decrease in systolic blood pressure
C. 5-mm Hg increase in diastolic blood pressure
D. 10-mm Hg increase in diastolic blood pressure

SITUATION

An elderly woman enters the ED limping. She informs the nurse that she slipped and fell 3 days ago, landing on her right side. An X-ray reveals a right impacted femoral neck fracture.

Questions 12 to 14 refer to the above situation.

12 Which assessment finding best indicates a fractured hip?

A. The affected leg is shortened and internally rotated
B. The affected leg is shortened and externally rotated
C. The affected leg is shortened but not rotated
D. The patient has no visible deformity but has pain on the affected side

13 Which finding would the nurse expect to see in a patient with an impacted femoral neck fracture?

A. Groin pain on the affected side and limited range of motion in the affected leg
B. Shortening and external rotation of the affected leg
C. Severe leg pain and inability to bear weight
D. Severe thigh swelling

14 Which application would be most appropriate for this patient?

A. Ice
B. Moist heat
C. Heating pad
D. Chemical cold pack

SITUATION

A patient arrives at the ED on a stretcher via an ambulance after involvement in a head-on automobile accident. The mechanism of injury was a force to the flexed knee with the hip in flexion. The patient reports that his knee struck the dashboard. During assessment, the nurse notes the affected leg is shortened, internally rotated, and adducted. The patient complains of severe hip pain on the affected side.

Questions 15 to 18 refer to the above situation.

15 Based on the assessment findings, the nurse suspects that this patient has:

A. A posterior hip dislocation
B. An anterior hip dislocation
C. A central acetabular fracture-dislocation
D. A pelvic fracture

16 The nurse knows that the prognosis for this patient will be good if the injury is reduced within the first:

A. 6 hours
B. 12 hours
C. 18 hours
D. 24 hours

17 Which nursing diagnosis is most appropriate for this patient?

A. Potential fluid volume deficit related to hemorrhage from pelvic fracture
B. Potential for injury related to sciatic nerve damage
C. Altered patterns of urinary elimination related to urethral trauma
D. Alteration in tissue perfusion of affected leg related to compartment syndrome

18 Which of the following is an expected outcome for the above nursing diagnosis?

A. The patient will have normal hemoglobin and hematocrit levels
B. The patient will have no sign of blood at the urethral meatus
C. The patient will maintain a urine output of at least 30 ml/hr
D. The patient will be able to move the affected leg with intact sensation

SITUATION

A 24-year-old man who is wearing a football uniform enters the ED. He is holding his right arm by his side and appears to be uncomfortable. He reports that he was injured during a game and developed sudden, severe right shoulder pain. The patient resists any passive movement and has a loss of shoulder symmetry.

Questions 19 to 22 refer to the above situation.

Orthopedic Emergencies
Questions

19 Based on the above assessment, the nurse suspects that the patient has:

A. An anterior shoulder dislocation
B. A posterior shoulder dislocation
C. A fractured clavicle
D. An acute tear of the rotator cuff

20 The nurse determines that no injury has occurred to the ulnar nerve based on which assessment finding?

A. Ability to oppose the thumb
B. Intact sensation to the smallest finger (pinky)
C. Intact sensation to the palmar aspect of the thumb
D. Intact sensation to the tip of the index finger

21 When relaying discharge instructions, the nurse should advise the patient to apply which treatment over the next 48 hours?

A. Ice
B. Moist heat
C. Heating pad
D. Ethyl chloride spray

22 Which statement indicates that the patient understands the nurse's discharge instructions for a shoulder dislocation?

A. "I should apply the treatment for 2 hours at a time"
B. "I should return to the hospital if my arm feels numb"
C. "I should expect the pain to get real bad"
D. "I should move my arm around as much as I can tolerate"

SITUATION

A 25-year-old man is transported to the ED after striking a lamppost while driving a motorcycle. His vital signs are stable, and he is alert and oriented. His right leg is splinted. The nurse examines the patient's leg and notes gross deformity. About 2" (5 cm) of the tibia is exposed, and dirt and shreds of denim are found in the open wound. The foot is warm, the dorsalis pedis and posterior tibial pulses are strong. Sensations are intact. X-rays reveal a comminuted fracture of the midshaft tibia and fibula.

Questions 23 and 24 refer to the above situation.

23 The nurse would expect the physician to order all of the following treatments for this patient *except:*

A. Antibiotic administration
B. Preparation for surgery
C. Cast application
D. Continuous leg splinting while the patient is in the ED

24 Which nursing diagnosis is most appropriate for the patient in this situation?

A. Fluid volume deficit related to vascular injury of the right lower leg
B. Altered tissue perfusion related to nerve damage of the right lower leg
C. Potential for infection related to wound contamination
D. Altered cerebral tissue perfusion related to cranial trauma

Answer Sheet

A B C D
1 ○ ○ ○ ○
2 ○ ○ ○ ○
3 ○ ○ ○ ○
4 ○ ○ ○ ○
5 ○ ○ ○ ○
6 ○ ○ ○ ○
7 ○ ○ ○ ○
8 ○ ○ ○ ○
9 ○ ○ ○ ○
10 ○ ○ ○ ○
11 ○ ○ ○ ○
12 ○ ○ ○ ○
13 ○ ○ ○ ○
14 ○ ○ ○ ○
15 ○ ○ ○ ○
16 ○ ○ ○ ○
17 ○ ○ ○ ○
18 ○ ○ ○ ○
19 ○ ○ ○ ○
20 ○ ○ ○ ○
21 ○ ○ ○ ○
22 ○ ○ ○ ○
23 ○ ○ ○ ○
24 ○ ○ ○ ○

1 Correct answer—**C**

The nurse should assess for development of fat embolism, caused by the mobilization of fat from the bone marrow into the vascular bed, and for shock—early complications in a patient with a femoral shaft fracture. Because the femur is the largest bone in the body and the shaft is extremely strong, the patient would have to sustain a violent, direct injury to fracture the femoral shaft. Internal hemorrhage and ensuing shock should be expected and must be treated expeditiously. The patient typically has a markedly swollen and deformed thigh with this type of fracture. Considerable soft tissue damage and blood loss of up to 1,000 ml is common.

Because a femoral shaft fracture is completely unstable, the leg should be immobilized with Thomas' splint during the emergency treatment phase. Splinting helps to relieve pain and prevent additional injury to the soft tissue. The patient is likely to have associated injuries in the same leg; X-rays of the joints above and below the injury must be taken. Persistent knee stiffness is a troublesome late complication. The quadriceps muscle or patella may adhere to the distal femur and require surgical release. Nonunion, delayed union, and infection are considered late complications. Nonunion without infection is rare. Delayed union is an indication for bone grafting.

2 Correct answer—**B**

In a child, the most serious complication of a femoral shaft fracture is Volkmann's ischemia of nerves and muscles, which typically results from femoral arterial spasm secondary to an intimal tear. Signs and symptoms include pain, pallor, puffiness, pulselessness, paresthesia, and paralysis. Analgesics typically mask these signs and should be avoided. The nurse should assess for severe, constant pain, especially in the calf. This pain may be worsened by excessive traction. If Volkmann's ischemia is suspected, encircling bandages should be removed, thereby restoring circulation.

Nonunion and progressive coxa vara may occur in a child with a femoral neck fracture. These complications typically result from nonuse or inadequate use of internal skeletal traction. Post-traumatic avascular necrosis, a complication that develops in about 30% of children with this type of injury, may result from disruption of the blood supply to the femoral head at the time of injury.

3 Correct answer—**C**

The nurse would expect a child between ages 2 and 9 to be treated with a double-hip spica cast after stabilization for 24 hours in Buck's traction. Bryant's skin traction, an overhead traction applied to both legs, is typically used for children under age 2. This type of traction is not used in older children because of the high risk of femoral arterial spasm and ensuing Volkmann's ischemia of nerves and muscles. Fixed (balanced-suspension) skeletal traction is typically used for children over age 9 or for whom a hip spica cast is impractical. Intramedullary nailing would be considered only after the child is skeletally mature, typically, by age 18, although skeletal maturity should be confirmed by X-rays.

4 Correct answer — **D**

A fracture of the ipsilateral rami is considered a stable (minor) pelvic fracture. Stable fractures, which are uncommon in patients with multiple trauma, commonly result from low-energy or well-localized injury to the pelvis. They typically fall into one of two categories: fractures involving individual bones without a break in the continuity of the pelvic ring (such as an avulsion fracture or a fracture of the pubic bone, ischium, iliac wing, sacrum, or coccyx) or fractures with a single break in the pelvic ring (such as a fracture of two ipsilateral rami or a fracture near or subluxation of the sacroiliac joint).

Unstable (major) pelvic fractures, most common in patients with multiple trauma, result in a double break of the pelvic ring. Such fractures include straddle fractures, which involve a break of the bilateral superior and inferior rami and are commonly associated with a high incidence of complications; Malgaigne's hemipelvis fracture-dislocation, which involves double vertical breaks in the pelvic ring; and combined hemipelvis fractures.

5 Correct answer — **A**

The nurse would not expect to prepare a patient with a bilateral pelvic fracture for surgery. This type of fracture is usually reduced by skeletal traction of the legs. Direct surgical management of pelvic fractures would be indicated for a patient with an open fracture or major vessel injury or for a patient in hypovolemic shock. An open fracture requires debridement, removal of contaminated material, and application of an external fixation device. Internal fixation may be performed later, after cardiopulmonary stability has been achieved. Major vessel injury, although uncommon in a patient with blunt pelvic trauma, is commonly associated with hypovolemic shock and thus requires surgical control. Severe shock after blunt trauma also requires endotracheal intubation, chest tube insertion, institution of two large-bore I.V. lines, application of medical antishock trousers (MAST, or a pneumatic antishock garment), and blood volume replacement once bleeding sites are identified and blood loss is estimated.

Orthopedic Emergencies Answers

6 Correct answer—**C**

The nurse would expect a 30-year-old man who was involved in a motorcycle accident to be at highest risk for a fractured pelvis. Any patient involved in a motorcycle or an automobile accident, either as a passenger or a pedestrian, should be considered at high risk for this type of fracture. Others at risk include those involved in crush injuries to the abdomen. A football-related injury usually involves the shoulders or knees. An injury sustained by an older person while walking usually involves the hip. Landing on the feet after falling from a window usually results in spinal trauma.

7 Correct answer—**D**

The most severe complication in a patient with a fractured pelvis would be bleeding from the iliac vessels. Other, less severe complications include damage to the gastrointestinal or genitourinary systems, such as intestinal perforation or ruptured bladder. Pneumothorax usually is not associated with pelvic fractures unless chest trauma has also been incurred.

8 Correct answer—**B**

Internal fixation would be inappropriate for stabilizing a severely displaced pelvic fracture in the early resuscitative period. Because a severely displaced pelvic or acetabular fracture typically involves massive hemorrhage (the patient may incur a blood loss of as much as 5,000 ml), appropriate methods of stabilization include external skeletal fixation (application of a Hoffman device), MAST application, or skeletal traction. External skeletal fixation, perhaps the optimal method of treating pelvic ring fractures, helps to decrease post-traumatic bleeding when the device is applied during the early resuscitative period. This type of fixation also relieves fracture pain and provides adequate immobilization. MAST immobilizes the fracture and prevents further damage to retroperitoneal tissues from sharp bony fragments. External compression of the pelvic ring forces bone fragments against one other and slows bleeding from cancellous bone. MAST may partially reduce the fracture and decrease intrapelvic volume, thereby resulting in tamponade of the retroperitoneal space.

Pelvic ring fractures also may be treated with skeletal traction, a pelvic sling, or a hip spica cast. Because these devices involve prolonged bed rest, late pulmonary, urologic, and soft tissue complications are possible. Open reduction and internal fixation should be carried out within the first week, after the patient is hemodynamically stable. This method is not used during the early resuscitative period because of the procedure's complexity and the likelihood of significant blood loss.

9 Correct answer—**B**

Blood at the tip of the urethral meatus in a male patient indicates urethral injury; therefore, indwelling urinary catheterization is contraindicated until the continuity of the urethra has been confirmed. Blood at the urethral meatus or vagina in a female patient may indicate an occult open fracture of the pelvis. Although pelvic fractures have been associated with injuries to the rectum, bladder, and male urethra, bladder trauma typically results in hematuria, not frank bleeding from the urethral meatus. Although retroperitoneal bleeding is difficult to assess, signs and symptoms may include ecchymoses, tenderness over the flank area, and signs of fluid loss.

10 Correct answer—**C**

Decreased venous return is not one of the clinical effects of MAST application for a patient with multiple injuries. Clinical effects include hemostasis (tamponade), autotransfusion, and increased peripheral vascular resistance. These combined effects produce decreased blood loss, increased venous return, and improved mean arterial pressure. Hemostasis occurs because the external pressure reduces the vessel wall pressure, allowing a clot to form. The volume of autotransfusion using MAST has been estimated at 250 to 1,000 ml.

11 Correct answer—**B**

The nurse knows that further deflation of the MAST would be contraindicated once the patient experiences a 10-mm Hg decrease in systolic pressure. Continuous blood pressure monitoring and gradual deflation are essential during MAST removal. Any decrease in systolic blood pressure greater than 10 mm Hg is a contraindication for further deflation, as this indicates that the patient is still hemodynamically unstable. The usual procedure for removing MAST is to deflate the abdominal portion first, then the leg compartments.

12 Correct answer—**B**

A patient with a fractured hip typically has an affected leg that is shortened and externally rotated as well as painful range of motion. Hip fracture, a common injury (especially in women between ages 70 and 80), may be classified as either femoral neck or intertrochanteric. A femoral neck fracture is intracapsular and does not usually lead to major blood loss because the hematoma is contained within the joint capsule. An intertrochanteric fracture, which is more common in older adults, typically causes more deformity and significant blood loss (approximately 500 to 750 ml within the first few hours). Swelling serves as a guide to the amount of blood loss. Nursing interventions include assessing the patient's circulation, sensation, and motor

Orthopedic Emergencies Answers

function. The patient should not be moved to the radiology department until she is immobilized or in traction. The fracture should be splinted. Sandbags should be applied to the affected leg, and 5 lb (2.25 kg) of Buck's traction (weighted skin traction, usually applied to one leg) should be used. The weights may be suspended over the end of the stretcher.

13 Correct answer—A

The nurse would expect to note groin pain on the affected side and limited range of motion in the affected leg of a patient with an impacted femoral neck fracture. The patient with this type of fracture typically complains of pain in the groin or medial knee and walks with a painless limp; he may feel slight discomfort with active or passive range of motion. Limited range of motion typically results from muscle spasms associated with this type of injury. No shortening or external rotation of the leg should be noted on physical examination.

Shortening and external rotation of the affected leg is commonly associated with displaced femoral neck fractures and intertrochanteric fractures. In a displaced femoral neck fracture, the patient typically has severe pain and cannot bear weight on the affected leg because of the instability of the fracture. Because blood infiltrates the joint rather than the soft tissue, swelling usually is not noted. In an intertrochanteric fracture, the thigh will appear swollen from extracapsular bleeding into the soft tissues.

14 Correct answer—C

Because the injury occurred over 48 hours ago, the most appropriate treatment for this patient would be the application of moist heat to reduce pain and stiffness. During the first 48 hours, cold therapy in the form of ice or chemical cold packs may help to reduce swelling and relieve pain. Dry heat, such as heating pads, is contraindicated because thermal burns may occur, especially in an elderly patient.

15 Correct answer—A

Based on the findings, the nurse would suspect that the patient has a posterior hip dislocation. This type of injury may occur when force is applied against the flexed knee with the hip in flexion, such as occurs when the knee strikes the dashboard during an automobile accident. The higher the degree of hip flexion, the greater the chance of a simple dislocation. Assessment typically reveals a shortened, internally rotated, and adducted leg. Associated knee and femur injuries are common. Major complications include sciatic nerve injury and avascular necrosis of the femoral head.

In an anterior hip dislocation, which occurs with forced abduction (as in a fall, an automobile accident, or a blow to the back while squatting), leg shortening is rare. Assessment typically reveals abduction, external rotation, and either flexion or extension of the affected leg, depending on the type of anterior dislocation. Early reduction is essential.

In a central acetabular fracture-dislocation, which occurs from a blow to the lateral side of the trochanter and pelvis with the force exerted on the femoral head, the patient typically has a slightly shortened affected leg, muscle spasms, and limited range of motion. This type of injury is commonly associated with other serious injuries, such as pelvic and abdominal trauma. Pelvic X-rays are recommended, because pelvic fractures are the second leading cause of traumatic death. The mechanism of injury for pelvic, sacral, and coccygeal fractures is direct trauma through the femur. The nurse should suspect a pelvic fracture if the patient has pain, crepitus, or tenderness over the symphysis pubis, anterior spine, iliac crest, sacrum, or coccyx. The patient must be observed for signs of shock and hemorrhage.

16 Correct answer—A

The prognosis for a patient with a dislocated hip without a fractured acetabulum will be good if the injury is reduced within the first 6 hours. A poor prognosis can be expected if the hip remains out of the acetabulum for more than 24 hours. If the patient suffers from sciatic nerve injury, only partial resolution may occur after reduction; typically, sensation to the bottom of the feet returns, but footdrop does not resolve.

17 Correct answer—B

The most appropriate nursing diagnosis in this situation is *Potential for injury related to sciatic nerve damage.* The nurse must assess sciatic nerve function and distal pulses in the patient with a hip dislocation because of the high risk of sciatic palsy associated with this type of injury. The other diagnoses are inappropriate because pelvic fractures and urethral trauma are more commonly seen with central acetabular fracture; in this situation, trauma to the knee forced the femoral head out of the acetabulum posteriorly. Also, the patient is at low risk for compartment syndrome with this type of injury.

18 Correct answer—D

The expected outcome for a patient with *Potential for injury related to sciatic nerve damage* is that the patient will be able to move the affected leg with intact sensation. This outcome indicates that nursing interventions to prevent sciatic nerve damage have been successful. Absence of footdrop would be another indication that injury has not occurred.

19 Correct answer—A

Based on the assessment findings, the nurse would suspect that the patient has an anterior shoulder dislocation. Approximately 50% of all major joint dislocations occur at the shoulder, 95% of which are anterior dislocations. An anterior dislocation occurs with abduction, extension, and external rotation of the shoulder. The patient typically resists passive and active abduction of the arm. Loss of shoulder symmetry is typically noted, and the humeral head can be palpated anteriorly. Assessing the patient's neurovascular status before reduction is important with this type of injury.

Posterior shoulder dislocations are difficult to diagnose. They typically occur with violent internal rotation, as occurs during a seizure. The patient may complain of shoulder pain and an inability to lift the arm. Examination typically reveals limited abduction and external rotation. The deformity is less noticeable than with an anterior dislocation. A neurovascular assessment is essential before reduction in this type of injury.

Clavicular fractures commonly result from falling onto a shoulder or an outstretched hand or from a direct blow to the clavicle. Diagnosis usually is based on the patient's history, the location of pain, and the degree of deformity noted during inspection and palpation. Acute tears of the rotator cuff commonly result from falling on a shoulder, throwing an object, or lifting a heavy object. Abduction of the shoulder may be impossible, and tenderness may be noted over the area where the rotator cuff is inserted into the tuberosities. Passive range of motion should be unrestricted with this type of injury. X-ray findings are normal in most cases.

20 Correct answer—B

Intact sensation to the smallest finger (pinky) is a good indication that no injury has occurred to the ulnar nerve. Intact sensation to the palmar aspect of the thumb reflects an intact radial nerve. Intact sensation to the tip of the index finger and ability to oppose the thumb reflect a functioning median nerve.

21 Correct answer—A

Cold therapy, such as ice, is indicated for the first 48 hours to reduce swelling and relieve pain. Heat applied to the injured area increases swelling. Cold sprays, such as ethyl chloride, are not recommended for home use; they should be applied only by a health care professional because of the risk of a cold thermal injury.

22 Correct answer — B

The patient's acknowledgment that he should return to the hospital if his arm feels numb indicates that he has understood the discharge instructions for a shoulder dislocation. Any patient with this type of injury should be advised to seek medical attention if numbness, tingling, or extreme pain occurs because prompt treatment can prevent neurovascular damage. Ice packs should be applied for 20 to 30 minutes at a time, to prevent frostbite. The arm should be kept immobile in a sling to reduce such complications as pain, neurovascular injury, and recurrence of the dislocation.

23 Correct answer — C

The nurse would not expect the physician to order cast application for this patient. The patient will require surgery to reduce and fixate the fracture. Antibiotics are necessary because of the gross contamination to the leg. Continuous leg splinting is necessary until the patient is in the operating room, to prevent neurovascular injury.

24 Correct answer — C

The most appropriate nursing diagnosis in this situation would be *Potential for infection related to wound contamination* because of the open wound and debris noted during assessment. The other diagnoses are inappropriate because there is no evidence of neurovascular injury or cranial trauma at this time.

Orthopedic Emergencies Answers

CHAPTER 12

Psychiatric and Psychological Emergencies

SITUATION

A 32-year-old man, accompanied by two police officers, is brought to the emergency department (ED) in handcuffs. He had been standing on the rooftop of a six-story office building, shouting obscenities and yelling, "You are all doomed to die for what you've done to me."

Questions 1 to 5 refer to the above situation.

1 The priority nursing action at this time would be to evaluate the patient's:

A. Orientation to time, place, and person
B. Vital signs
C. Threat to the safety of self and others
D. History of psychiatric illness

2 The patient is agitated and complains about the handcuffs and the presence of the police officers. The most helpful approach for the nurse to take in this situation is one that is:

A. Calm and firm, but nonthreatening
B. Relaxed, casual, and friendly
C. Authoritarian and directive
D. Permissive and comforting

3 After the patient is evaluated by the nurse and the psychiatric resident, the officers remove the handcuffs. Which statement would be most appropriate at this time?

A. "If you promise to be good, we won't have to restrain you anymore"
B. "We will remove the handcuffs now; you will not be restrained as long as you can control yourself"
C. "I know that the handcuffs are uncomfortable, so we will take them off now"
D. "Because you have calmed down, we will remove the handcuffs"

4 The patient appears anxious and guarded during the interview. The nurse knows that such anxiety may be reduced by:

A. A detailed explanation of the entire admission procedure
B. Approaching the patient confidently and offering simple, direct explanations
C. Limited interaction and focus on physical assessment rather than conversation
D. A warm attitude and the use of touch to demonstrate caring

5 Admitting this patient for psychiatric observation would most likely be made on the basis of:

A. The patient's history of previous psychiatric hospitalizations
B. The patient's anxiety level
C. The need to evaluate the patient's homicidal and suicidal ideation more thoroughly
D. The fact that the patient was brought in by the police

SITUATION

A 30-year-old woman is brought to the ED by her husband, who reports that she has not eaten or slept in 7 days and that she has become progressively elated over the past 3 weeks. The patient is wearing only shorts, a T-shirt, and sneakers, despite that fact that it is 20° F (−6.7° C) outside.

Questions 6 to 10 refer to the above situation.

6 The nurse notes that the patient is shivering and confronts her about her clothing. The patient says, "Well, it must be summer somewhere, and that's where I want to be." Which response would be most appropriate?

A. "It is obvious that your judgment is impaired. You are dressed inappropriately"
B. "Where would you like to be, instead of here?"
C. "Please put this robe on. You don't want to catch pneumonia, do you?"
D. "You are shivering and appear chilled. Put this robe on"

7 While waiting to be examined, the patient begins singing loudly and walking around "entertaining" the other patients. The best approach at this time is to:

A. Assign three available nursing assistants to keep the patient from annoying others
B. Recognize that this behavior is characteristic of bipolar disorder
C. Lead the patient to a quiet area
D. Obtain an order for medication to control her behavior

8 During the admission interview, the nurse asks the patient about her sleeping and eating patterns. The patient replies, "I live on love. I thank the stars above. Sleep is cheap. Food ruins the mood." The nurse knows that this response is indicative of:

A. Grandiose delusion
B. Auditory hallucination
C. Word salad
D. Clang association

9 The physician diagnoses the patient as having a manic bipolar disorder. The nurse is aware that signs and symptoms supporting this diagnosis include:

A. Looseness of association, agitation, suspiciousness, and irregular menses
B. Flight of ideas, hyperactivity, social isolation, and increased appetite
C. Rhyming, grandiosity, insomnia, and decreased appetite
D. Pressured speech, anxiety, delusions and persecution, and refusal to eat or drink

10 While waiting for the patient to be admitted to the medical-surgical unit, the nurse would expect the physician to order:

A. Chlorpromazine hydrochloride (Thorazine) 100 mg P.O.
B. Lithium carbonate (Eskalith) 300 mg P.O.
C. Imipramine hydrochloride (Tofranil) 50 mg I.M.
D. Chlordiazepoxide hydrochloride (Librium) 25 mg P.O.

SITUATION

A 40-year-old woman walks into the ED and says to the admissions secretary, "Are there any doctors here who can take the radio out of my brain?" The secretary tells the patient to have a seat and calls for the nurse.

Questions 11 to 15 refer to the above situation.

11 While sitting in the waiting area, the patient strikes herself in the head, saying, "Somebody has to help me. I can't take this any longer." Which action is most appropriate at this time?

A. Alert the security team that the patient may become agitated, and ask them watch her closely

B. Approach the patient with two other staff nurses, and ask, "What seems to be the problem?"

C. Walk over to the patient and say, "I understand you think there is a radio in your brain. How did that happen?"

D. Sit next to the patient and say, "I'm a nurse. I saw you hitting your head. Can you tell me what you are experiencing right now?"

12 The patient becomes increasingly agitated and begins pacing the floor, hitting her head harder and yelling, "Stop it. I'm a good girl. Stop saying those things about me." The nurse suspects that the patient is experiencing:

A. Auditory hallucinations

B. Delusions of persecution

C. Obsessive ideation

D. Looseness of association

13 The nurse should plan to focus further assessment on the patient's:

A. Vital signs

B. Orientation to time, place, and person

C. Receptivity to treatment

D. Content of thought

14 Which nursing action would be most appropriate if the patient were to become uncontrollable and require restraint?

A. Address the patient in a warm, reassuring manner

B. Administer medication while the patient is being restrained by two security guards

C. Restrain the patient with the help of at least three other trained personnel

D. Administer medication to avoid restraint

15 The nurse knows that safe nursing care for a restrained patient includes:

A. Allowing the patient to rest undisturbed until calm

B. Talking to the patient about what precipitated the restraint

C. Continuous observation and monitoring of vital signs

D. Performing range-of-motion exercises every ½ hour until the patient is released from the restraints

SITUATION

A 30-year-old man is brought to the ED by his mother, who states that she can no longer manage him at home. According to the mother, the patient, who has been in and out of psychiatric hospitals since age 19, acts infantile; he refuses to dress or wash without her help and has frequent episodes of urinary and fecal incontinence.

Questions 16 to 20 refer to the above situation.

16 In the examining room, the patient grimaces and poses in front of a glass cabinet. He does not respond when his name is called. The nurse determines that the best way to approach this patient would be to:

A. Walk over to him, place a hand on his shoulder, and repeat his name
B. Ask him what he is doing
C. Tell him to stop making faces and to explain what is wrong
D. Repeat his name louder, then move closer and wait for a sign that he is aware of her presence

17 When the patient is questioned about why his mother brought him to the hospital, he replies, "I had to go on a trip. The sky is empty now. The man's name is Big Bob." The nurse knows that this response demonstrates:

A. Looseness of association
B. Flight of ideas
C. Neologism
D. Echolalia

18 During the admission interview, the patient has an episode of urinary incontinence. The best way to handle this situation would be to:

A. Ignore the incontinence to avoid embarrassing the patient
B. Firmly remind the patient that men do not urinate in their pants
C. Have the patient remove his wet pants and put on a gown and a diaper to prevent further urine leakage
D. Say, "You are wet. Let me help you change into this dry gown"

Psychiatric and Psychological
Emergencies Questions

19 The patient says to the nurse, "Is it better to eat or to drink? To sleep or to wake? To sing or to dance? Which is better?" The nurse knows that these questions indicate:

A. Ambivalence
B. Confusion
C. Autism
D. Regression

20 The mother informs the nurse that she feels guilty about bringing her son back to the hospital. She says, "He doesn't like to be here; he always begs me to take him home once he's here. Why can't I take care of him at home?" Which statement offers the best support for the mother?

A. "Don't feel guilty. You've certainly done your best for him. Let us help him now"
B. "I understand how much you care about your son and can see that you're able to recognize when you need help in managing him"
C. "Patients like your son never really recover; they typically require repeated hospitalizations"
D. "It must have been an awful strain taking care of your son all these years. Perhaps you should consider a group home"

SITUATION

A 45-year-old man is brought to the ED by his wife, who reports that he had been well until 2 months ago, when he began to exhibit changes in personality, mood, and thought processes. On admission, the patient appears disheveled and assumes bizarre postures. He does not respond to questions and cannot describe his feelings; his speech is only partly understandable. His thoughts seem to be dominated by delusions of being controlled by Jesus Christ. He states that he has heard Jesus and the president of the United States speaking to him. He believes that the FBI is following him and that the nurses are secret agents who plan to destroy him. The physician diagnoses paranoid schizophrenia.

Questions 21 to 25 refer to the above situation.

21 The nurse is aware that schizophrenia is one of a group of psychotic reactions characterized by:

 A. Marked psychomotor disturbance, which may involve stupor, negativism, excitement, rigidity, or posturing
 B. Incoherence, grossly disorganized actions, prominent delusions, and hallucinations
 C. Alternating episodes of psychosis and apparent normalcy
 D. Basic disturbances in relationships with others and an inability to communicate and think clearly

22 Nursing assessment of this patient requires careful inquiry and observation of the patient's:

 A. Reality perception and ability to communicate on multiple levels
 B. Ability to communicate and interact with others during periods of total self-absorption
 C. Ability to think, perceive, symbolize, communicate, and make decisions
 D. Ability to interact in established relationships

23 When assessing the patient's thought content, the nurse should focus primarily on:

 A. Delusions
 B. Complex fantasies and self-absorption
 C. The degree of negative verbalization toward significant others
 D. Objective data elicited from the patient's psychiatric history

24 During the interview, the nurse should ask such questions as "Do you dream vividly? Do you see light flashes or figures that others cannot see? Do you hear voices when no one is present? If so, whose voices? Are the voices clear? Abusive? Accusatory? Can you stop the voices?" These questions are important because:

 A. The patient's major defense mechanisms are an indication of his level of psychosis
 B. Assessing for hallucinations is integral to determining the patient's perception
 C. Elicited emotional responses provide an assessment of the appropriateness of the patient's affect (mood)
 D. The psychotic patient can never distinguish between what is real and unreal

Psychiatric and Psychological Emergencies Questions

25 When caring for a psychotic patient, the ED nurse must be:

A. Nonthreatening, to enable the patient to express emotions appropriately

B. Goal-directed, to ensure the gathering of data necessary for the treatment plan

C. Nonjudgmental, to provide an atmosphere of trust and open communication

D. Flexible, to enable the nurse to adjust the care as the situation demands

SITUATION

A 36-year-old woman is brought to the ED anxious, trembling, and crying. She states that she began feeling depressed and disinterested in life 1 year ago, after learning that her husband wanted a divorce because of his relationship with another woman. The couple had been married for 10 years. The patient claims that she was not angry with her husband and blames herself for his infidelity. During the marriage, she developed few personal interests, having little time between her career and domestic responsibilities. After her husband began divorce proceedings, she became aware of intense feelings of sadness, fatigue, grief, hopelessness, and worthlessness and had recurrent thoughts of death. Family history reveals that the patient's mother had suffered from chronic illness and depression. A diagnosis of distorted grief reaction, major depression, is made.

Questions 26 to 31 refer to the above situation.

26 The nurse understands that a maladaptive or pathologic response to loss is likely to occur when a person:

A. Does not successfully complete the normal grieving process associated with loss

B. Does not resolve the social situations that precipitated feelings of powerlessness and low self-esteem

C. Cannot use coping mechanisms and ego strengths successfully

D. Does not balance intrapersonal and interpersonal needs successfully

27 The nurse is aware that a patient with a delayed or distorted grief reaction must experience the feelings and thoughts she initially avoided if she is ever to complete the grieving process and accept her loss. In this situation, the most appropriate way to help the patient through the grieving process would be to:

A. Encourage the patient to undergo psychotherapy with her former husband to work through her loss
B. Gently encourage the patient to discuss her loss, then support her during the grieving process
C. Encourage the patient to increase her social contacts and accept her ego strengths
D. Explain to the patient that grieving is time-limited and that the emotional pain eventually will resolve

28 The patient tells the nurse that she is afraid to face her feelings and express emotion; she fears that her condition will worsen if she remembers the past and its accompanying pain. When teaching this patient about the grieving process, the nurse should:

A. Reassure the patient that she will not cry forever, lose permanent control, or go crazy if she grieves
B. Reassure the patient that the expression of active feelings is a natural part of the grieving process
C. Discourage the patient from blaming herself for the divorce
D. Encourage the patient to express repressed feelings toward herself and her former husband through role-playing

29 Which test is commonly used to help diagnose depression?

A. Serotonin level test
B. Serotonin suppression test
C. Dexamethasone suppression test
D. Monoamine oxidase inhibitor suppression test

30 The nurse knows that sadness is the major affect associated with grief and depression. Other characteristic affects include:

A. Euphoria with varying degrees of dysphoria
B. Self-absorption, crying, and psychomotor agitation or retardation
C. Irritability, agitation, hostility, anger, apathy, lethargy, shame, self-doubt, and anhedonia (total lack of pleasure)
D. Low energy level; withdrawal; and demanding, regressive, and infantile behavior with periodic crying

31 The physician prescribes phenelzine sulfate (Nardil) 15 mg P.O. stat and advises the patient to set up an appointment with the outpatient mental health department in 2 weeks. Which information should the nurse include in the discharge instructions for this patient?

A. Follow-up instructions, including the need to undergo a thorough physical examination and psychotherapy
B. Signs and symptoms of potential adverse effects, including blurred vision, constipation, tachycardia, and delayed micturition
C. Signs and symptoms of potential adverse effects, including hypothalamic crisis and hyperglycemia
D. Dietary precautions

SITUATION

A 41-year-old man is brought to the ED by two police officers, who report that the patient had been standing on a busy street corner, throwing rocks at pedestrians and passing automobiles. The patient states that he was acting this way because he was just fired from his job. He also states that his wife recently left him because he had hit her on several occasions. He is angry about being brought to the hospital and verbally abusive to the nursing and medical staff. He belligerently demands to be discharged.

When the nurse asks the patient to remove his jacket for a vital signs assessment, he throws a chair against the wall. He threatens those who approach him, saying, "I'll break every bone in your body." A team of five staff members calmly enters the room and escorts him to a seclusion room, where he is given haloperidol (Haldol) 5 mg I.M. and is isolated from other patients until he regains control. Two hours later, still visibly angry but no longer verbally or physically violent, the patient reenters the waiting room. During the patient interview, he tells the nurse, "I hope I didn't hurt anyone before. At times my mind loses control, and I can't help myself. I don't mean to be violent; it just happens from time to time."

Questions 32 to 39 refer to the above situation.

32 The nurse knows that assaultive or violent behavior is a common manifestation of:

A. A psychotic state, an organic condition, a depressive state, or a disorder of impulse control
B. Repressed frustration, psychotic manifestations, or substance abuse
C. Psychosis, lack of impulse control, or history of child abuse
D. Alcohol intoxication, depression, or loss of ego and superego control

33 A patient in an acute psychotic or organic state who demonstrates assaultive, violent, or homicidal behavior typically does so because he:

A. Possesses an explosive personality
B. Imagines being threatened by outside forces
C. Acts out of rage, frustration, or anger because he cannot think before acting
D. Succumbs to violent impulses and reenacts old conflicts to get what he wants

34 Which patient is most likely to exhibit violence?

A. A patient with organic brain syndrome
B. A criminal
C. A substance abuser
D. A psychotic patient

35 The nurse knows that the best means of predicting the threat of violent behavior is via:

A. The patient's psychomotor activity
B. The patient's affect and accompanying changes in speech and motor activity
C. The degree of violence to which the patient has been subjected
D. Observation and intuition

36 Upon which criteria would the nurse determine that a patient is potentially assaultive?

A. Disorientation, visual and auditory hallucinations, and memory impairment
B. Diagnosis of psychosis and a history of violent behavior, particularly violence that resulted in a recent criminal incarceration
C. Diagnosis of manic depression with psychotic features and possession of a weapon, such as a gun or knife
D. Increased motor agitation, threatening statements or gestures, intensification of affect, and use of alcohol or addictive drugs

37 The immediate goal when caring for an assaultive or homicidal patient is to:

A. Administer a fast-acting sedative, as ordered
B. Help the patient to regain or prevent further loss of control
C. Restrain the patient according to hospital policy and help him to regain control
D. Provide the patient with opportunities for appropriate release of frustrations

Psychiatric and Psychological
Emergencies Questions

38 Which is the most effective means of managing an overtly violent patient?

A. Speaking to the patient calmly but firmly
B. Using a team approach
C. Calling in the psychiatric resident or a supportive family member to speak to the patient
D. Restraining the patient, then administering a psychotropic medication

39 Most state mental health laws are specific about the length of time a patient legally may be restrained, commonly stipulating that restraints:

A. Cannot be used for longer than 24 hours
B. Cannot be used if the patient has cardiac or respiratory disease or insufficiency
C. Can be used only after the patient is evaluated by a psychiatrist
D. May be applied if the patient poses a danger to himself or others, provided the risk of danger is reevaluated every few hours

SITUATION

A 52-year-old secretary is brought to the ED after attempting suicide. Divorced 5 years, she has been living in an apartment that she shared with her sister until her sister's death 1 year ago. She has seen several internists during the past several months for various somatic complaints, which gradually caused her to lose much time from work. During this period, she began to lose interest in her appearance and job. After being placed on probation by her supervisor last week, the patient went home and has not left her apartment. Her supervisor alerted the police after several unsuccessful attempts at reaching her. When found by the police, the patient was lying on the floor of her apartment, slashing at her wrists with a razor blade.

Examination on arrival at the ED reveals superficial cuts and stable vital signs. While the nurse applies sterile dressings to the wounds, the patient says, "It makes sense. I don't have anybody. I want to put myself out of this misery. Next time, I'll succeed."

Questions 40 to 46 refer to the above situation.

Psychiatric and Psychological Emergencies Questions

40 Which nursing action would be essential during the initial interview of this patient?

A. Help the patient to reevaluate her life and to make immediate, realistic changes

B. Inform the patient that a professional mental health practitioner will be assigned to care for and watch over her

C. Assess the need for psychotropic medications

D. Listen carefully to what the patient says about the nature of the suicidal intent

41 When assessing this patient's behavior, the nurse should pay particular attention to the suicide method because:

A. Certain suicide methods are gestures, a means of engaging in attention-seeking behavior, and not meant to be taken seriously

B. Most nonlethal methods reflect the patient's intrapsychic hope that someone will rescue her from self-destruction

C. Although all suicide threats and attempts must be taken seriously, more vigorous and vigilant nursing attention is indicated when the patient plans or attempts a highly lethal means

D. Most nonlethal methods reflect the patient's wish to discover whether anyone cares enough to prevent his self-destruction

42 All of the following statements about suicide are true *except:*

A. Most people who talk about committing suicide do not go through with their plan

B. Suicide occurs equally among all levels of society

C. Most suicides occur within 3 months after the beginning of improvement, when the person has the energy to put morbid thoughts and feelings into action

D. Although a suicidal person is extremely unhappy, he is not necessarily mentally ill

43 Because a severely depressed patient is at high risk for suicide, the nurse must carefully investigate all factors that may contribute to depression, including the patient's medication regimen. Which commonly prescribed drugs can cause depression?

A. Chlordiazepoxide hydrochloride, diazepam (Valium), doxepin hydrochloride (Sinequan), imipramine hydrochloride

B. Clonidine hydrochloride (Catapres), methyldopa (Aldomet), propranolol (Inderal), reserpine (Serpasil)

C. Clonidine hydrochloride, diazepam, methylphenidate hydrochloride (Ritalin), protriptyline hydrochloride (Vivactil)

D. Amitriptyline hydrochloride (Elavil), chlorpromazine hydrochloride, phenelzine sulfate, tranylcypromine sulfate (Parnate)

Psychiatric and Psychological
Emergencies Questions

44 The physician and the nurse concur that the patient should be hospitalized because she cannot control her destructive impulses without medical assistance. Which is the most appropriate intervention to include in the plan of care to ensure the patient's physical safety?

A. Provide the patient with a quiet room to decrease stimuli
B. Institute suicide precautions
C. Keep the patient in a locked room
D. Administer psychotropic medications, as ordered, to help the patient gain better control and reduce her self-destructive impulses

45 Which characteristic is shared by most suicidal patients?

A. Psychosis
B. Guilt
C. Ambivalence
D. Anger

46 Which groups are at highest risk for self-destructive behavior?

A. Alcoholics, previous suicide attempters, terminally ill patients, members of minority groups, and psychotic patients
B. Adolescents, psychotic patients, substance abusers, and newlyweds
C. Psychotic patients, previous attempters, clergy members, adolescents, and terminally ill patients
D. Psychotic patients, depressed individuals, and preadolescents

SITUATION

A 12-year-old girl is admitted to the ED with dysuria, scant vaginal bleeding, and a 2-cm linear laceration on the posterior aspect of her left thigh. She has not had menarche. The mother reports that her daughter has a poor relationship with her peers and that she has recently become more withdrawn. The parents are divorced; the patient and her mother recently moved in with a maternal uncle to help ease financial difficulties. The nurse suspects that the patient is a victim of child abuse.

Questions 47 to 61 relate to the above situation.

47 The nurse knows that child abuse is most prevalent among children of which age-group?

A. Infants
B. Toddlers
C. School-age children (ages 5 to 12)
D. Adolescents

48 The nurse would expect a hospitalized child-abuse victim to exhibit all of the following behaviors *except:*

A. Always wanting to know what will happen next
B. Seeming constantly alert to potential danger
C. Looking to adults for reassurance
D. Seeming less afraid of other children

49 All of the following factors increase a child's risk for abuse *except:*

A. Mental retardation
B. Physical handicap
C. Prematurity
D. First-born status

50 The nurse should suspect child abuse or neglect if a 2-year-old child presents with:

A. Symmetrical bruises on both knees
B. A finger laceration and clinging behavior
C. Bruises in various stages of healing on both arms
D. A partial-thickness burn to the fingers of one hand

51 Which cause of death is most commonly associated with child abuse?

A. Abdominal trauma
B. Asphyxiation
C. Head trauma
D. Malnutrition

52 The nurse would suspect which child of suffering from neglect?

A. An uneducated older child
B. A young child whose parents provide little or no supervision
C. An infant who is diagnosed with failure to thrive
D. All of the above

53 Which statement about sexual abuse is *true?*

A. Incest that begins and ends before adolescence is more difficult to manage than incest that occurs during adolescence
B. A child typically recovers more easily from sexual abuse when the abuser is a family member
C. Boys have more difficulty adjusting to sexual abuse than girls do
D. Boys receive more family support than girls when incest is discovered

54 Which assessment findings best support a diagnosis of child abuse?

A. Occasional accidents from lack of adult supervision
B. Sexually transmitted disease in a young child
C. Pregnancy in late adolescence
D. Excessive anger by a daughter toward her father

55 Which of the following should be the nurse's primary concern when caring for an abused child?

A. Helping the child to establish peer relationships
B. Ensuring the continuation of parental contact
C. Demonstrating acceptance of and affection for the child
D. Recommending appropriate behavior modification for the child

56 Which factor should be the nurse's primary consideration when planning the care of a child admitted to the hospital because of child abuse?

A. The nurse's personal feelings about the parents and their expectations for the child
B. The child's developmental level
C. The child's peer relationships
D. Community support and foster parent needs

57 Which nursing action is most appropriate in cases of suspected child abuse?

A. Assume that the physician caring for the child will suspect abuse and report it to the appropriate agency
B. Confront the parents directly and report findings to the appropriate agency
C. Assume responsibility for reporting suspected abuse to the appropriate agency
D. Assign responsibility for reporting suspected abuse to a social worker

58 The nurse is aware that parents who abuse their children typically:

A. View violence as an acceptable method of behavior modification
B. Are socially involved with their neighbors
C. Have had good relationships with their parents
D. Are self-sufficient

59 Which statement about abuse or neglect is *true?*

A. A neglectful parent is likely to restrict a child's social activities
B. An abusive parent is unlikely to restrict a child's social activities
C. Only a small percentage of neglected children are also abused
D. All of the above

60 All of the following treatment objectives for an abused child and his family are appropriate *except:*

A. Helping the parents to understand their needs
B. Teaching the child to express his needs in a direct manner
C. Encouraging the parents and child to increase their isolation and focus upon themselves
D. Redistributing power within the family so that no one assumes total control

61 Which observation should the ED nurse report when referring an 8-year-old girl who has been sexually abused to the community health nurse?

A. The child received 50,000 units/kg of procaine penicillin I.M.
B. Results of the Venereal Disease Research Laboratory test revealed that no further studies are indicated
C. A urine specimen for human chorionic gonadotropin levels was obtained for pregnancy testing
D. Pelvic examination revealed an intact hymen

Answer Sheet

	A	B	C	D			A	B	C	D			A	B	C	D
1	○	○	○	○		31	○	○	○	○		61	○	○	○	○
2	○	○	○	○		32	○	○	○	○						
3	○	○	○	○		33	○	○	○	○						
4	○	○	○	○		34	○	○	○	○						
5	○	○	○	○		35	○	○	○	○						
6	○	○	○	○		36	○	○	○	○						
7	○	○	○	○		37	○	○	○	○						
8	○	○	○	○		38	○	○	○	○						
9	○	○	○	○		39	○	○	○	○						
10	○	○	○	○		40	○	○	○	○						
11	○	○	○	○		41	○	○	○	○						
12	○	○	○	○		42	○	○	○	○						
13	○	○	○	○		43	○	○	○	○						
14	○	○	○	○		44	○	○	○	○						
15	○	○	○	○		45	○	○	○	○						
16	○	○	○	○		46	○	○	○	○						
17	○	○	○	○		47	○	○	○	○						
18	○	○	○	○		48	○	○	○	○						
19	○	○	○	○		49	○	○	○	○						
20	○	○	○	○		50	○	○	○	○						
21	○	○	○	○		51	○	○	○	○						
22	○	○	○	○		52	○	○	○	○						
23	○	○	○	○		53	○	○	○	○						
24	○	○	○	○		54	○	○	○	○						
25	○	○	○	○		55	○	○	○	○						
26	○	○	○	○		56	○	○	○	○						
27	○	○	○	○		57	○	○	○	○						
28	○	○	○	○		58	○	○	○	○						
29	○	○	○	○		59	○	○	○	○						
30	○	○	○	○		60	○	○	○	○						

Psychiatric and Psychological Emergencies Answer Sheet

1 Correct answer—**C**

Ensuring the safety of the patient and others is always the top priority. Evaluating the patient's orientation to time, place, and person; vital signs; and psychiatric history are part of the total assessment.

2 Correct answer—**A**

The most helpful approach would be one that is calm and firm, but nonthreatening. Taking this approach should help to lessen the patient's fear and anxiety. The patient may view the other approaches as suspicious or threatening.

3 Correct answer—**B**

The most appropriate statement would be "We will remove the handcuffs now; you will not be restrained as long as you can control yourself." This statement clearly informs the patient about what will be done and sets appropriate limitations. The nurse should avoid asking the patient to make promises that he may be unable to keep.

4 Correct answer—**B**

Anxiety interferes with a patient's ability to concentrate and comprehend complex information. Therefore, the nurse should approach the patient confidently and offer simple, direct explanations. Performing a physical assessment and touching the patient may be interpreted as intrusive and threatening and, therefore, should be avoided at this time.

5 Correct answer—**C**

Because the patient had been threatening others, he must undergo a thorough evaluation for homicidal and suicidal ideation. The patient's history of previous psychiatric hospitalizations and the fact that he was brought in by the police would be insufficient grounds to warrant admission for further psychiatric evaluation.

6 Correct answer—**D**

The most appropriate response would be "You are shivering and appear chilled. Put this robe on." Such a response allows the nurse to comment on her observation and to suggest an appropriate behavior in a matter-of-fact, nonjudgmental way. Telling the patient that her judgment is impaired degrades the patient; asking where she would like to be provides no meaningful information.

7 Correct answer—**C**

The best approach in this situation would be to lead the patient to a quiet area, thereby decreasing environmental stimuli and reducing hyperactivity. The patient should receive constant supervision; however, assigning three nursing assistants may be overstimulating for the patient. The nurse should avoid obtaining an order for medication until the patient has been thoroughly evaluated.

8 Correct answer—**D**

This response is indicative of clang association, a form of clanging rhyme that is common in manic disorders. Auditory hallucinations and word salad (meaningless combination of words) are seen in schizophrenia. The patient does not show evidence of grandiose delusions.

9 Correct answer—**C**

Rhyming, grandiosity, insomnia, and decreased appetite are signs and symptoms of a manic disorder. The other signs and symptoms are not characteristic of this disorder.

10 Correct answer—**A**

The nurse would expect the physician to order chlorpromazine hydrochloride, an agent commonly prescribed to control hyperactivity. Lithium carbonate, which is used to prevent or control mania, takes 7 to 10 days to achieve therapeutic blood levels. Imipramine hydrochloride, an antidepressant, would not be prescribed in this situation.

11 Correct answer—**D**

The appropriate action would be to sit next to the patient and say, "I'm a nurse. I saw you hitting your head. Can you tell me what you are experiencing right now?" This enables the nurse to acknowledge the patient's distress and to reassure the patient that someone understands and wishes to help. Measures that place the patient on the defensive, such as alerting the security team, approaching the patient with two other staff nurses, or confronting the patient head-on, should be avoided.

12 Correct answer—**A**

The nurse would suspect auditory hallucinations because the patient appears to be responding to what she is hearing.

13 Correct answer—D

The nurse should plan to focus on the patient's content of thought. Such assessment should reveal the nature of the hallucinations and enable the nurse to protect the patient and others from potential violent outbursts.

14 Correct answer—C

If the patient were to become uncontrollable and require restraint, the appropriate action would be to restrain the patient with the help of at least three other trained personnel. Restraints are used to protect the safety of the patient and staff. At least four persons trained in restraining patients can do this safely and efficiently. Medication should have been given earlier in an attempt to prevent any escalation of the patient's agitated behavior to the point where restraints were required.

15 Correct answer—C

A restrained patient requires continuous observation and close monitoring of vital signs. Talking about the event at this point will further agitate the patient rather than calm her. Range-of-motion exercises are not as important as checking for circulation, respirations, and hydration; also, performing range-of-motion exercise would require the release of restraints, which may be unsafe.

16 Correct answer—D

The nurse should repeat the patient's name louder, then move closer and wait for a sign that the patient is aware of her presence. The nurse should avoid startling the patient by not touching him or asking questions before she identifies herself and establishes a relationship.

17 Correct answer—A

This type of response indicates looseness of association, a thought process characterized by obscure links in thought content. In flight of ideas, the links, although weak, are more evident. In this situation, the patient is not demonstrating neologisms (fabricated words) or echolalia (repetitious speech).

18 Correct answer—D

The best response in this situation would be to say, "You are wet. Let me help you change into this dry gown." The nurse should be aware that the patient's self-esteem may be fragile during such regressive episodes and that sensitively helping the patient change his clothes is the best approach. Having the patient put on a diaper may embarrass him. Ignoring the incontinence may be interpreted as not caring.

19 Correct answer—A

These questions demonstrate ambivalence, which is characterized by statements of opposing or dual behaviors.

20 Correct answer—B

The most supportive statement would be "I understand how much you care about your son and can see that you're able to recognize when you need help in managing him." This acknowledges the mother's concern and decision to bring her son to the hospital. The nurse should not deny the mother's feelings, imply that there is no hope, or promote feelings of guilt.

21 Correct answer—D

Schizophrenia is one of a group of psychotic reactions characterized by basic disturbances in relationships with others and an inability to communicate and think clearly. The patient's thoughts, feelings, and behavior are often evidenced by withdrawal, fluctuating moods, disordered thinking, and regressive tendencies.

22 Correct answer—C

Nursing assessment of a patient with psychosis requires careful inquiry and observation of the patient's ability to think, perceive, symbolize, communicate, and make decisions. Such assessment should focus on alterations in thought content and processes, perception, affect (mood), and psychomotor behavior; changes in personality, coping styles, and sense of self; lack of self-motivation; psychosocial stressors; and degeneration of adaptive functioning.

23 Correct answer—A

Delusions typically constitute the major disturbance in thought content of a patient with psychosis and therefore should be the nurse's primary focus. Although some patients report delusions spontaneously, specific questioning commonly is required. During the interview, the nurse should look for clues suggestive of delusions, such as evasiveness, suspicion, and oversensitivity.

24 Correct answer—B

The nurse should include such questions in the patient interview to assess for hallucinations, the most common perceptual disturbance manifested in psychosis. Such hallucinations may be auditory or visual. During auditory hallucinations, the patient may hear the voices of family members or strangers making derogatory or insulting remarks. The patient also may hear voices telling him to do something (command hallucinations) that may be dangerous to himself or others.

25 Correct answer—D

The emergency department (ED) nurse must be flexible when caring for any patient who behaves in a suspicious, withdrawn, or regressed way or who has a thinking disorder. Because such a patient typically communicates in an unpredictable fashion and is in control of himself at various times, the nurse must adjust the care as the situation demands.

26 Correct answer—A

A maladaptive or pathologic response to loss implies that something has prevented the patient from completing the normal grieving process associated with loss. Pathologic grief reactions may take on one of two forms: a distorted reaction or a delayed reaction. A distorted reaction is characterized by failure to successfully engage in the physical and psychological distress normally associated with loss. In this situation, the patient is suffering from depression, a type of distorted grief reaction characterized by the abnormal extension or overelaboration of sadness and grief.

27 Correct answer—B

The most appropriate way to help this patient would be to gently encourage her to discuss her loss, then support her during the grieving process. Those who fail to grieve sometimes do so because they have no available and supportive social matrix. The nurse can direct this patient to various support groups within the hospital and community.

28 Correct answer—A

When teaching the patient about the grieving process, the nurse should reassure the patient that she will not cry forever, lose permanent control, or go crazy if she grieves. She should explain that such untoward consequences typically occur only when a patient fails to grieve. If the patient complains that the past is the past and should remain buried, the nurse should reply that the past is very much in the present because it has not really been buried. Grieving is necessary to put the past in proper perspective.

29 Correct answer — C

The dexamethasone suppression test has gained considerable attention as a diagnostic marker for endogenous depression, as well as for its implications for treatment and prognostic factors. Most studies have found that 40% to 50% of patients suffering from endogenous depression or from major depressive disorders with melancholia demonstrate early recovery from cortisol suppression after the administration of dexamethasone.

30 Correct answer — C

Besides sadness, other characteristic affects associated with grief and depression include irritability, agitation, hostility, anger, apathy, lethargy, shame, self-doubt, and anhedonia (total lack of pleasure). Assessment of a depressed patient typically involves a thorough mental examination that includes a careful evaluation of affect. The nurse should assess for ambivalence and hopelessness, which may indicate dire feelings of emptiness, worthlessness, and a lack of self-respect and confidence. Self-blame and low self-esteem are also present. The patient may be emotionally labile, crying easily one moment and laughing the next.

31 Correct answer — D

When giving discharge instructions to a patient with a prescription for phenelzine sulfate, the nurse must include information about necessary dietary precautions. Because of the dangers of hypertensive reactions resulting from the tyramine content of this monoamine oxidase inhibitor, the patient should be advised to avoid ingesting aged cheese, sour cream, beer, wine (especially Chianti), yogurt, yeast, pickled herring, aged meat, meat tenderizer, and chicken liver. Chocolate and caffeine also have been implicated in blood pressure elevation and therefore should be avoided. The nurse also should advise the patient to note and report early signs of an impending hypertensive reaction, including headache, palpitations, neck stiffness, sweating, nausea, and photophobia.

32 Correct answer — A

Assaultive or violent behavior is primarily a manifestation of a psychotic state, an organic condition, a depressive state, or a disorder of impulse control or acting out.

33 Correct answer — B

In an acute psychotic or organic state, assaultive, violent, or homicidal behavior typically occurs because the patient imagines being threatened by outside forces. He cannot correctly perceive the reality of his environment and acts in response to real or imagined threats.

34 Correct answer—D

A psychotic patient is most likely to exhibit violence. Such a patient typically suffers from acute attacks of paranoia (psychotic episodes) that may result from a functional mental disorder or an organic brain syndrome. The patient's thought pattern is projective (the patient projects his thoughts to those around him) and leads to the development of delusions, which are typically persecutory in nature. The patient's reality perception is impaired; if uncorrected, this could lead to persistent delusions that cause the patient to perceive his environment as hostile and destructive. Violence may ensue as the patient attempts to protect himself in such an environment.

35 Correct answer—D

The nurse's best means of predicting the threat of violent behavior is via observation and intuition. By observing the patient's behavior and mannerisms, the nurse can gauge whether the patient is acting strangely or in a potentially destructive way. For example, the nurse might note a patient suddenly beginning to pace, mumble angrily, and make threatening gestures—all warning signs of potential violence. Although direct observation of dangerousness is a good indication of potential violence, the nurse also needs to rely on intuition to evaluate the potential for violence. Such intuition commonly is based on the nurse's gut instincts and feelings in a particular situation as well as on previous experience in similar situations. Thus, a nurse who witnessed the same warning signs in a previous situation is likely to sense the possibility of danger more readily than an inexperienced nurse would.

36 Correct answer—D

The criteria for determining whether a patient is potentially assaultive include increased motor agitation, threatening statements or gestures toward real or imagined objects, intensification of affect, and use of alcohol or addictive drugs, as well as a history of assaultive behavior or diagnosis of acute organic brain syndrome.

37 Correct answer—B

The immediate goal when caring for an assaultive or homicidal patient is to help the patient regain or prevent further loss of control. The other interventions may be appropriate but are not the immediate goal.

352

38 Correct answer—B

The most effective means of managing an overtly violent patient is a team approach. The team, whose presence serves as a constant reminder of discipline and external control, aims to help the patient to understand his feelings. This is accomplished by helping him to control or set limits on impulsive aggressive behavior, examine the immediate situation that prompted the impulse reaction, and learn alternative methods of reacting in similar situations or other ways to discharge aggressive energies on an ongoing basis.

39 Correct answer—D

Most state mental health laws stipulate that restraints may be applied if the patient poses a danger to himself or others, provided the risk of danger is reevaluated every few hours and the restraints are continued only until more humane methods (such as sedative administration) become effective. In some instance, however, more humane methods are impossible. For example, when treating a violent patient who is intoxicated or who has overdosed on drugs, administering a sedative is impossible until the alcohol or drug is metabolized; restraints with continued observation may be necessary.

In many states, the only legal form of restraint is a camisole (straitjacket) or restraining sheet. Four-point restraint (both wrists and ankles tied separately) is illegal in many states. However, when no other method works, four-point restraint may be used, provided that one limb is untied at a specified interval and the restraints are rotated, much in the manner of rotating tourniquets. Handcuffs, which are commonly used by the police to restrain violent patients brought to the ED, may *never* be used by health professionals.

40 Correct answer—D

During the initial interview, the nurse should listen carefully to what the patient says about the nature of the suicidal intent. After evaluating the information, the nurse should assess the patient's feelings of adequacy in coping with immediate and chronic stressors, her degree of hope, and her overall view of life and the immediate situation.

41 Correct answer—C

When assessing suicide behavior, the nurse should place heavy emphasis on the lethality of the suicide method chosen or used by a patient who has threatened or attempted suicide. Although all suicide threats and attempts should be taken seriously, more vigorous and vigilant nursing attention is indicated when the patient plans or tries a highly lethal means, such as shooting, hanging, or jumping from a high place. Less lethal means include carbon monoxide poisoning and drug overdose, which allow time for discovery once the suicidal action has been taken.

Such assessment also should focus on whether the patient has made a specific plan and whether the means to carry out the plan is readily available. Typically, the patient at highest risk for suicide is one who plans a violent death (such as a gunshot to the head), has a specific plan of action (for example, shooting himself as soon as his wife leaves the house to go shopping), and has the means readily available (such as a loaded handgun in a desk drawer).

42 Correct answer — **A**

One of the misconceptions about suicide is that most people who talk about committing suicide do not actually follow up on their plan. In reality, 8 out of 10 persons who commit suicide give definite warnings of their suicidal intentions. Almost no one commits suicide without letting others know how he is feeling. Another misconception is that those who attempt suicide are fully intent on dying. The fact is that most people who attempt suicide are undecided about living and dying and gamble with death, relying on others to save them.

43 Correct answer — **B**

When investigating the source of a patient's depression, the nurse must not overlook the possibility that the patient's medication regimen may be responsible. Commonly prescribed drugs that may cause depression include clonidine hydrochloride, methyldopa, propranolol, and reserpine. Other common depression-causing drugs include asparaginase (Elspar), baclofen (Lioresal), carisoprodol (Soma), chloramphenicol (Chloromycetin), dantrolene sodium (Dantrium), diazepam, diethylstilbestrol (DES), gentamicin sulfate (Garamycin), guanethidine sulfate (Ismelin), hydralazine hydrochloride (Apresoline), indomethacin (Indocin), pentazocine hydrochloride (Talwin), phenytoin (Dilantin), tamoxifen citrate (Nolvadex), and trimethobenzamide hydrochloride (Tigan), as well as anorectants, barbiturates, estrogen-containing products, and sulfonamides.

44 Correct answer — **B**

The most appropriate intervention to include in the plan of care to ensure the patient's safety is to institute suicide precautions. Such precautions include searching the patient's personal effects for toxic agents, such as drugs or alcohol; removing any sharp instruments from the room, including razor blades, knives, letter openers, and glass bottles; removing all cords and sheets from the room and all straps, belts, neckties, stockings, and pantyhose from the patient's clothing; and instituting one-on-one observation.

45 Correct answer — C

A common characteristic shared by most suicidal patients is ambivalence. Within each of these patients is a struggle between self-preserving and self-destructing forces. This is most apparent when patients threaten or attempt suicide, then try to get help. When discussing the possible outcomes of suicide, many patients focus on life-related outcomes, such as relief from an unhappy situation, rather than on death.

46 Correct answer — A

The groups at highest risk for self-destructive behavior include alcoholics, previous suicide attempters, terminally ill patients, members of minority groups, psychotic patients, police officers, physicians, adolescents, and elderly people. Of those who attempt suicide, three times as many men as women die; although more women attempt to kill themselves, they typically choose less effective means than men do.

47 Correct answer — A

Child abuse is most prevalent among infants because they are typically defenseless, nonverbal, and at times difficult to manage.

48 Correct answer — C

The nurse would not expect a hospitalized child-abuse victim to look to adults for reassurance. In most cases, the abused child shows a wariness and distrust of adults because adults are the most common abusers. The nurse would expect the abused child to attempt to gain some control over the environment by wanting to know what will happen next and remaining alert to potential danger. Other children are typically nonthreatening to the abused child, who may easily settle into the hospital environment.

49 Correct answer — D

A child's first-born status does not increase his risk for abuse. Maltreatment is commonly noted in children who are mentally retarded or physically handicapped. A contributing factor in both of these cases appears to be the increased difficulty in caring for these children. The increased incidence of abuse among premature children is attributed to ensuing medical problems, financial stress, and interruption of the bonding process.

50 Correct answer — **C**

One of the hallmarks of chronic physical abuse is the appearance of bruises in various stages of healing on a child's arms or legs. When assessing for possible abuse, the nurse should keep in mind that ecchymotic areas normally appear reddish purple (initially), then green (within 5 to 7 days), and then yellowish brown (within 1 to 3 weeks) before they finally disappear (in about 4 weeks).

The nurse would not suspect abuse in the other situations because symmetrical bruises on both knees commonly result from a 2-year-old's tendency to fall on his knees; lacerations are an atypical finding in an abused child, especially one who demonstrates clingy behavior suggestive of the need for parental support; and intentionally burned areas typically are symmetrical and full-thickness and usually involve the feet and buttocks, not the fingers of one hand.

51 Correct answer — **C**

Head trauma, especially involving a subdural hematoma, is the most common cause of death in child abuse. Abdominal trauma with bruising or rupture of the abdominal viscera is the second leading cause of death in abused children. Asphyxiation, although reported as the cause of death in some situations, seldom occurs. Malnutrition, a commonly reported finding in abuse, rarely is a cause of death, except in children who are isolated from society.

52 Correct answer — **D**

Lack of education or supervision and failure to thrive are recognized forms of child neglect. Other categories include abandonment; nutritional, medical, or dental neglect; and inappropriate or insufficient clothing.

53 Correct answer — **C**

Boys have more difficulty adjusting to sexual abuse than girls do because this type of abuse is more common among girls, for whom support networks have been established. Incest that begins and ends before adolescence is less difficult to manage than incest that occurs during adolescence, possibly because younger children are not as cognizant of society's norms. A child typically recovers more easily from sexual abuse when the abuser is outside the family, because the child does not have to face the abuser on an ongoing basis. Also, the child's family typically assumes a protective role when the abuser is a nonfamily member.

Psychiatric and Psychological
Emergencies Answers

54 Correct answer — B

Sexually transmitted disease in a young child indicates child abuse. Child abuse can take many forms: physical, sexual, and emotional. Physical and behavioral indicators may include bruises, welts, burns, fractures, dislocations, lacerations, abrasions, dysuria, vaginal or penile discharge, wariness of physical contact with adults, feeding disorders, self-stimulation, withdrawal, or unusual sexual knowledge or behavior. Frequent accidents because of lack of adult supervision may indicate neglect. Pregnancy in early adolescence is indicative of sexual abuse; commonly, the child fails to disclose the paternal source. Excessive anger from a daughter directed toward the mother may be another indicator of sexual abuse; this results from the perceived failure of the mother to protect the daughter.

55 Correct answer — C

The nurse's primary concern when caring for an abused child should focus on demonstrating acceptance of and affection for the child through consistent caregiving. The nurse should keep in mind, however, that the abused child may not readily return acceptance and affection because his previous efforts had been met with frustration, neglect, or abuse. As a result, the abused child will not easily establish a trusting relationship with an adult. The nurse must demonstrate affection while attempting to modify negative methods of interaction and discipline and to provide the child with appropriate ways to display anger and frustration. An abused child typically has little difficulty establishing peer relationships. Depending on the nature and severity of the abuse, parental rights and contact may be terminated.

56 Correct answer — A

The most important factor to consider when planning the care of a child who has been admitted to the hospital because of child abuse is the nurse's personal feelings about the parents and their expectations for their child. The nurse, the primary health care professional responsible for the abused child's care, must be careful to examine her feelings toward the parents and refrain from expressing any negative feelings. Once the nurse has come to terms with her feelings, she can proceed with planning interventions. Appropriate interventions should focus on helping the parents to establish realistic expectations for the child and promoting adequate parental problem-solving skills with appropriate discipline.

In many cases, parents have unrealistic expectations for the child and thus need information about appropriate growth and development. Self-help groups may benefit abusive families by helping the parents to gain personal insight and learn appropriate methods of releasing frustration. Crisis centers or hotlines may decrease the incidence of child abuse, but only on a short-term basis.

An abused child typically adjusts well to new environments and makes friends without difficulty. Poor peer relationships, when they occur, tend to be more common among sexually abused children. If foster care is necessary, the foster parents should be encouraged to visit the hospitalized child and participate in care. They should be encouraged to show affection for and acceptance of the child to help the child develop a sense of trust.

57 Correct answer—C

In many states, nurses are legally responsible for reporting all cases of suspected child abuse to the appropriate agency. The nurse is typically the primary health care professional caring for an abused child in the hospital setting. Because of the intimate nature of the nurse-patient relationship, the nurse may have more insight into the child's relationship with his parents. Consequently, the nurse is in a better position to recognize the signs of possible abuse and typically assumes an active role in reporting and preventing child abuse. Direct confrontation with the parents is not recommended, because this may escalate the anger and fear of the parents, who may remove the child from the hospital before the proper authorities arrive.

58 Correct answer—A

Parents who abuse or neglect their children typically view violence as an acceptable method of behavior modification. Various factors can precipitate or fuel violence in such parents, including mental or physical handicaps, low self-esteem, and poor coping mechanisms. Abusive parents tend to be socially isolated and have minimal support systems. Most are not in a position to be self-sufficient; this, coupled with their social isolation, fosters a nonsupportive environment that can lead to abuse. Studies indicate that parents who abuse their children commonly were abused themselves.

59 Correct answer—C

Only a small percentage of neglected children are also abused. A child suffering from neglect typically is ignored; therefore, abuse is less likely to occur. An abusive parent tends to restrict the child's social interactions to minimize the risk of discovery, whereas a neglectful parent typically allows the child to interact freely.

60 Correct answer—C

The parents and child should be encouraged to expand their relationships, thereby improving support mechanisms. The child must be taught to express his needs directly, thus eliminating confusion and fostering realistic expectations. Helping the parents to understand themselves, redistribute power within the family, and share responsibilities helps to strengthen the family unit.

61 Correct answer — D

When referring this patient to the community health nurse, the ED nurse should report that a pelvic examination revealed an intact hymen. Although the condition of the hymen neither proves nor disproves penetration, this information has legal significance and must be reported. A child's hymen may rupture as a result of various noncoital activities or accidents, or it may have enough elasticity for penetration without laceration. Nevertheless, a pelvic examination must be performed whenever penetration is suspected. Hair sampling and swabs for spermatozoa and gonorrhea also must be obtained. A serologic Venereal Disease Research Laboratory test for syphilis is required and should be repeated 1 to 2 months after the initial examination. The administration of 100,000 units/kg of procaine penicillin I.M. for a child and 4.8 million units for an adolescent is recommended. After menarche, urine should be obtained for human chorionic gonadotropin testing to determine possible pregnancy.

CHAPTER 13

Respiratory Emergencies

1 In a patient with atelectasis, the nurse would expect to hear bronchial breath sounds over the:

A. Carina
B. Middle of the right lung lobe
C. Right main-stem bronchus
D. Left main-stem bronchus

2 While percussing a patient's lung fields, the nurse notes consolidated areas. These areas typically produce which sound?

A. Tympany
B. Flatness or dullness
C. Hollowness
D. Hyperresonance

3 The nurse knows that bronchovesicular breath sounds are normally auscultated over the:

A. Large bronchi
B. Lung periphery
C. Entire lung surface area
D. Trachea

4 When auscultating a patient, the nurse notes decreased vesicular breath sounds. This is an indication of:

A. Pulmonary fibrosis
B. Pleural effusion
C. Chronic obstructive pulmonary disease
D. All of the above

5 Which technique is commonly used to determine the degree of respiratory excursion?

A. Cardiothoracic ratio on chest X-ray
B. Percussion
C. Palpation
D. Auscultation

6 Which of the following is the most common cause of upper airway obstruction in an unconscious adult?

A. Food
B. Dentures
C. Bronchospasm
D. Relaxed tongue

7 Which assessment finding is a symptom of complete upper airway obstruction?

A. Hoarseness
B. Inability to speak
C. Forceful cough
D. Wheezing

8 Which nursing action is most appropriate in the initial management of a conscious adult with complete upper airway obstruction by a foreign body?

A. Administering four quick back blows with the heel of the hand between the victim's scapulae
B. Administering abdominal thrusts
C. Allowing the victim to expel the foreign body through vigorous coughing
D. Administering artificial respiration

9 Which action would be the nurse's highest priority if a patient suddenly goes into respiratory arrest?

A. Auscultate for breath sounds
B. Feel for a carotid pulse
C. Insert an oropharyngeal airway
D. Open the patient's airway

10 Which statement about endotracheal intubation for a patient in respiratory arrest is *true?*

A. It is necessary to ensure adequate ventilation
B. It should be performed as the initial step in airway management
C. It should be attempted only after other oxygenation methods have failed
D. It should be performed within 2 minutes of the onset of respiratory arrest

11 Which statement about esophageal obturator airway management is *true?*

A. It may damage the trachea
B. It requires visualization of the airway for insertion
C. It should be removed before endotracheal intubation is performed
D. Its removal is commonly followed by immediate regurgitation

12 The nurse assesses a patient at risk for respiratory failure. All of the following are early signs of respiratory failure *except:*

A. Restlessness
B. Tachycardia
C. Cyanosis
D. Tachypnea

13 When assessing a patient with acute respiratory failure resulting from impaired ventilation, the nurse would initially expect to note:

A. Hypoxia
B. Hypoxia and hypercapnia
C. Hypercapnia
D. Hypocapnia

14 Acute respiratory failure in a patient with essentially normal lung tissue usually is indicated by:

A. Shortness of breath, a PaO_2 of 80 mm Hg, and a $PaCO_2$ of 40 mm Hg
B. Diaphoresis, chest pain, and shortness of breath
C. A $PaCO_2$ greater than 50 mm Hg and a PaO_2 less than 50 mm Hg
D. A $PaCO_2$ less than 40 mm Hg and a PaO_2 greater than 50 mm Hg

15 Naloxone (Narcan) effectively reverses the respiratory depression associated with overdose of all the following medications *except:*

A. Methadone hydrochloride (Dolophine) and oxycodone with aspirin (Percodan)
B. Diazepam (Valium)
C. Morphine sulfate and meperidine hydrochloride (Demerol)
D. Chloral hydrate (Noctec)

16 Which statement about the aspiration of gastric contents is *true?*

A. An unconscious patient is at low risk for aspiration because regurgitation is impossible in this state
B. Aspiration of gastric contents is more common in adults than children
C. Adult respiratory distress syndrome can occur as a result of aspiration because of the high pH of gastric contents
D. Aspiration of gastric contents commonly results from attempts to ventilate an obstructed airway

17 Which factor should be the nurse's most important consideration in efforts to prevent aspiration?

A. Level of consciousness
B. Body position
C. Degree of gastric distention
D. Cardiac sphincter integrity

18 A 34-year-old woman is found unconscious in the emergency department (ED) waiting room. She is diaphoretic and apneic, with a slightly irregular pulse rate of 88 beats/minute. She is ventilated effectively with oxygen. Which drug treatment would the nurse expect the physician to order next?

A. Lidocaine (Xylocaine)
B. Naloxone
C. Epinephrine
D. Dextrose

19 Which statement about airway management is *true?*

A. Nasotracheal intubation is a logical choice in a patient with maxillofacial injury
B. Cricothyroidotomy is the formation of an opening for an artificial airway above the vocal cords
C. Tracheotomy is a less hazardous procedure than cricothyroidotomy
D. The carina is the landmark by which proper depth of endotracheal intubation should be measured

20 Which is the most common cause of impaired gas exchange after blunt chest trauma?

A. Apnea or hypopnea
B. Flail chest
C. Pulmonary contusion
D. Phrenic nerve paralysis

21 Fracture of the scapula or first or second rib indicates a serious force of injury and a high probability of underlying tissue damage. The nurse knows that, in the emergent phase of care, pulmonary contusion is best indicated by:

A. Auscultation
B. Arterial blood gas analysis
C. Radiographic studies
D. Dyspnea assessment

22 Which assessment finding is indicative of hypoxia?

A. Deterioration in level of consciousness
B. Change in urine output
C. Peripheral vasoconstriction
D. Delayed capillary refill time

23 The nurse knows that an increase in negative pressure inside the pleural space will result in:

A. Lung collapse
B. Tension pneumothorax
C. Normal inspiration
D. Normal expiration

24 The nurse would suspect dyspnea in a patient with a stab wound in the left upper abdominal quadrant to result from:

A. Pain and anxiety
B. Peritoneal irritation
C. Gastric rupture
D. Associated chest injury

25 Development of sudden subcutaneous emphysema and a crunching or crackling sound associated with auscultation of the apical heart rate is indicative of:

A. Empyema
B. Mediastinal air leak
C. Pericarditis
D. Fat embolism

26 The nurse's discharge instructions for a patient with a rib contusion and a minor rib fracture include information on the need to report fever, dyspnea on exertion, sputum production, or chest pain should any of these symptoms occur. These symptoms are indicative of:

A. Pneumonia or costochondritis
B. Empyema
C. Pulmonary hypertension
D. Pneumothorax

27 Which size chest tube should be prepared for a suspected hemothorax in an adult?

A. #20 French
B. #28 French
C. #36 French
D. #44 French

28 Autotransfusion usually is indicated for a patient with which condition?

A. Left-sided hemothorax with hypotension
B. Hypotension secondary to spinal cord injury
C. Avulsion amputation of the left thigh and leg
D. Hepatic hemorrhage secondary to a gunshot wound

29 A woman with a history of coronary artery disease is standing outside a supermarket when she suddenly complains of chest pain and collapses in full cardiac arrest. Bystanders initiate basic life support measures until emergency medical technicians (EMTs) arrive. The EMTs properly intubate and ventilate the patient; an automatic chest compressor also is used. One of the EMTs radios the ED nurse that the patient is not responding. Which factor is probably *not* contributing to the patient's unresponsiveness?

A. Pericardial tamponade
B. Hypocapnia
C. Tension pneumothorax
D. Volume deficit

30 A 25-year-old man drives to the ED after falling off a roof and landing on his right side on a concrete abutment. His chief complaints are dyspnea and significant chest pain. All of the following nursing actions would ensure proper ventilation and perfusion in this patient *except:*

A. Splinting the affected side with a pillow
B. Encouraging slow, deep breathing
C. Positioning the patient on his right side
D. Positioning the patient on his left side

31 Which injury constitutes flail chest?

A. Single fractures of the fourth, fifth, sixth, and seventh left lateral ribs

B. Single fractures of the seventh and eighth left and right anterior ribs

C. Fractured xiphoid process

D. Fractured sternum

32 The nurse knows that flail chest is easiest to assess:

A. When the thoracic fracture occurs posteriorly

B. When the thoracic fracture occurs anteriorly

C. In a conscious patient with well-developed musculature

D. Immediately after the injury

33 In a patient with a massive flail chest, all of the following factors are indications for ventilatory support *except:*

A. Advanced age and obesity

B. Progressive breathing fatigue

C. Hypercapnia, hypoxia, and dyspnea

D. Imminent abdominal surgery

34 In a patient with multiple rib fractures, which nursing intervention would be appropriate to encourage optimal ventilation?

A. Binding the chest wall

B. Frequently administering low-dose narcotics, as ordered

C. Performing postural drainage and incentive spirometry

D. Encouraging forceful coughing after chest percussion

SITUATION

A 50-year-old man is admitted to the ED with a diagnosis of suspected pulmonary embolus. He is dyspneic and anxious. The physician plans to start heparin therapy.

Questions 35 to 39 refer to the above situation.

35 Which laboratory test results are consistent with a diagnosis of pulmonary embolism?

A. A PaO_2 of 70 mm Hg and an elevated lactic dehydrogenase (LDH) level

B. A normal LDH level and a PaO_2 of 70 mm Hg

C. A white blood cell (WBC) count of 10,000/mm³ and a PaO_2 of 85 mm Hg

D. A WBC count of 20,000/mm³ and a PaO_2 of 85 mm Hg

36 Which nursing diagnosis would be the highest priority for this patient?

A. Anxiety related to hypoxia and pain

B. Pain related to pulmonary ischemia

C. Potential for injury related to hemorrhage from anticoagulant therapy

D. Impaired gas exchange related to altered pulmonary tissue perfusion

37 When the nurse dorsiflexes the patient's foot, the patient complains of calf pain. The nurse correctly interprets this response as an indication of a positive:

A. Trousseau's sign

B. Homans' sign

C. Kehr's sign

D. Babinski's reflex

38 Which electrocardiographic finding would the nurse expect to find in a patient with pulmonary embolism?

A. Sinus tachycardia

B. Increased R waves in lead V_2

C. First-degree atrioventricular block

D. Left axis deviation

39 The physician orders the nurse to begin the patient's heparin therapy. Which statement about the use of heparin therapy for pulmonary embolism is *true*?

A. Heparin helps to dissolve existing clots

B. Heparin reduces the risk of secondary thrombi formation

C. The heparin dosage is based on the patient's prothrombin time

D. Bolus administration is preferred for the high-risk patient

SITUATION

A 69-year-old man is admitted to the ED with difficulty breathing. He has a 50-pack-year history of smoking. Upon examination, the nurse notes the patient's reliance on accessory muscles for breathing and his barrel chest.

Questions 40 and 41 refer to the above situation.

40 The nurse would anticipate initial emergency treatment for a patient with respiratory distress secondary to chronic obstructive pulmonary disease (COPD) to include:

A. Administration of 30% oxygen via face mask and bronchodilator therapy

B. Administration of 50% oxygen via humidity mask and bronchodilator therapy

C. Administration of 100% oxygen via face mask and 2 mg of morphine sulfate I.V. push to decrease anxiety

D. Endotracheal intubation and positive-pressure ventilation

41 Which nursing intervention would be appropriate for a patient with respiratory distress secondary to COPD?

A. Place the patient in a supine position in preparation for endotracheal intubation

B. Place the patient in high-Fowler's position or leaning upright over an overbed table

C. Administer morphine sulfate, as ordered, to decrease anxiety

D. Perform postural drainage and chest percussion

SITUATION

A 56-year-old accountant arrives at the ED, complaining of dyspnea and anxiety that seemed to have progressively worsened while he and his family were at the movies. A smoker for more than 35 years, the patient had been treated for chronic bronchitis, which became increasingly severe with each attack. He claims that this is his worst episode. The physician diagnoses COPD resulting from exacerbation of chronic bronchitis with mild emphysema.

Questions 42 to 54 refer to the above situation.

42 Which history finding is the most significant factor contributing to this patient's condition?

A. Anxiety
B. Smoking
C. Occupation
D. Activity level

43 The nurse knows that chronic bronchitis is classified as COPD because of which pathogenic occurrence?

A. Increased goblet cell production and disappearance of cilia
B. Hyperplasia of bronchiolar mucus-secreting glands
C. Hyperplasia and inflammation of goblet cells and increased production of thick mucus
D. Increased production and stimulation of neutrophils and macrophages

44 The nurse would expect the physician to order all of the following treatments for a patient with COPD *except:*

A. Fluid restriction
B. Bronchodilator therapy
C. Chest physiotherapy
D. Diuretic therapy

45 The patient wonders aloud whether it is too late to quit smoking. The nurse correctly explains that if the patient stops smoking now:

A. His symptoms will disappear and he will be cured
B. His cough and sputum production will decrease and his pulmonary function tests will improve
C. His symptoms will not improve because too much damage has been done
D. He will suffer much stress because of his illness

46 Which term best describes the condition of a patient with the above medical history and evidence of alveolar destruction?

A. Pink puffer
B. Blue bloater
C. Hyperreactive airway
D. None of the above

47 The nurse knows that cor pulmonale is a complication of COPD secondary to:

A. Atrophy of the right ventricle caused by heart failure
B. Stimulation of erythropoiesis, which decreases blood viscosity
C. Decreased intravascular blood volume with arterial congestion
D. Pulmonary hypertension caused by vasoconstriction in response to hypoxia

48 When assessing a patient with cor pulmonale resulting from COPD, the nurse would expect to note:

A. Bibasilar crackles
B. Capillary refill time of 4 seconds
C. Poor skin turgor
D. Jugular vein distention

49 In which condition is small-airway obstruction usually irreversible?

A. Asthma
B. Atelectasis
C. Pneumonia
D. Emphysema

50 Which information should the nurse plan to include in the discharge instructions for this patient?

A. The importance of an annual chest X-ray and spirometry testing
B. The need for weight control and vitamin supplements
C. The need for influenza and pneumonia vaccines
D. The benefits of living in a warm, dry climate with air conditioning

51 Nursing assessment of a patient with emphysema typically reveals barrel chest, which results from:

A. Hyperinflation and overdistention of alveoli
B. Distention and destruction of the primary lobules
C. Hyperventilation in response to hypoxemia and hypocapnia
D. Hypoventilation in response to hypoxemia and hypercapnia

52 Which nursing intervention is useful early in the management of a patient with dyspnea caused by emphysema?

A. Inspiratory muscle training
B. Postural drainage
C. Pursed-lip breathing exercises
D. Chest percussion and vibration

53 Chronic cough is common in COPD. When planning the discharge instructions for a patient with COPD, the nurse should remember to advise the patient to avoid:

A. Hydration and aerosol humidification
B. Spicy foods
C. Cough suppressants and self-medication with antihistamines
D. Chest physiotherapy and postural drainage

54 Which nursing diagnostic category would be appropriate for a patient with COPD?

A. Altered nutrition: More than body requirements
B. Ineffective individual coping
C. Potential for injury
D. Fluid volume excess

SITUATION

At 3 a.m., a 13-year-old girl is brought to the ED by her mother because of coughing and severe dyspnea. Her medical history reveals allergic rhinitis and eczema since early childhood. The nurse notes that the patient is wheezing and talking with effort. When questioned about precipitating factors, the mother states that her daughter had put on a new acrylic sweater to go to a makeup demonstration at a friend's house the previous evening and that she also had worn a new down jacket, which she is wearing now. The physician diagnoses acute asthmatic attack.

Questions 55 to 61 refer to the above situation.

55 Which term best describes the type of asthma precipitated by a known allergen?

A. Intrinsic
B. Extrinsic
C. Mixed
D. Idiopathic

56 The nurse suspects that the patient's asthma attack was precipitated by the:

A. Season
B. Makeup
C. Acrylic sweater
D. Down jacket

57 The patient complains of increased dyspnea and tightness in her chest. The nurse knows that these symptoms may result from all of the following *except:*

A. Bronchospasm
B. Mucus production in response to mucosal edema
C. Bronchiolar constriction during expiration
D. Alveolar constriction during respiration

58 Which additional findings would the nurse expect to note during assessment of this patient?

A. Rhonchi and labored inspiratory breathing
B. Coughing and pursed-lip breathing
C. Prolonged wheezing on expiration with a nonproductive cough
D. Shallow wheezing on inspiration with a productive cough

59 Which early treatment is likely to improve this patient's condition most rapidly?

A. Administration of prednisone (Deltasone) orally and terbutaline sulfate (Brethine) orally
B. Administration of cromolyn sodium (Intal) by inhalation and terbutaline sulfate S.C.
C. Administration of metaproterenol sulfate (Alupent) by inhalation and aminophylline (Phyllocontin) I.V.
D. Administration of oxygen via a face mask and lactated Ringer's solution I.V.

60 Which nursing intervention would be most appropriate when treating this patient's asthma attack?

A. Maintaining a calm, reassuring attitude while with the patient
B. Teaching the patient about measures to prevent future attacks
C. Keeping the patient's mother away from the bedside
D. Providing diversional therapy to avoid panic or anxiety

61 When writing discharge instructions for this patient, the nurse should include information on the importance of:

A. Obtaining prompt treatment for all upper respiratory tract infections
B. Attending an aerobic exercise program on a regular basis
C. Participating in outdoor activities to improve respiratory aeration
D. Eliminating any exercise regimen to prevent undue exertion

SITUATION

The nurse is examining a 21-year-old man in the ED. His temperature is 103.6° F (39.8° C) rectally; pulse rate, 88 beats/minute; and respiratory rate, 28 breaths/minute. He complains of chills and a productive cough with rust-colored sputum. The physician diagnoses bacterial pneumonia.

Questions 62 and 63 refer to the above situation.

62 The nurse knows that the most common type of bacterial pneumonia is caused by:

A. *Staphylococcus aureus*
B. *Streptococcus pneumoniae*
C. *Streptococcus pyogenes*
D. *Bacillus anthracis*

63 Which diagnostic studies would the nurse expect the physician to order for this patient?

A. Bronchoscopy and electrolyte studies
B. Pulmonary function tests and arterial blood gas measurements
C. Gram stain of sputum and chest X-rays
D. Lung scan and sputum cultures

SITUATION

A 4-year-old boy is brought to the ED because of dysphagia, excessive salivation, mild respiratory distress, orthopnea, and fever. The child's father reports an abrupt onset of symptoms, with the child refusing to lie down for a nap. The physician diagnoses epiglottitis and arranges for the child to be admitted to the pediatric unit.

Questions 64 to 67 refer to the above situation.

64 Which assessment findings are commonly associated with epiglottitis?

A. Cherry red, edematous epiglottis and muffled voice sounds
B. Cyanotic, edematous epiglottis and muffled voice sounds
C. Grayish, edematous epiglottis and muffled voice sounds
D. Pink, edematous epiglottis and aphonia

65 When a child in the acute stage of epiglottitis begins to exhibit airway obstruction, the nurse's main priority would be to:

A. Request the parents to leave the room
B. Secure intubation and tracheotomy equipment
C. Obtain the parents' consent to perform a tracheotomy
D. Administer oxygen via a face mask

66 Which factor should the nurse consider when planning this patient's care?

A. The possibility of agitation and combative behavior
B. Bacteremia, which occurs in almost all cases of epiglottitis
C. The possibility of a productive cough and vomiting
D. Laryngospasm, which may occur upon attempted visualization of the child's epiglottis

67 Which is the primary reason for administering chloral hydrate to an intubated child with epiglottitis?

A. To produce mild sedation and prevent seizure activity from fever
B. To produce mild sedation without drying respiratory secretions
C. To promote rest through respiratory muscle paralysis
D. To reduce epiglottic edema and promote rest

SITUATION

A 19-month-old boy with respiratory distress is being examined by the ED nurse. The child's mother reports that he has had a temperature of 101° F (38.3° C), fatigue, and hoarseness for the past 2 days, during which time the hoarseness and fatigue have progressively increased. The patient developed a barking cough during the night. The physician diagnoses laryngotracheobronchitis croup.

Questions 68 to 72 refer to the above situation.

68 Upon assessment, the nurse would expect to note which early signs of hypoxemia in this patient?

A. Use of accessory respiratory muscles and development of a resonant cough
B. Expiratory stridor and cyanosis
C. Lethargy and tachypnea
D. Restlessness and a rapidly increasing heart rate

69 The nurse knows that management of a child with croup is primarily directed toward:

A. Maintaining the patient's airway and adequate respiratory exchange
B. Maintaining acid-base balance
C. Increasing the humidification of inspired air
D. Liquefying respiratory secretions

70 The nurse's care plan for this patient should include a notation to inform the parents about the importance of avoiding the administration of:

A. Antitussives
B. Acetaminophen
C. Acetylsalicylic acid
D. Decongestants

71 The nurse knows that, to ensure adequate respiratory exchange, this child should be placed in:

A. Semi-Fowler's position with the neck slightly extended
B. Semi-Fowler's position with the neck slightly flexed
C. Supine position
D. Prone position

72 The nurse initiates I.V. therapy, as ordered, and monitors the child's hydration status by assessing:

A. Weight, fluid intake and output, and serum electrolyte levels
B. Weight, fluid intake and output, and fontanelle tension
C. Skin turgor, fluid intake and output, and fontanelle tension
D. Skin turgor, fluid intake and output, and urine specific gravity

SITUATION

A 64-year-old man with emphysema is admitted to the ED because of a sudden attack of dyspnea. Auscultation reveals no breath sounds over the right lung. The physician diagnoses spontaneous pneumothorax and inserts a chest tube.

Questions 73 and 74 refer to the above situation.

73 The patient's chest tube is ordered to be on suction, at 20 cm of water pressure. When checking the chest tube drainage system at the start of the shift, the nurse notices continuous bubbling in the suction chamber. The nurse correctly interprets this to mean:

A. The tubing or system is leaking
B. Bronchial disruption has developed
C. Esophageal fistula has developed
D. The system is functioning normally

74 The patient's lung is well-expanded, and the chest tube is positioned to allow for water-seal drainage without suction. The nurse should anticipate that the water-seal level will:

A. No longer be needed
B. Rise upon spontaneous inspiration
C. Rise with positive-pressure ventilation
D. Fall during forceful coughing

SITUATION

A 26-year-old man diagnosed with spontaneous pneumothorax is being monitored in the holding room overnight. Because the patient had limited symptoms and lung involvement, decompression of the pleural cavity was not initiated.

Questions 75 and 76 refer to the above situation.

75 Which assessment finding should the nurse report immediately to the physician?

A. Pain on deep inspiration
B. Expanding hyperresonance on lung percussion
C. Respiratory rate of 20 breaths/minute, moderate depth, and easy arousal
D. Heart rate of 64 beats/minute

76 The next morning, an expiratory upright chest X-ray shows full lung expansion. The patient is instructed to report to his physician any findings indicative of recurrence. Which finding would be least useful in evaluating recurrence of a pneumothorax?

A. Activity intolerance
B. Fever and chills
C. Sudden, sharp chest pain
D. Diaphoresis and dyspnea

Respiratory Emergencies Questions

SITUATION

A paramedic radios data to the base station regarding the status of a 64-year-old man who is showing signs and symptoms of an acute tension pneumothorax after involvement in an automobile accident. The paramedics are instructed to perform a needle thoracotomy.

Questions 77 to 80 refer to the above situation.

77 The nurse anticipates that the paramedic will correctly insert the needle:

A. Under the fourth rib at the anterior axillary line
B. Over the third rib at the midclavicular line
C. On the side toward which the trachea deviates
D. On the right side to avoid puncturing the heart

78 Which signs and symptoms are characteristic of tension pneumothorax?

A. Cyanosis, chest pain, and vasodilation
B. Tachycardia, subcutaneous emphysema, and dullness on percussion
C. Paradoxical chest movement, bradycardia, and high cardiac output
D. Dyspnea, jugular vein distention, hypotension, and tracheal deviation

79 After thoracotomy, the patient's condition does not improve despite assisted ventilation with 100% oxygen and rapid infusion of crystalloids. Which other condition causes similar symptoms?

A. Large diaphragmatic hernia
B. Cardiac contusion
C. COPD
D. 10% hemothorax

80 When the patient arrives in the ED, a chest tube is inserted. The tube is connected to a water-seal bottle that has a moderate air and fluid leak seen on expiration. When the patient is taken to the radiology department, the bottle is accidently broken. Which nursing action should be taken?

A. Remove the chest tube immediately to prevent aspiration of glass particles

B. Apply a clamp to the chest tube near the insertion site, and instruct the patient to exhale deeply

C. Pinch the chest tube, place the end of the tube in a bottle of sterile saline solution or water, and encourage the patient to cough and breathe deeply

D. Use the phone in radiology to order a new bottle, and do not manipulate the chest tube

Answer Sheet

	A B C D		A B C D		A B C D
1	○ ○ ○ ○	31	○ ○ ○ ○	61	○ ○ ○ ○
2	○ ○ ○ ○	32	○ ○ ○ ○	62	○ ○ ○ ○
3	○ ○ ○ ○	33	○ ○ ○ ○	63	○ ○ ○ ○
4	○ ○ ○ ○	34	○ ○ ○ ○	64	○ ○ ○ ○
5	○ ○ ○ ○	35	○ ○ ○ ○	65	○ ○ ○ ○
6	○ ○ ○ ○	36	○ ○ ○ ○	66	○ ○ ○ ○
7	○ ○ ○ ○	37	○ ○ ○ ○	67	○ ○ ○ ○
8	○ ○ ○ ○	38	○ ○ ○ ○	68	○ ○ ○ ○
9	○ ○ ○ ○	39	○ ○ ○ ○	69	○ ○ ○ ○
10	○ ○ ○ ○	40	○ ○ ○ ○	70	○ ○ ○ ○
11	○ ○ ○ ○	41	○ ○ ○ ○	71	○ ○ ○ ○
12	○ ○ ○ ○	42	○ ○ ○ ○	72	○ ○ ○ ○
13	○ ○ ○ ○	43	○ ○ ○ ○	73	○ ○ ○ ○
14	○ ○ ○ ○	44	○ ○ ○ ○	74	○ ○ ○ ○
15	○ ○ ○ ○	45	○ ○ ○ ○	75	○ ○ ○ ○
16	○ ○ ○ ○	46	○ ○ ○ ○	76	○ ○ ○ ○
17	○ ○ ○ ○	47	○ ○ ○ ○	77	○ ○ ○ ○
18	○ ○ ○ ○	48	○ ○ ○ ○	78	○ ○ ○ ○
19	○ ○ ○ ○	49	○ ○ ○ ○	79	○ ○ ○ ○
20	○ ○ ○ ○	50	○ ○ ○ ○	80	○ ○ ○ ○
21	○ ○ ○ ○	51	○ ○ ○ ○		
22	○ ○ ○ ○	52	○ ○ ○ ○		
23	○ ○ ○ ○	53	○ ○ ○ ○		
24	○ ○ ○ ○	54	○ ○ ○ ○		
25	○ ○ ○ ○	55	○ ○ ○ ○		
26	○ ○ ○ ○	56	○ ○ ○ ○		
27	○ ○ ○ ○	57	○ ○ ○ ○		
28	○ ○ ○ ○	58	○ ○ ○ ○		
29	○ ○ ○ ○	59	○ ○ ○ ○		
30	○ ○ ○ ○	60	○ ○ ○ ○		

1 Correct answer — **B**

Atelectasis is indicated when bronchial breath sounds are heard over the right middle lung lobe. Bronchial sounds normally are heard only over the manubrium of the sternum and along the sternal borders, which are located over the trachea. They are characteristically high-pitched, loud, and harsh in quality, with a pause between the inspiratory and expiratory phases. Bronchial breath sounds heard over the lung periphery may indicate abnormal sound transmission because of consolidated lung tissue, as in atelectasis.

2 Correct answer — **B**

Consolidated lung areas typically produce a flat or dull sound on percussion because of the increased mass. Percussion over a normal lung produces a resonant or hollow sound that is of low pitch and intensity. An overinflated lung, such as in emphysema, typically produces a sustained hyperresonant sound. Tympanic sounds are high-pitched and are produced by air-containing organs, such as the stomach.

3 Correct answer — **A**

Bronchovesicular breath sounds normally are auscultated over the large bronchi, below the clavicles and between the scapulae. These sounds are of moderate amplitude and medium to high in pitch, representing a mixture of bronchial and vesicular sounds. In other lung areas, bronchovesicular sounds may indicate consolidation or other abnormalities. Bronchial sounds, which typically are loud and high-pitched, normally are auscultated over the trachea.

4 Correct answer — **D**

Any condition that produces disruption of alveolar function, consolidation, or compression (such as pulmonary fibrosis, pleural effusion, or chronic obstructive pulmonary disease [COPD]) may result in decreased or absent vesicular sounds. Vesicular sounds, produced by the opening of alveoli on inspiration and the movement of air through the larynx (glottic hiss) during expiration, are of low amplitude and medium to low pitch; they may be described as swishing or rustling.

5 Correct answer — **C**

Palpation is commonly used in respiratory assessment to determine the degree of respiratory excursion as well as to identify areas of tenderness, to assess for abnormalities, and to elicit fremitus. The nurse assesses respiratory excursion by determining if each lung expands to the same degree at different chest locations. This is accomplished by placing the hands, with thumbs together and fingers spread, over the center of the chest. As the patient takes a deep breath, the nurse notes if the fingers and thumbs move apart to an equal degree. Each lung lobe, or its equivalent area on the chest wall, should be assessed in this manner. Unequal excursion may be caused by such conditions as atelectasis or pneumothorax.

6 Correct answer—**D**

A relaxed tongue is the most common cause of upper airway obstruction in the unconscious adult. Because of insufficient muscle tone, the relaxed tongue can fall over the back of the throat, obstructing the pharynx and larynx. Since the tongue is attached to the lower jaw, moving the lower jaw forward (as in the head-tilt-chin-lift maneuver) lifts the tongue away from the back of the throat and opens the airway. Performing this maneuver may restore spontaneous respirations in an apneic patient.

7 Correct answer—**B**

Complete airway obstruction is marked by the absence of air movement and coughing and by the inability to speak. Partial airway obstruction may produce good or poor air exchange. A patient with good air exchange typically is able to cough forcefully but may experience wheezing between coughs. A patient with poor air exchange typically has an ineffective, weak cough, inspiratory stridor, and cyanosis.

8 Correct answer—**B**

The American Heart Association recommends administering abdominal thrusts (the Heimlich maneuver) as the initial management for relieving foreign-body airway obstruction. This procedure involves the delivery of repeated subdiaphragmatic thrusts, each one delivered with enough force to remove a sufficient volume of air from the lungs and produce an artificial cough capable of expelling a foreign body from the airway. The procedure should be repeated, as necessary, until the object is expelled from the victim. The efficacy of back blows in relieving airway obstruction is not well documented. An adult with complete airway obstruction would be unable to cough to expel a foreign body. Administering artificial respiration would be of no help in ventilating the victim if the obstruction has not been relieved.

9 Correct answer—**D**

If a patient suddenly goes into respiratory arrest, the nurse's highest priority would be to open the patient's airway. In an emergency, the nurse should always follow the ABCs of airway management, ensuring the patient's Airway, Breathing, and Circulation sequentially. The airway may be opened using a head-tilt-chin-lift or jaw-thrust maneuver. This action allows the victim to resume spontaneous respirations without the need for further intervention.

10 Correct answer—C

Endotracheal intubation should be attempted only after other oxygenation methods have failed; it should never be used as the initial procedure for ventilation in respiratory arrest. The lungs should be well-oxygenated before any intubation attempt; adequate ventilation can be provided with the use of a bag-valve-mask device. Intubation requires the skill of a trained individual who can efficiently complete the procedure in 20 to 30 seconds.

11 Correct answer—D

Esophageal obturator airway removal commonly is followed by immediate regurgitation of stomach contents; therefore, suction equipment must be readily available. The patient who does not have an endotracheal tube in place should be turned on the left side before removal of the esophageal obturator airway to prevent aspiration of stomach contents.

The esophageal obturator airway consists of a tube approximately 14½" (37 cm) long that is open at the top and has a blind end at the bottom. The blind end is inserted into the esophagus; the airway is not visualized. An inflatable cuff is located just above the blind end, and several side holes located near the upper end allow passage of air from the interior of the tube into the pharynx. Possible hazards associated with the use of this airway include laceration and rupture of the esophagus, not the trachea. Performing endotracheal intubation with an esophageal obturator airway in place is possible.

12 Correct answer—C

Cyanosis is not an early sign of respiratory failure. Restlessness, tachycardia, and tachypnea are early signs of hypoxia and hypoxemia that occur in respiratory failure. Cyanosis, which occurs secondary to unoxygenation of hemoglobin in the capillaries, is imperceptible until 5 g of unoxygenated hemoglobin/100 ml of blood is detected. Therefore, cyanosis is a later sign of respiratory failure. Cyanosis may not present in a patient with a decreased hematocrit.

13 Correct answer—B

Acute respiratory failure resulting from impaired ventilation initially produces hypoxia and hypercapnia. Ventilation impairment (such as

occurs in atelectasis, emphysema and the late stages of asthma)
prevents gas exchange, leading to decreased oxygen and carbon
dioxide retention in the blood. Oxygenation impairment (such as
occurs in lung tumors and pulmonary edema) initially produces only
hypoxia. Although oxygen reaches the alveoli, it is either not absorbed
or not used. Carbon dioxide is not retained because it is 20 times more
diffusable than oxygen. Hypocapnia and hypoxia are seen in the early
stages of asthma because of the blowing off of carbon dioxide that
results from tachypnea.

14 Correct answer — C

In a patient with no underlying lung disease and essentially normal
lung tissue, respiratory failure usually is indicated by a $PaCO_2$ greater
than 50 mm Hg and a PaO_2 less than 50 mm Hg (oxygen saturation
below 85%). Respiratory failure is defined as any condition in which
the blood oxygen content is insufficient to fulfill tissue demands for
oxygen secondary to decreased lung function. A diagnosis of
respiratory failure must be based on the patient's history, clinical
appearance, and changes in serial arterial blood gas (ABG) studies. A
patient with an obstructive disorder, such as COPD, will function with
abnormal blood gas levels, such as those indicative of hypoxia and
hypercapnia.

15 Correct answer — D

Chloral hydrate, a sedative-hypnotic drug, has no known response to
naloxone, a pure opioid antagonist. Naloxone effectively reverses the
respiratory depression associated with overdose of such opioid
analgesics as methadone hydrochloride, oxycodone with aspirin,
morphine sulfate, and meperidine hydrochloride within 1 to 2 minutes
of administration. It also effectively reverses the sedative effects and
depressed blood pressure produced by these agents. Antagonism of
some depressant effects of diazepam has been shown in people.

16 Correct answer — D

Aspiration of gastric contents commonly results from attempts to
ventilate an obstructed airway. Excessive air pressure is needed to
inflate a partially or completely obstructed airway. Since air follows
the path of least resistance, a large volume of air travels down the
esophagus and into the stomach, resulting in gastric distention and a
high risk of regurgitation and aspiration. To decrease the risk of
distention, the American Heart Association has issued new basic life
support guidelines that alter the recommended speed of airflow
delivery during mouth-to-mouth or mouth-to-mask resuscitation. An
unconscious patient is at high risk for aspiration because of depressed
or absent gag and cough reflexes. Aspiration of gastric contents is

more common in children than adults. Children have a greater tendency for aerophagia (air swallowing) when crying or frightened; this increases the risk of gastric distention and aspiration. Adult respiratory distress syndrome (ARDS) can occur as a result of aspiration because of the low pH of gastric contents.

17 Correct answer—A

Level of consciousness should be the nurse's most important consideration when determining a patient's risk of aspiration. An alert, cooperative patient with intact cerebral, brain stem, and spinal input typically can swallow with concurrent glottic closure while maintaining cough and gag reflexes; such a patient is at decreased risk for aspiration. A sedated or unconscious patient, however, has reduced protective reflex mechanisms and therefore is at increased risk for aspiration. Appropriate nursing interventions for preventing aspiration include ensuring proper positioning (semi-Fowler's or side-lying), including the positioning of the alert patient who is immobilized for spinal precautions; ensuring that suction equipment is accessible; and monitoring for gastric distention and patency of nasogastric tubes. The cardiac sphincter is the lower esophageal sphincter near the opening of the stomach; its integrity cannot be assessed easily in the clinical setting.

18 Correct answer—D

In this situation, the nurse would expect the physician to order dextrose administration because the patient's symptoms suggest severe hypoglycemia. Because neurons, which are glucose-dependent, become irreversibly damaged when deprived of glucose, administering dextrose I.V. can help prevent any further damage. If possible, the nurse should draw a blood specimen before administering dextrose to document the serum glucose level. After administration, the nurse should observe the patient's reaction to the drug. Usually, naloxone is given along with dextrose early in therapy to reverse possible respiratory depression from a drug overdose. However, since the patient's airway is not being maintained, administering this medication is not the highest priority. Lidocaine and epinephrine are not indicated because the patient has no lethal arrhythmias.

19 Correct answer—D

The carina is the landmark by which proper depth of endotracheal intubation should be measured. Placement of the tip of the endotracheal tube too near or below the carina can result in right main-stem bronchus intubation or atelectasis of the left lung. Placement too far above the carina increases the risk of vocal cord damage or inadvertent extubation.

Nasotracheal intubation is not necessarily a logical choice in a patient with a maxillofacial injury. Despite the association of facial injury with spinal cord injury and the fact that nasotracheal intubation is safer than endotracheal intubation in a patient with a suspected spinal cord injury (it requires less extension and manipulation of the patient's neck), nasotracheal intubation is hazardous because of the risk of nasal fracture, frontal skull and cribriform plate damage, and sinus or intracranial infection. Cricothyroidotomy is an emergency procedure involving the formation of an opening for an artificial airway in the cricothyroid membrane, which is below the thyroid cartilage (Adam's apple) and above the cricoid cartilage. The vocal cords are above these landmarks. Because cricothyroidotomy involves catheterization with a needle, it is less invasive and traumatic than a tracheostomy.

20 Correct answer—C

Pulmonary contusion is the most common cause of impaired gas exchange after blunt thoracic trauma. Blunt or penetrating trauma to the lung characteristically results in the accumulation of blood and fluid in the involved interstitial tissue, alveoli, and small bronchi. The reduced vital capacity and pulmonary compliance together with increased secretions from the injured lung produce increasing atelectasis. This combination of atelectasis, disrupted tissue, and extravasated blood results in impaired gas exchange. Flail chest is a type of penetrating chest trauma. Apnea, hypopnea, and phrenic nerve paralysis may occur after spinal cord injury.

21 Correct answer—C

During the emergent phase of care, pulmonary contusion is best indicated by radiographic studies. Pulmonary contusion, a bruise on the lung that causes interstitial edema and hemorrhage, may appear as patchy infiltrates initially on chest X-ray; later X-rays typically show consolidation. Auscultation may not initially reveal abnormalities unless other injuries are present. ABG test results, although checked serially, may not demonstrate intrapulmonary shunting in the emergent phase. Hypoxemia may be delayed; therefore, dyspnea may not be evident. Signs and symptoms depend on the severity of contusion and associated injuries. Pulmonary contusion may evolve into ARDS.

22 Correct answer—A

Changes in level of consciousness, such as restlessness, confusion, irritability, and decreased responsiveness, indicate serious hypoxia. Peripheral vasoconstriction, changes in urine output, and delayed

386

Respiratory Emergencies Answers

capillary refill are related primarily to reduced vascular volume and
inadequate perfusion.

23 Correct answer – C

An increase in negative pressure inside the pleural space results in
normal inspiration. Airflow into the lungs normally travels from an
area of higher pressure to an area of lower pressure. As the
diaphragm contracts, the thorax enlarges and the visceral and
parietal pleura move with it. Healthy lungs will recoil and pull away
from the chest wall, which pulls the parietal pleural layer, creating
negative (subatmospheric) pressure within the intrapleural space. The
more the thorax enlarges, the more the lung stretches and tries to
recoil, creating more and more negative pressure. Outside air at
atmospheric pressure flows into the lungs during this inspiratory
process. Positive pleural pressure will collapse the lung, resulting in a
pneumothorax.

24 Correct answer – D

Dyspnea in this situation is most likely caused by an associated chest
injury. The lungs extend to the sixth rib anteriorly and the eighth rib
laterally, and may descend to the twelfth rib posteriorly on deep
inspiration. The nurse should suspect a chest injury in any patient
with a blunt or penetrating injury to the upper abdomen or a gunshot
wound in the same area because of the possible trajectory of the knife
or bullet.

25 Correct answer – B

These findings are indicative of a mediastinal air leak. Subcutaneous
emphysema may occur in pneumothorax or any condition that causes
a sudden increase in intrathoracic pressure that results in alveolar
rupture. Air dissects to the loose mediastinal tissues and gravitates
up to the neck, face, and supraclavicular area, where it may be first
detected. A mediastinal air leak, which may arise from the esophagus
or lungs, can be heard during auscultation of the apical rate as the air
is compressed by the contraction of the heart with each beat
(Hamman's sign).

26 Correct answer – A

These symptoms may indicate pneumonia (inflammation or infection of
the lung) or costochondritis (inflammation of the cartilage
surrounding the ribs). Pneumothorax, a rare occurrence after a rib
contusion or rib fracture, usually is associated with all of the
symptoms except fever and sputum production. Empyema may develop

after penetrating chest trauma. Pulmonary hypertension does not develop after a rib fracture.

27 Correct answer – C

A large chest tube, with or without a trocar, is used to evacuate blood from the chest cavity to prevent obstruction from clots. The typical size used is a #36 French or #40 French for a hemothorax, a #28 French for pneumothorax.

28 Correct answer – A

Hemothorax is the most common reason for autotransfusion in an emergency setting. Most basic autotransfusion devices are attached to the chest tube, which evacuates accumulated blood. Evacuating blood from other sites, such as the liver or thigh, places the patient at increased risk for bacterial contamination and development of clotting and particulate matter; autotransfusing blood from these sites would not be advantageous unless the patient were exsanguinating and blood products were unavailable. Hypotension from a spinal cord injury does not result from hemorrhage; therefore, transfusion is not required.

29 Correct answer – B

Hypocapnia, which may result from aggressive ventilation, would be of least concern because this results in a mild respiratory alkalosis that is offset by metabolic acidosis. Ventilatory efforts will prevent hypoxia. Other contributing factors, such as pericardial tamponade, volume deficit, or pneumothorax, will seriously hinder resuscitation but can be rapidly corrected.

30 Correct answer – C

Positioning the patient on his injured (right) side would cause great pain and might cause further internal injury. Placing him on his left side would be optimal. This position would allow for insertion of chest tubes, as necessary, while providing the best ventilation and perfusion to the uninjured lung, since pulmonary blood flow follows gravity, and ventilation (per unit of lung volume) is greater in the dependent area of the lung. Positioning the patient on his left side also would help to drain secretions from his affected side.

31 Correct answer – D

Flail chest is defined as two or more ribs fractured in two or more places, or with one fracture plus costochondral separation, or a fractured sternum. A flail segment or free-floating piece of thoracic cage must be present. This piece causes the chest wall to move paradoxically because of the defect in thoracic skeletal structure. The chest wall is pulled toward the negative intrapleural pressure during inspiration and pushed away from positive intrapleural pressure on expiration. Changes in ventilation and perfusion are most closely linked with underlying pulmonary damage rather than paradoxical motion.

32 Correct answer — B

Flail chest is easiest to assess when the thoracic fracture segments occur anteriorly, as anterior thoracic structures are least supported by muscle and easiest to visualize. Flail chest is most difficult to visualize in a muscular patient or a patient with posterior thoracic fracture segments because contracted muscle splints the area. Flail chest is moderately easy to assess when segments occur laterally. An alert patient typically splints the area to relieve the pain, making the flail less evident until fatigue sets in. Because an unconscious patient does not react to discomfort and does not splint the area, flail chest is typically easy to detect.

33 Correct answer — A

Although advanced age and obesity can contribute to reduced ventilatory reserve, they do not necessarily indicate the need for ventilatory support in a patient with a massive flail chest. A patient with flail chest may need assisted ventilation if breathing fatigue progressively worsens and if signs and symptoms of inadequate oxygen and carbon dioxide exchange (hypercapnia, hypoxia, and dyspnea) are evident. All trauma patients are intubated and ventilated during surgery. When associated injuries are present, assisted ventilation may be provided on a temporary basis to ensure proper oxygenation.

34 Correct answer — B

The appropriate nursing intervention in this situation would be to frequently administer low-dose narcotics, as ordered. This will relieve the patient's pain without causing significant respiratory depression. The most effective method of pain control is through physician-initiated intercostal nerve blocks or thoracic epidural analgesia. These allow for optimal chest wall movement and ventilation; then incentive spirometry may be used. The other interventions are inappropriate in the early stages of injury because the patient will be unable to tolerate chest percussion or postural drainage because of his pain and unstable condition. Also, binding and taping the chest wall will limit chest excursion and air exchange.

35 Correct answer—A

A decreased oxygen tension or room air (PaO$_2$ less than 80 mm Hg) and elevated lactic dehydrogenase (LDH) levels are the most common laboratory findings in pulmonary embolism. The white blood cell (WBC) count may be elevated or normal (normal is 5,000 to 10,000/ mm^3). A PaO$_2$ greater than 80 mm Hg is inconsistent with pulmonary embolism. Elevated LDH levels are common in many diseases; this finding alone is not specifically diagnostic for pulmonary embolus.

36 Correct answer—D

The priority nursing diagnosis would be *Impaired gas exchange related to altered pulmonary tissue perfusion* because, at this time, the patient is at highest risk for complications from pulmonary embolism. Although *Anxiety related to hypoxia and pain* and *Pain related to pulmonary ischemia* are important diagnoses, they are not the priority at this time. *Potential for injury related to hemorrhage from anticoagulant therapy* would not be a concern because heparin therapy has not yet been started.

37 Correct answer—B

Calf pain on dorsiflexion of the foot is considered a positive Homans' sign, which is indicative of deep vein thrombosis. Trousseau's sign is a carpal spasm elicited by compressing the upper arm, causing ischemia of the distal nerves; a positive sign is indicative of tetany. Babinski's reflex is dorsiflexion of the great toe and fanning of the smaller toes in response to a strong stimulus on the sole of the foot. A positive Babinski's sign in a patient over age 2 indicates an upper motor neuron lesion. Kehr's sign, radiating shoulder pain that occurs when the diaphragm is irritated from blood loss in the peritoneum, usually is seen in a patient with a ruptured spleen.

38 Correct answer—A

Pulmonary embolism rarely causes specific electrocardiographic (ECG) changes. However, sinus tachycardia caused by apprehension, pain, and a decreased PO$_2$ is the most common ECG finding. Some ECG findings that may suggest a pulmonary embolus include enlarged P waves, depressed ST segments, inverted T waves, and atrial fibrillation. If a massive pulmonary embolism has occurred, the ECG may show right axis deviation, indicating right ventricular failure.

39 Correct answer—B

Heparin impedes clotting by preventing thrombi formation. It does not act on existing clots. Because adequate anticoagulation is based on the partial thromboplastin time (PTT), the dosage is adjusted to achieve a PTT from 55 to 85 seconds. Continuous I.V. heparin administration is preferred for a high-risk patient because it maintains a steady therapeutic blood level. Heparin bolus administration produces peak levels for a short time, but subtherapeutic levels are evident before the next dose is due.

40 Correct answer—A

The initial emergency treatment for a patient in acute respiratory distress secondary to chronic obstructive pulmonary disease (COPD) includes administering 30% oxygen via face mask and bronchodilator therapy. Unless the patient has severe acidosis or is obtunded, a conservative approach to treatment is initially recommended. Most patients with COPD are dependent on the hypoxic drive to maintain adequate ventilation. Uncontrolled or high-flow oxygen therapy may precipitate severe carbon dioxide narcosis and respiratory arrest. Precise oxygen therapy delivered by face mask may allow time for use of other therapeutic measures, such as bronchodilator therapy, thereby avoiding the need for intubation and mechanical ventilation. Morphine sulfate would be inappropriate in this situation because of its ensuing respiratory depressant effects.

41 Correct answer—B

An appropriate intervention for a patient in acute respiratory distress secondary to COPD would be to place the patient in a high-Fowler's position or leaning upright over an overbed table to ensure optimal ventilation. In a less acutely ill patient, having the patient sit in a chair is also beneficial. All these positions assist in lowering the diaphragm, thereby increasing respiratory excursion. Placing the patient in a supine position would diminish optimal ventilation and worsen the respiratory failure. Endotracheal intubation is not indicated at this time. Respiratory depressants, such as morphine sulfate, are not indicated at this time as they will further inhibit the stimulus to breathe.

42 Correct answer—B

Cigarette smoking appears to be the single most important factor leading to chronic airway obstruction. In most cases, cigarette smoking also interacts with virtually every other contributing factor. Anxiety may affect breathing patterns, typically by causing hyperventilation and exacerbation of dyspnea during respiratory distress. In certain occupational groups, such as auto mechanics and miners, the incidence of COPD is high; however, this is not the case with the patient in this situation. Although increased activity in a patient with lung disease may exacerbate symptoms, the patient in this situation had been sedentary during the attack.

43 Correct answer—C

Chronic bronchitis is classified as COPD because of hyperplasia and inflammation of goblet cells and increased production of thick mucus. The constant irritation of the bronchioles leads to hypertrophy of mucus-secreting glands, goblet cell hyperplasia, and increased mucus production, which leads to bronchial plugging and narrowing and diminished airflow.

44 Correct answer—A

The nurse would not expect the physician to order fluid restriction for a patient with COPD. Instead, intake should be encouraged to help mobilize secretions.

45 Correct answer—B

In the early stages of COPD, cessation of cigarette smoking is probably the most significant factor in halting the disease's progression. After discontinuation of smoking, the accelerated decline in pulmonary function slows and the patient's pulmonary function returns to the more normal level of a nonsmoker. Therefore, if the patient stops smoking now, his cough and sputum production will decrease and his pulmonary function tests will improve.

46 Correct answer—B

A patient with severe bronchial abnormalities and mild emphysema is commonly labeled a blue bloater. In this condition, hypoventilation leads to hypoxemia and hypercapnia. A patient with severe emphysema and mild bronchitis is commonly labeled a pink puffer. In this condition, hyperventilation assists in adequate oxygenation; therefore, cyanosis is absent. Asthmatic symptoms are caused by a hyperreactive airway.

47 Correct answer—D

Cor pulmonale is a complication of COPD secondary to pulmonary hypertension caused by vasoconstriction in response to hypoxia; acidosis further potentiates the vasoconstriction. Chronic alveolar hypoxia causes ventricular hypertrophy and stimulates erythropoiesis, which increases the blood viscosity. Clinical manifestations are related to dilation and failure of the right ventricle, with subsequent intravascular volume expansion and systemic venous congestion.

48 Correct answer—D

A patient with cor pulmonale resulting from COPD typically develops pulmonary hypertension and signs of right-sided heart failure, including jugular vein distention, hepatosplenomegaly, and edema. Bibasilar crackles are typically seen in left-sided heart failure. A capillary refill of 4 seconds indicates impaired circulation or an inadequate circulatory volume. Poor skin turgor indicates a fluid volume deficit.

49 Correct answer—D

Small-airway obstruction usually is irreversible in such chronic diseases as emphysema and bronchitis; however, this same obstruction usually is reversible in asthma. Pneumonia is an inflammation of the lung, not of the small airways. Atelectasis can be reversed by improving ventilation.

50 Correct answer—C

The nurse should plan to include information on the importance of receiving influenza vaccines at the prescribed times and to seek medical advice about receiving a vaccine against streptococcal pneumonia. A patient with COPD is more prone to respiratory infections, which subsequently intensify the pathologic destruction of lung tissue and the progression of COPD. The most common causative organisms are *Haemophilus influenzae* and *Streptococcus pneumoniae*. Retained secretions provide a good medium for the proliferation of these organisms. Chest X-rays are not recommended annually. Vitamin supplements are not usually recommended unless the patient also has a vitamin deficiency or poor dietary intake. Dry climates could be harmful for a patient who is expectorating sputum that is not liquefied.

51 Correct answer—A

Barrel chest results from hyperinflation and overdistention of alveoli. In a patient with emphysema, elastin and collagen, the supporting structures of the lung, are destroyed. Without this support, the bronchiolar walls tend to collapse and air becomes trapped in the distal alveoli, resulting in hyperinflation and overdistention of the alveoli. This trapped air gives the patient a barrel chested appearance.

52 Correct answer—C

Pursed-lip breathing slows expiration and prevents collapse of lung units. It also helps the patient to control the rate and depth of respirations and to relax, which decreases dyspnea and feelings of panic. Use of inspiratory muscle training devices must be judiciously monitored by a health care professional. Indiscriminate use can produce inspiratory muscle exhaustion and acute ventilatory failure. Postural drainage, chest percussion, and vibration are indicated for patients with increased sputum production.

53 Correct answer — C

Although the use of expectorants is not uniformly recommended for a patient with COPD, cough suppressants must be avoided. Antihistamines cause drying of the respiratory mucosa, which can result in mucus thickening and possible airway obstruction. Hydration, aerosol humidification, chest physiotherapy, and postural drainage loosen and remove thick secretions. The patient with COPD does not need to avoid spicy foods.

54 Correct answer — B

Ineffective individual coping is a common diagnostic category used by nurses caring for patients with COPD. Developing healthy psychological coping mechanisms is perhaps the most difficult task the patient must master. Because a patient with COPD typically must learn to cope with and manage various life-style changes, he may find himself in a vicious cycle of emotional entrapment. The nurse may need to help him learn to communicate honestly with supportive family and friends and to avoid anxiety-producing situations. Learning these skills is more difficult than learning facts about the nutritional and therapeutic aspects of COPD.

55 Correct answer — B

Extrinsic asthma is precipitated by a known allergen or allergy. Patients with extrinsic asthma usually have a family history of allergies and a medical history of infantile eczema or allergic rhinitis. Intrinsic asthma is exacerbated by cold air, air pollution, and primary infection. Mixed asthma is associated with some allergic tendencies. Idiopathic asthma has unknown causative factors.

56 Correct answer — D

Because extrinsic asthma attacks are precipitated by exposure to certain allergens, such as pollen, dander, feathers, mold, dust, and some foods, the nurse would suspect that the down jacket precipitated the attack. The other answer choices are not likely to be respiratory allergens.

57 Correct answer — C

Normally, the bronchioles constrict during expiration. However, expiration becomes more difficult when the bronchioles are already constricted, edematous, and filled with mucus. Bronchospasm and mucus production typically occur during asthma attacks. The alveoli are not constricted during respiration.

58 Correct answer — C

Besides the dyspnea and chest tightness, the nurse would expect to note the characteristic clinical manifestations of asthma — wheezing and coughing. Expiration is more difficult than inspiration; therefore, prolonged, wheezing expirations are characteristic. The cough may be nonproductive, possibly indicating widespread bronchiolar plugging. Production of thick, tenacious, white, gelatinous mucus also may occur, typically only after treatment has begun.

59 Correct answer — C

Administration of metaproterenol sulfate and aminophylline should improve the patient's condition most rapidly. To relieve bronchospasm, treatment is aimed at decreasing mucosal edema and facilitating secretion removal. Beta-adrenergic agents and bronchodilators, such as aminophylline, epinephrine, and terbutaline, administered by inhalation or direct I.V. therapy, offer rapid relief. Corticosteroids usually are effective 6 to 9 hours after administration. Cromolyn sodium is used prophylactically but should not be used for an acute attack. Oxygen and I.V. fluids will not reverse bronchospasm.

60 Correct answer — A

An important nursing goal during an acute asthma attack is to decrease the patient's sense of panic. The best approach would be to maintain a calm, quiet, reassuring attitude to help the patient relax. Staying with the patient and being available provides additional comfort. Teaching is most effective after the attack subsides. However, diversional therapy is not the best approach. Although visitors should be restricted, a parent may be helpful in alleviating anxiety in an adolescent. Although diversional therapy is a commonly used tactic, it would be inappropriate in this situation because the patient is having difficulty breathing and probably would not be able to concentrate on the diversion.

61 Correct answer — A

Prompt diagnosis and treatment of upper respiratory tract infections may prevent exacerbations. Physical exercise within the patient's tolerance level is beneficial. Staying indoors when the air pollution index is high is helpful.

62 Correct answer — B

The most common type of pneumonia is pneumococcal, caused by *Streptococcus pneumoniae*. *Staphylococcus* pneumonia occurs more commonly in hospitalized patients than in people in the community. *Bacillus* pneumonia is associated with agricultural or industrial exposure to *Bacillus* microorganisms. Pneumonia caused by *Streptococcus pyogenes* is known to occur in military populations after influenza epidemics.

63 Correct answer — C

The nurse would expect the physician to order a Gram stain of the patient's sputum and chest X-rays. A Gram stain of sputum provides the information on which the initial therapy is based. Immediate identification of the infecting organism permits the institution of appropriate antimicrobial therapy. Sputum and blood cultures take 24 to 72 hours. Chest X-rays frequently show a pattern characteristic of the infecting organisms; lung scans do not show this. Bronchoscopy may be necessary if the patient cannot voluntarily produce a sputum specimen. Arterial blood gas measurements and electrolyte studies, although helpful, usually are not critical unless the patient is tachypneic and diaphoretic.

64 Correct answer — A

Epiglottitis, which typically occurs betwen ages 3 and 7, is associated with a large, cherry red, edematous epiglottis; muffled voice sounds or aphonia; dysphagia; drooling; and a croaking or froglike sound on inspiration. The patient may have a rapid onset of symptoms and complain of a sore throat. Typically, the patient will not struggle to breathe, but rather prefers to remain still for better air exchange. He may assume an upright position and lean with his chin thrust forward (tripod position). A younger child may protrude his tongue. Temperatures may range from 100° to 105° F (37.8° to 40.6° C).

65 Correct answer — B

Intubation or tracheotomy equipment must be available whenever epiglottitis is suspected because complete airway obstruction can occur suddenly. Suction equipment and humidified oxygen also should be accessible. Epiglottitis requires immediate intervention, and the child should be admitted to the pediatric intensive care unit. He should never be left unattended. Separation from the parents may increase the child's anxiety and agitation, thereby increasing his oxygen need. The need for a tracheotomy consent varies according to the institution. Usually, the physician is responsible for obtaining an informed consent for surgical procedures or medical care. Oxygen may not be needed once an airway is established.

66 Correct answer—D

Attempts to directly visualize the epiglottis with a tongue blade can precipitate sudden laryngospasm and result in complete airway obstruction. A nurse should never attempt to visualize the epiglottis. Such visualization should occur within the operating room, with intubation or tracheotomy equipment available. An I.V. infusion should be started before the procedure. To prevent trauma, the endotracheal tube should be smaller than that normally used. To prevent laryngospasm, a throat culture should be obtained after the airway is established; *Haemophilus influenzae* is the most common bacterial agent found. Because bacteremia is present in 50% of cases, blood cultures should be obtained. The white blood cell count typically is greater than 15,000/mm^3. A child with epiglottitis typically is quiet because he has better air exchange with little activity. Coughing and vomiting do not occur with epiglottitis, although occasionally a child may have some retching.

67 Correct answer—B

Chloral hydrate is commonly administered to produce mild sedation without respiratory depression or drying of secretions. Restlessness, agitation, or anxiety can increase the respiratory rate and oxygen demand. Sedation may be required to prevent the child from removing the artificial airway, as restraints typically produce increased agitation and are not used. Steroids may be administered to reduce epiglottal edema. Chloral hydrate has no anticonvulsant effect.

68 Correct answer—D

The earliest signs of hypoxemia in children are restlessness, tachypnea, and a rapidly increasing heart rate. Accessory respiratory muscle use, retractions, and nasal flaring are intermediate signs of hypoxemia. Cyanosis and lethargy are late signs and require immediate intervention. The cough is brassy or barking and resonant. Inspiratory stridor is caused by partial upper airway obstruction. In a child, any increase in metabolism will increase oxygen consumption, thereby increasing the respiratory rate (the normal respiratory rate for a 19-month-old is 24 to 40 breaths/minute). A fever can increase the respiratory rate by 4 breaths/minute for each Fahrenheit-degree rise in temperature above normal.

69 Correct answer — **A**

Management of a child with croup is primarily directed toward maintaining the patient's airway and adequate respiratory exchange. These two goals are of prime importance and are typically more difficult to achieve in children than adults. A child's airway is smaller than an adult's and contains more soft tissue; thus, it is more susceptible to obstruction from edema or secretions. Because a child's respiratory mucous membranes are more susceptible to irritation, any irritation can result in edema or cough. The larynx of a young child is located two to three cervical vertebrae higher than in an adult. Its location allows for greater proximity of the esophagus and trachea, resulting in a greater risk of aspiration. Also, the tongue is proportionately larger, increasing the possibility of airway obstruction. Because of the obstruction, respiratory alkalosis is possible from tachypnea. Treatment for croup consists of high humidity with cool mist; this decreases mucosal edema and prevents drying of secretions. Oxygen and intubation are indicated for anoxia and obstruction.

70 Correct answer — **C**

Acetylsalicylic acid (aspirin) should not be administered to a child with croup. Acetylsalicylic acid has been correlated with Reye's syndrome, which can cause fatal encephalopathy. Reye's syndrome commonly follows acute upper respiratory tract viral infections. Laryngotracheobronchitis, the most common form of croup, results from a viral infection and usually occurs in the fall and winter. It is more prevalent in males between ages 3 months and 3 years. The nurse should keep in mind that a child with potential respiratory distress should never be given a sedative because it may mask restlesness, an early indicator of hypoxemia.

71 Correct answer — **A**

Placing the patient in a semi-Fowler's position with the neck slightly extended will ensure adequate respiratory exchange, as semi-Fowler's position aids in lung expansion, and slight neck extension opens a child's narrow airway. A prone position helps to compress distended lungs during expiration, but this is not a problem in croup. During auscultation, the child should be sitting to facilitate accurate assessment. Auscultation of the entire chest is necessary; because the chest is small, breath sounds frequently are referred to other aspects of the chest.

72 Correct answer — **D**

Skin turgor, fluid intake and output, and urine specific gravity are the most important measures of hydration status. Hydration is particularly important in infants and young children because their total water body composition differs from that of adults. The composition does not become similar to that of an adult until about age 2. Until that time, the child's weight is a more important parameter for hydration assessment. In a child over age 2, the other parameters are of greater importance.

Skin turgor is a good indication of hydration in a child as well as an adult. A dehydrated child's skin turgor typically is poor. I.V. fluid replacement may be necessary to decrease the child's physical exertion, respiratory rate, and risk of aspiration. Fluid intake and output measurements are essential to monitor the hydration status, especially to prevent overhydration with I.V. therapy. Urine specific gravity is an excellent indicator of hydration because the kidneys' ability to concentrate and dilute urine increases with age (because an infant's kidneys are immature, specific gravity is not a good indicator of renal function at such an early age). Although serum electrolyte levels provide an indirect measurement of hydration status, they are more valuable as indicators of electrolyte status. Fontanelle tension would not be an appropriate indicator in this situation because the posterior fontanelle usually closes by age 2 to 3 months; the anterior fontanelle, by age 12 to 18 months.

73 Correct answer—D

The suction chamber should be bubbling constantly if connected to suction; this indicates that the system is functioning normally. Continuous bubbling in the water-seal chamber would indicate fluctuation with respiration or an air leak on expiration; the patient may have a significant air leak caused by bronchial damage, or a leak may have developed in the chest tube connection or in the drainage holes in the end of the tube extending outside the chest wall. Gastric drainage in the chest drainage system may indicate an esophageal fistula.

74 Correct answer—C

The water-seal level should rise with positive-pressure ventilation or upon forceful coughing because of the increase in intrapleural pressure. During spontaneous respiration, the intrapleural pressure becomes more negative (or subatmospheric), which pulls fluid in the water-seal chamber toward the patient and causes a fall in the water-seal level.

75 Correct answer—B

The nurse should report expanding hyperresonance on lung percussion. Extension of the pneumothorax rather than the desired reabsorption would be detected by auscultation of diminished breath sounds and a larger area of hyperresonance on percussion over the affected lung. Percussion creates vibration in the lung and chest wall; when it is performed over the air-filled intrapleural space, a tympanic sound results because of an increase in the normal resonance of the lung. The patient will have constant pain, tachypnea, and tachycardia.

76 Correct answer — B

Fever and chills may indicate atelectasis; however, with full lung expansion and a short duration of pulmonary abnormality, atelectasis is unlikely. The patient's symptoms are more likely caused by a viral infection. The other symptoms listed are characteristic of pneumothorax and place the patient at a higher risk of recurrence.

77 Correct answer — B

The nurse would anticipate insertion of the needle over the third rib at the midclavicular line. The needle should be inserted over the third rib because the intercostal artery and vein are located under the rib. Placement at the superior border should avoid vascular trauma. The procedure may be done at the second intercostal space midclavicular line or the fourth or fifth intercostal space midaxillary line.

Tension pneumothorax is caused by excessive pressure on the injured side. This will eventually shift the mediastinal contents to the uninjured side, affecting vascular flow and ventilation. Treatment should be aimed at the side of origin of injury, the side opposite the tracheal deviation. Needle thoracotomy can be performed correctly on the left side of the chest without inducing cardiac injury.

78 Correct answer — D

Signs and symptoms of a tension pneumothorax include dyspnea, jugular vein distention, hypotension, and tracheal deviation. In tension pneumothorax, the injured lung is collapsed and the contralateral lung is partially collapsed. This creates severe dyspnea from ineffective gas exchange. The mediastinal contents (large vessels, trachea, and heart) are shifted or deviated and compressed, depending on the pressure created. This results in ineffective cardiac contraction and reduced venous return, resulting in jugular vein distention and low cardiac output. Tachycardia is a compensatory mechanism and hypotension would be present.

79 Correct answer — A

A large diaphragmatic hernia caused by a rupture or laceration of the diaphragm allows abdominal contents to enter the thoracic cavity. Pressure within the abdominal cavity is higher than intrathoracic pressure. Diaphragmatic hernias occur most often on the left side because the right side is better protected by the liver. Excursion of the bowel and other abdominal structures into the thorax creates excessive pressure that can also compress and shift the thoracic structures. A 10% hemothorax and chronic obstructive pulmonary disease will not cause such severe symptoms. Cardiac contusion does not produce respiratory symptoms.

80 Correct answer — C

The best action is to pinch the tubing to prevent atmospheric air from entering the pleural space until a temporary water seal can be obtained. In this situation, the nurse may be creative in seeking a new form of water seal and enlist the help of other personnel in the immediate area. Use of a clean urinal filled with water would be better than sustained clamping. Pinching is suggested rather than clamping because the nurse is less likely to forget to release the tube. This patient required a needle thoracotomy to relieve a tension pneumothorax. The current chest tube, if clamped, is ineffective in allowing escape of intrapleural air or fluid. It should not be removed or the tension will recur.

CHAPTER 14

Shock

1 Which sign would the nurse expect to note in a patient who has undergone multiple blood transfusions?

A. Brudzinski's sign
B. Chvostek's sign
C. Cullen's sign
D. Babinski's sign

2 The nurse knows that administering a vasopressor, such as dopamine hydrochloride (Intropin) is least beneficial for a patient in:

A. Cardiogenic shock
B. Distributive shock
C. Septic shock
D. Hypovolemic shock

3 The nurse would anticipate a patient with which condition to develop hypovolemic shock?

A. Drug overdose
B. Postpartum fever
C. Intestinal obstruction
D. Cardiac tamponade

4 Which patient is at lowest risk for developing cardiogenic shock?

A. A 24-year-old patient with cardiac tamponade from a stab wound to the heart
B. A 72-year-old patient with a history of heart disease who has developed an arrhythmia
C. A 55-year-old patient with acute pericarditis who underwent cardiac surgery 3 weeks ago
D. A 44-year-old patient with an anterolateral wall myocardial infarction (MI)

5 Clinical manifestations of cardiogenic shock include all of the following *except:*

A. Distended neck veins
B. Pulmonary congestion
C. S_3 heart sounds
D. Low central venous pressure (CVP)

Shock Questions

6 Which treatment for a patient in cardiogenic shock is least effective in protecting the myocardium from further damage?

A. Decreasing peripheral vascular resistance
B. Decreasing ventricular preload
C. Increasing left ventricular afterload
D. Increasing cardiac output

7 When caring for a patient with an acute MI, which early assessment finding may indicate the development of cardiogenic shock?

A. S_3 heart sounds
B. Bilateral crackles heard during inspiration
C. Warm, diaphoretic skin
D. Urine output of 30 ml/hour

8 The nurse knows that the evaluation of renal function in a patient with early circulatory failure does not reveal:

A. An increased blood urea nitrogen (BUN) level
B. An increased serum creatinine level
C. A decreased urine specific gravity
D. A decreased urine sodium level

9 Which of the following is a beneficial effect of vasodilator therapy in a patient in cardiogenic shock?

A. Increased systemic vascular pressure
B. Reduced preload and afterload
C. Increased pulmonary vascular pressure
D. Increased peripheral vascular resistance

10 Which of the following is a therapeutic outcome following use of inotropic agents in a patient in cardiogenic shock?

A. Vasodilation
B. Improved tissue perfusion
C. Increased heart rate
D. Decreased force of myocardial contractility

11 While assessing a patient, the nurse notes a sharp decrease in systolic pressure, dyspnea, and bilateral crackles. Which nursing action holds the highest priority at this time?

A. Beginning a vasopressor drip
B. Rapidly infusing 0.45% saline solution to maintain the patient's blood pressure
C. Placing the patient in a supine position and elevating his legs to increase the blood pressure
D. Elevating the patient's head and administering oxygen

12 Based on the following admission histories, which patient is least likely to develop septic shock?

A. A patient with multiple sclerosis who has an indwelling urinary catheter in place and a temperature of 100° F (37.8° C)
B. A patient with a lung carcinoma who is receiving chemotherapy and radiation therapy
C. A patient with a permanent pacemaker that was inserted 1 week ago
D. A patient who severed two fingers while using garden machinery

13 During the initial treatment phase of a patient with septic shock, which nursing action holds the highest priority?

A. Obtaining an allergy history
B. Obtaining blood for cultures, then administering antibiotic therapy
C. Initiating antibiotic therapy after obtaining urine culture results
D. Inserting an indwelling urinary catheter to monitor urine output

14 The nurse would expect a patient who is admitted to the emergency department (ED) in the early stages of septic shock to present with:

A. Weak, thready pulses and low blood pressure
B. Decreased urine output and an elevated serum creatinine level
C. Warm, flushed, and moist skin
D. Hyperventilation and pulmonary congestion

15 In a patient with early septic shock, which respiratory symptom would the nurse expect to note?

A. Increased mucus production
B. Bilateral crackles
C. Hyperpnea
D. Respiratory acidosis

Shock Questions

16 The nurse knows that a patient with septic shock typically is depleted of intravascular fluid (hypovolemia). Which factor does *not* cause hypovolemia in septic shock?

A. Leakage of fluid into tissues from an increase in vessel permeability
B. Fluid loss associated with infection, such as sweating during fever, and respiratory losses during hyperventilation
C. Sequestration of plasma fluid in extravascular spaces
D. Increased vascular resistance compromising blood flow to vital areas

17 Which of the following is least likely to introduce the pathogens responsible for septic shock?

A. Bladder instrumentation
B. Childbirth
C. Appendectomy
D. Gingival abscess

18 All of the following pharmacologic agents are appropriate treatments for a patient with septic shock *except:*

A. Beta-adrenergic blockers
B. Corticosteroids
C. Salicylates
D. Vasopressors

19 Which of the following explains the cause of altered mental status during septic shock?

A. Increased cerebral perfusion resulting from the low flow state
B. Elevation of metabolic waste products, such as BUN and creatinine, because of decreased kidney perfusion
C. Alkalosis that results from hyperventilation, causing cerebrovascular constriction
D. Endotoxins acting directly on the central nervous system (CNS)

20 Which pathophysiologic alteration is responsible for the clinical manifestations of neurogenic shock?

A. Compression of the CNS within the spinal cord
B. Interruption of neural transmissions of the afferent spinal tracts
C. Inhibition of motor reflexes of the cerebral cortex
D. Disrupted transmission of the sympathetic nerve impulses from the vasomotor center

21 The nurse knows that all of the following conditions contribute to the development of neurogenic shock *except:*

A. Encephalitis
B. General anesthesia
C. Head trauma
D. Spinal cord injury

22 Which assessment findings indicate neurogenic shock?

A. Increased heart rate and low blood pressure
B. Shallow breathing and diaphoresis
C. Warm, dry skin and bradycardia
D. Weak, thready pulse and hypotension

23 Which nursing action is inappropriate during the management of a patient with neurogenic shock resulting from a spinal cord injury?

A. Elevating the head of the bed 20 degrees to promote oxygenation
B. Inserting a nasogastric tube to prevent aspiration caused by paralytic ileus
C. Keeping the patient supine at all times
D. Inserting an indwelling urinary catheter to prevent urine retention

SITUATION

A 26-year-old man was involved in an automobile accident. Approximately 20 minutes elapsed between the time of the accident and the arrival of the paramedics. He sustained severe abdominal injuries, spinal cord injury, and multiple fractures. On arrival at the ED, the patient's vital signs are blood pressure 80/50 mm Hg; heart rate, 120 beats/minute; and respiratory rate, 30 breaths/minute.

Questions 24 to 29 refer to the above situation.

24 Which nursing action is inappropriate during the initial stabilization of this patient?

A. Administering oxygen therapy
B. Applying medical antishock trousers (MAST, or pneumatic antishock garment)
C. Placing the patient in the Trendelenburg (head-down) position
D. Infusing lactated Ringer's solution via a large-bore I.V. line

25 At the time of admission, which assessment finding may be indicative of hypovolemic shock?

A. Pulsus paradoxus
B. A hemoglobin of 10 mg/dl and a hematocrit of 38%
C. A widening pulse pressure
D. A central venous pressure (CVP) of 4 mm Hg

26 Which assessment finding suggests that hypovolemia may be a cause of shock in this patient?

A. A decreased CVP and distended neck veins only while the patient is prone
B. An increased urine sodium level and a urine specific gravity of 1.010
C. A positive tilt-test result and a decreasing pulse pressure
D. Tachycardia with ventricular gallop (S_3 heart sounds)

27 Which statement best describes shock?

A. It is the inability of the body to excrete metabolic waste products
B. It refers to the collapse of the respiratory system
C. It refers to the collapse of the sympathetic nervous system
D. It is a state of inadequate tissue perfusion

28 The nurse would expect a patient in early shock to have:

A. Metabolic acidosis
B. Metabolic alkalosis
C. Respiratory acidosis
D. Respiratory alkalosis

29 Which assessment finding indicates that the compensatory response mechanisms for shock are failing?

A. An increase in capillary refill time
B. Cool, clammy skin
C. Pale, moist skin
D. Mottled skin

Shock
Questions

SITUATION

An 18-year-old man sustained musculoskeletal and abdominal injuries when he crashed into a tree and was thrown from his motorcycle. He is brought to the ED by paramedics with MAST in place.

Questions 30 to 33 relate to the above situation.

30 Which statement about MAST is *false?*

A. It is a single-unit apparatus with three compartments
B. Each compartment may be pressurized and deflated individually or in combination
C. When inflated, it achieves pressures ranging from 0 to 160 mm Hg
D. Once optimal pressure is achieved, automatic release valves prevent further pressure increases

31 The therapeutic effects of MAST on a hypovolemic patient include:

A. Augmentation of preload to increase stroke volume
B. Increased peripheral vascular resistance in unpressurized areas
C. Decreased functional residual capacity and tidal volume
D. Decreased cerebral perfusion pressure

32 MAST would be least beneficial for a patient with:

A. Spinal shock
B. Pelvic fractures
C. Severe intra-abdominal bleeding
D. Bilateral hemothorax

33 Which procedure is correct when using MAST to stabilize a patient?

A. Inflate it to the highest pressure, then slowly deflate it until the desired response is obtained
B. When deflation is indicated, the leg segments should be depressurized one at a time followed by the abdominal segment
C. During deflation, if the patient's systolic blood pressure drops more than 5 mm Hg, stop deflating and infuse fluids
D. If cyanosis of the feet occurs, even though dorsalis pedis pulses are palpable, decrease the MAST pressure by 10 mm Hg

SITUATION

Paramedics are transporting a 32-year-old woman with a severe anaphylactic reaction. The estimated time of arrival in the ED is 11 minutes.

Questions 34 to 39 refer to the above situation.

34 The nurse knows that anaphylaxis most commonly is precipitated by:

A. Insect venom
B. Food ingestion
C. Antibiotic use
D. Blood transfusions

35 After exposure to an allergen, a patient typically develops symptoms of anaphylaxis within:

A. 2 to 20 minutes
B. 20 to 60 minutes
C. 48 hours
D. 3 days

36 Which anaphylactic manifestation is the nurse's lowest priority when treating a patient with altered gas exchange?

A. Inspiratory wheezing
B. Stridor
C. Hoarseness
D. Angioneurotic edema

37 All of the following treatments are used in the initial management of anaphylaxis *except:*

A. Corticosteroids
B. I.V. fluids
C. Epinephrine (Adrenalin)
D. Diphenhydramine hydrochloride (Benadryl)

38 Which pharmacologic agent is least likely to be used to treat a patient with anaphylaxis?

A. Hydrocortisone (Cortef)
B. Dobutamine hydrochloride
C. Aminophylline (Aminophyllin)
D. Antihistamine

Shock
Questions

39 Which principle holds the highest priority when caring for a patient with a history of allergies?

A. Avoid known allergens and unnecessary patient exposure by administering drugs only when indicated
B. Observe any patient who receives penicillin in the ED for at least 30 minutes before discharge
C. Initiate current skin-testing procedures to identify allergens
D. Obtain an accurate and thorough drug history, which includes identifying and describing previous drug reactions

Answer Sheet

	A	B	C	D			A	B	C	D
1	○	○	○	○		31	○	○	○	○
2	○	○	○	○		32	○	○	○	○
3	○	○	○	○		33	○	○	○	○
4	○	○	○	○		34	○	○	○	○
5	○	○	○	○		35	○	○	○	○
6	○	○	○	○		36	○	○	○	○
7	○	○	○	○		37	○	○	○	○
8	○	○	○	○		38	○	○	○	○
9	○	○	○	○		39	○	○	○	○
10	○	○	○	○						
11	○	○	○	○						
12	○	○	○	○						
13	○	○	○	○						
14	○	○	○	○						
15	○	○	○	○						
16	○	○	○	○						
17	○	○	○	○						
18	○	○	○	○						
19	○	○	○	○						
20	○	○	○	○						
21	○	○	○	○						
22	○	○	○	○						
23	○	○	○	○						
24	○	○	○	○						
25	○	○	○	○						
26	○	○	○	○						
27	○	○	○	○						
28	○	○	○	○						
29	○	○	○	○						
30	○	○	○	○						

1 Correct answer — **B**

The nurse would expect to note Chvostek's sign in a patient who has undergone multiple transfusions. Hypocalcemia is a potential problem during massive transfusions because citrate preservatives may bind ionized calcium. In fact, alkalosis may develop after multiple transfusions, as sodium citrate is converted to sodium bicarbonate. A patient with these electrolyte and acid-base imbalances may demonstrate Chvostek's sign, a facial twitching that occurs when the side of the face is tapped. Brudzinski's sign indicates meningeal irritation; both the upper legs at the hips and the lower legs at the knees are flexed in response to the path of flexion of the head and the neck on the chest. Babinski's sign, which is the dorsiflexion of the big toe upon scratching the bottom of the foot, indicates upper motor neuron dysfunction. Cullen's sign, which is ecchymosis around the umbilicus, usually is seen in hemorrhagic pancreatitis.

2 Correct answer — **D**

The administration of a vasopressor, such as dopamine, would be least beneficial to a patient in hypovolemic shock. Natural vasoconstriction compensates for a hypovolemic state during the early shock phase. Giving a vasopressor in early shock increases vasoconstriction, possibly closing arterioles and further halting blood flow. Hypovolemia must be treated before dopamine can be given. For the patient in cardiogenic shock or septic shock (distributive shock), a vasopressor is appropriate because it increases myocardial contractility and raises cardiac output and systolic blood pressure.

3 Correct answer — **C**

The nurse should anticipate manifestations of hypovolemic shock in a patient admitted to the emergency department (ED) with an intestinal obstruction. Such an obstruction could cause altered fluid movement, resulting in the trapping of fluid in the interstitial space within the intestinal lumen and the depletion of intravascular volume (third-space fluid shift). The nurse should suspect neurogenic shock in a patient with a drug overdose; septic shock in a postpartum patient with a fever; and cardiogenic shock in a patient with cardiac tamponade.

4 Correct answer — **C**

A postoperative cardiac patient with acute pericarditis is least likely to develop cardiogenic shock. Cardiogenic shock is a vicious cycle that involves loss of myocardial contractility; resultant hemodynamic and metabolic reflex mechanisms cause further ischemia and the deterioration of contractility. Acute pericarditis, inflammation of the pericardium, has a self-limiting, short-term clinical course when related to an acute myocardial infarction (MI) or cardiac surgery. The cause is not irritation but, rather, an autoimmune response that lasts 2 to 6 weeks. Pericardial effusion usually does not develop. Pain, the most characteristic symptom of acute pericarditis, usually can be alleviated by leaning forward. Pericardial friction rub is the most important physical finding in this condition.

Most commonly, cardiogenic shock occurs as a complication of an MI, especially when at least 40% of the left ventricle is necrotic and ischemic. When the heart's ability to pump blood declines, the risk of cardiogenic shock increases. This occurs in conditions that produce deficient cardiac filling, such as cardiac tamponade and arrhythmias in a compromised patient.

5 Correct answer — D

Low central venous pressure (CVP) is not one of the manifestations of cardiogenic shock. The clinical manifestations of cardiogenic shock result from impaired contractility of the heart, which decreases cardiac output and elevates left ventricular end-diastolic pressure (LVEDP). The reduced cardiac output impairs perfusion to the vital organs and peripheral tissues. Thus, the patient exhibits changes in sensorium, such as restlessness, anxiety, or confusion. The skin is cold and clammy because of peripheral vasoconstriction. As the cardiac output declines, the pulse pressure narrows; peripheral pulses are rapid and thready. Systemic arterial pressure drops and hypotension ensues. Urine output decreases as kidney perfusion declines. A rise in LVEDP increases left atrial and pulmonary pressures, resulting in pulmonary congestion. Tachypnea, dyspnea, and pulmonary edema develop; S_3 heart sounds can be heard as the left ventricle fails and becomes overdistended during diastole. Increased pressure on the left side of the heart progresses back through the pulmonary venous system into the right side of the heart. This increase in pulmonary pressure decreases right ventricular performance and may result in right ventricular failure, which in turn produces an elevated CVP and jugular vein distention with hepatomegaly.

Shock Answers

6 Correct answer — C

The treatment that is least effective in protecting the myocardium from further damage in a patient in cardiogenic shock involves increasing left ventricular afterload. The goals of therapy in this situation are to improve myocardial contractility, increase cardiac output, and reduce the myocardial demand for oxygen. Improvement of cardiovascular function is primarily managed by pharmacologic therapies. Nitroprusside sodium (Nipride) and nitroglycerin (Tridil) are commonly used to decrease both preload (ventricular end-diastolic pressure) and afterload (vascular resistance). These vasodilators reduce blood return to the heart and decrease systemic peripheral vascular resistance. Cardiac output is further increased by a decrease in cardiac work load and oxygen demand and by complete emptying of the ventricles during systole. Vasodilator therapy is used with sympathomimetic drugs, such as dopamine hydrochloride and dobutamine hydrochloride (Dobutrex). These vasopressors have an inotropic effect that enhances myocardial contractility and increases cardiac output.

7 Correct answer—**A**

S_3 heart sounds are an early assessment finding that may indicate the development of cardiogenic shock in a patient with an acute MI. The patient with an acute MI is at high risk for developing cardiogenic shock because of a decrease in the contractile function of the left ventricle. Early recognition of signs and symptoms of left ventricular failure, which may lead to shock, are vital. Initially, the failing ventricle causes a decrease in cardiac output. The body compensates by increasing sympathetic stimulation to increase the heart rate and to shunt blood to vital organs via peripheral vasoconstriction. The skin is typically cool and clammy. Tachycardia and increased afterload from vasoconstriction increase the cardiac work load and oxygen consumption. Decreased ventricular emptying during systole occurs, preload increases, and S_3 sounds may be heard. Pulmonary congestion then follows from the backward transmission of left-sided pressure, resulting in dyspnea, orthopnea, and bilateral crackles. As left ventricular failure progresses, pulmonary congestion increases and cardiogenic shock ensues.

8 Correct answer—**C**

An evaluation of renal function in a patient with early circulatory failure typically does not reveal a decreased urine specific gravity. In the context of shock, the kidneys are peripheral organs. Thus, their perfusion declines from the onset of shock. Renal vessels are initially among the most constricted. As renal perfusion declines, the kidneys respond by conserving water; concentrating urine causes an increase in the urine specific gravity. Also, when the blood supply to the kidneys is decreased, the tubules respond by reabsorbing sodium. This results in a decreased urine sodium level. An increase in blood urea nitrogen (BUN) level and serum creatinine levels occurs because of a decrease in the rate at which the kidneys clear metabolic end products, such as urea and creatinine, from plasma.

9 Correct answer—**B**

A beneficial effect of vasodilator therapy in the management of cardiogenic shock is reduced preload and afterload. Vasodilator

414

Shock Answers

therapy reduces venous tone and increases venous capacitance. This decreases blood return to the heart, thereby lowering LVEDP. Vasodilator therapy also reduces arterial vascular tone, which results in decreased impedance to left ventricular ejection (afterload); cardiac work load is decreased, and cardiac output is increased.

10 Correct answer – B

Inotropic agents improve tissue perfusion in a patient with cardiogenic shock. They increase the force of myocardial contraction, resulting in increased cardiac output from enhanced contractility. Dopamine, a sympathomimetic drug, has positive inotropic properties. Its vasopressor effects result in increased coronary blood flow, which improves tissue perfusion. Dopamine's positive chronotropic effects result in an increased heart rate; this potential adverse effect may limit dopamine's use because tachycardia increases myocardial oxygen consumption.

11 Correct answer – D

Initial nursing measures in this situation include positioning the patient with his shoulders and head elevated to decrease pulmonary congestion and administering oxygen to increase the myocardial oxygen supply. This will protect the myocardium from further damage. After implementing necessary measures to ensure improvement in airway and breathing, the nurse should help to stabilize the patient's arterial pressure. Any infusion of I.V. fluids or vasopressor drips requires a physician's order. The rapid infusion of a hypotonic solution, such as 0.45% saline solution, may result in a sudden decrease in serum osmolarity. This can cause a shift of fluid into the cells, resulting in intravascular depletion and symptoms of increased intracranial pressure. Dextran, glucose, normal saline, and albumin solutions can be used in patients with cardiogenic shock.

12 Correct answer – D

A patient who severed two fingers while using garden machinery is least likely to develop septic shock. Factors that increase a patient's risk include any invasive procedure or foreign body insertion, such as an I.V. line, an indwelling catheter line, or a pacemaker; diseases affecting the reticuloendothelial system (RES), such as leukemia; and any therapy that suppresses the RES, such as radiation therapy and cytotoxic or immunosuppressant drug therapy.

13 Correct answer – A

Obtaining an allergy history holds the highest priority in this situation because antibiotics, which are essential in treating septic shock, cause anaphylaxis more often than any other substance. Afterward, the nurse should obtain blood for cultures before administering the first antibiotic dose. Initiating antibiotics before collecting cultures is a serious error. Accurately identifying the infecting organism is essential to provide optimal antibiotic treatment. A switch to a more appropriate therapy can help ensure patient survival.

14 Correct answer—C

The nurse would expect a patient who is admitted in the early (hyperdynamic) stages of septic shock to present with warm, flushed, and moist skin; tachycardia with full bounding pulses; tachypnea; confusion; normal or slightly increased urine output; and normal or slightly decreased blood pressure.

15 Correct answer—C

Hyperpnea is common in early sepsis. Sometimes bordering on respiratory alkalosis, this symptom is caused by the respiratory response to lactic acidosis as well as by stimulation of the medullary respiratory control center by the release of endotoxins. Advanced shock is characterized by pulmonary edema, which produces bilateral crackles. Also, adult respiratory distress syndrome has been associated with gram-negative sepsis.

16 Correct answer—D

Several factors account for the hypovolemia that occurs in septic shock; however, increased vascular resistance compromising blood flow to vital areas is not among them. Fluid and electrolytes can leave the body through events associated with infection, such as sweating during fever, diarrhea, vomiting, and respiratory losses during tachypnea. Also, plasma fluid can be sequestered in the extravascular spaces because of a local or generalized increase in vessel permeability secondary to the production of histamine, bradykinin, and other agents. Vessel permeability is increased in septic shock; thus there is an increased tendency for fluid leakage into tissues.

17 Correct answer—D

Gingival abscess is least likely to introduce the pathogens responsible for septic shock. Septic shock is more common in men than women because of the greater number of urinary tract infections and genitourinary procedures occurring in men. Women are most vulnerable to septic shock after pregnancy. The ED nurse must determine whether the patient has undergone a recent pelvic examination, appendectomy, or catheterization, especially during childbirth. These procedures are common methods for induction of causative organisms. Indwelling urinary tubes, intrauterine devices, instrumented abortions, and peritonitis from a ruptured appendix are additional ways in which gram-negative bacilli may be introduced.

18 Correct answer—A

Beta-adrenergic blockers are used rarely in septic shock because they depress myocardial function. The use of steroids is still controversial, although studies have shown that, overall, pharmacologic doses of steroids appear to be efficacious in the treatment of septic shock. Multiple mechanisms of action have been proposed to explain their reported therapeutic effects. The most common explanations involve the intracellular action of steroids in stabilizing lysosomal membranes. Stabilization of lysosomal membranes decreases the release of vasoactive substances and interrupts the pathogenesis of the shock syndrome. Vasopressors, such as dopamine hydrochloride, dobutamine hydrochloride, and norepinephrine (Levophed) are also used during shock because of their ability to improve the patient's hemodynamic status. Salicylates are used to decrease body temperature.

19 Correct answer—D

Endotoxins acting directly on the central nervous system are responsible for the altered mental status that occurs in septic shock. Early in septic shock, a patient's sensorium may change from awake, alert, and oriented to confused, agitated, and restless. This results from decreased cerebral perfusion caused by the low flow state produced by endotoxin-induced vasodilation, which increases pooling of blood within the venous system. The elevated BUN and creatinine levels and respiratory alkalosis seen in septic shock are not responsible for changes in mental status.

20 Correct answer—D

The primary problem in neurogenic shock is altered blood vessel capacity caused by disrupted transmission of sympathetic nerve impulses from the brain's vasomotor center. The unopposed parasympathetic stimulation causes a loss of vasomotor tone, resulting in massive vasodilation. The result is relative hypovolemia, decreased venous return, and decreased cardiac output.

21 Correct answer—A

Encephalitis does not contribute to the development of neurogenic shock. Neurogenic shock may result from any condition that shuts down the entire vasomotor system, including spinal anesthesia, the most common cause of neurogenic shock; deep general anesthesia, which may severely depress the brain's vasomotor center and lead to vasomotor collapse; head trauma; and spinal trauma.

22 Correct answer—C

Assessment findings indicative of neurogenic shock include warm, dry, and flushed skin; normal to low blood pressure; full, regular pulses; profound bradycardia; and an increased respiratory rate. These result from blocked sympathetic vasomotor regulation.

23 Correct answer—A

Elevating the head is inappropriate for a patient with neurogenic shock resulting from a spinal cord injury. Such a patient should be maintained in a supine position to avoid further spinal cord damage and prevent orthostatic hypotension, which may result from relative hypovolemia caused by increased vascular capacity. I.V. fluids should be instituted to expand the intravascular volume. Fluids must be administered cautiously, as they may cause fluid overload when vasomotor tone is restored. An indwelling urinary catheter should be inserted to permit frequent measurement of urine output. Catheterization also helps prevent urine retention if the patient has a spinal cord injury that has paralyzed the bladder.

24 Correct answer—C

Placing the patient in the Trendelenburg (head-down) position would be inappropriate during the initial stabilization of this patient. The initial management of a patient in shock involves ensuring an adequate airway and ventilation; maintaining blood volume, pressure, and circulation; and maintaining cellular oxygen consumption. Specific measures include administering oxygen and I.V. fluids, preferably lactated Ringer's solution via a large-bore I.V. line, as ordered. Medical antishock trousers (MAST, or pneumatic antishock garment) also may be used on a patient with lower-extremity or abdominal injuries who has signs and symptoms of hypovolemic shock. This will redirect approximately 1,000 ml of blood, reduce blood loss by application of direct pressure, and immobilize injuries of the lower extremities. The patient in shock should lie flat with only the legs elevated. The Trendelenburg position, once favored, has been abandoned because it allows the diaphragm to migrate upward, thus compromising ventilation. Also, this position may cause a reflex inhibition of the pressoreceptor activity, thereby decreasing sympathetic stimulation and further compromising arterial blood pressure.

25 Correct answer—A

Pulsus paradoxus is indicative of hypovolemic shock. It is characterized by an abnormal drop (greater than 10 mm Hg) in systolic blood pressure during inspiration. The systolic sound disappears during inspiration because of pulmonary vascular pooling caused by increased lung expansion and increased intrathoracic negative pressure. When intravascular depletion is present, such as in hypovolemic shock, the drop in systolic blood pressure during inspiration is exaggerated when venous blood return to the heart is compromised. The patient also may demonstrate a narrowing pulse pressure, indicating a fall in cardiac output, and a central venous pressure (CVP) reading below 4 mm Hg, indicating intravascular depletion. A single hematocrit or hemoglobin value is an unreliable indicator of the patient's condition. Either an increase or a decrease in hemoglobin values may signal hypovolemia; dropping values suggest whole blood loss, whereas rising values suggest plasma loss. Acute blood loss may cause a significant drop in hemoglobin over 1 to 2 hours; however, in older patients, acute blood loss may not cause a significant drop for at least 12 hours.

26 Correct answer—C

An abnormal tilt-test result and a decreasing pulse pressure may suggest that hypovolemia is the cause of shock in this patient. The tilt test is an assessment tool that indicates circulating blood volume loss by measuring blood pressure and pulse rate changes during patient position changes. Abnormal tilt-test findings include improved blood pressure levels when the patient's legs are raised above heart level or a 10-mm Hg or greater drop in systolic blood pressure between supine and sitting positions. Pulse pressure is a far better indicator of early shock than is blood pressure. Pulse pressure is related to cardiac stroke volume; thus, changes provide a good indication of blood flow. During the early stages of shock, the systolic pressure usually drops faster than the diastolic pressure, thereby narrowing or decreasing the pulse pressure.

A hypovolemic patient typically has flat neck veins when prone, a low CVP, a decreased urine sodium level, and a high urine specific gravity. S_3 heart sounds are heard when the patient experiences an increase in left-ventricular end-diastolic pressure, as occurs in congestive heart failure or cardiogenic shock. Tachycardia, which occurs in all forms of shock, results from the heart's attempt to increase cardiac output.

27 Correct answer—D

Shock is a complex clinical syndrome characterized by impaired cellular metabolism from decreased blood flow. It is a state of

Shock
Answers

inadequate tissue perfusion. The major pathophysiologic problem occurs in the microcirculation at the capillary level. Inadequate tissue perfusion and decreased oxygen delivery result in a constellation of physiologic responses. As shock develops, a fall in cardiac output triggers compensatory mechanisms as pressoreceptors are stimulated to cause vasoconstriction. The net effect is an increase in mean arterial pressure and a restriction of peripheral blood flow. The available circulating volume is shunted to perfuse vital organs. As peripheral vasoconstriction progresses, a marked reduction in oxygen delivery to the cells forces a switch from aerobic to anaerobic metabolism. Increased lactic acid is produced, resulting in respiratory compensation; body-acid load is reduced by blowing off carbon dioxide.

As a shock state continues, respiratory compensation fails and the progressive decline in pH from excessive lactate levels ensues. Metabolic acidosis causes impaired cellular function and impaired capillary permeability. Intravascular volume is further decreased as blood flows into capillary beds. At this point, the patient is in a progressive state of shock as compensatory mechanisms fail to maintain an adequate cardiac output.

28 Correct answer — D

Respiratory alkalosis develops in the initial phase of shock. A compensatory mechanism of tachypnea is initiated as a decrease in peripheral tissue perfusion occurs, resulting in hypoxia. In early shock, the patient hyperventilates to increase oxygenation, thus blowing off carbon dioxide. During progressive stages, excessive and prolonged vasoconstriction causes lactic acid levels to increase within the body, producing systemic acidosis.

29 Correct answer — D

Mottled skin would indicate that compensatory mechanisms for shock are failing. During the compensatory stage of shock, the skin is typically cool, pale, and clammy as a result of peripheral vasoconstriction and increased sweat gland activity. If the cause of shock is not corrected and compensatory mechanisms continue, the same physiologic events that were initiated to compensate for decreased cardiac output will lead to detrimental effects. Impaired cellular function leads to acidosis; the resultant decrease in cardiac contractility and loss of vasomotor tone produce mottled skin. The capillary refill time decreases in shock.

30 Correct answer — C

MAST is a single-unit device with three compartments: an abdominal compartment and two individual leg compartments. It may achieve pressures ranging from 0 to 104 mm Hg. Each of the three compartments may be pressurized and deflated individually or in combination. Once a pressure of 104 mm Hg is achieved, automatic release (or pop-off) valves prevent further pressure increases.

31 Correct answer—A

The therapeutic effects of MAST on a hypovolemic patient include augmentation of preload, thereby increasing blood return to the heart. This results in a greater cardiac output because of increased contractility and stroke volume. MAST increases peripheral vascular resistance in pressurized areas, decreases peripheral vascular resistance in the remainder of the body, and increases cerebral perfusion pressure. Although use of MAST also decreases the patient's functional residual capacity and tidal volume, these effects are not considered therapeutic.

32 Correct answer—D

MAST would be least beneficial for a patient with a bilateral hemothorax, as this device is contraindicated in shock secondary to hemorrhage above the diaphragm. Indications for MAST use include hypotension secondary to hypovolemia, as occurs in acute trauma; nontraumatic bleeding and nonhemorrhagic hypovolemia; hypotension secondary to volume maldistribution, as occurs in spinal shock, drug effects, and septic shock; and hypotension secondary to low cardiac output, as occurs in cardiac tamponade and cardiogenic shock. MAST is beneficial in stabilizing patients with pelvic and lower-extremity fractures. MAST not only supports the fracture site and decreases unwanted movement, but it also decreases bleeding. It is useful in lower-extremity hemorrhage and intra-abdominal bleeding.

33 Correct answer—C

At no time should suit deflation continue if the patient's systolic blood pressure drops more than 5 mm Hg. Such a drop implies an inadequate circulating volume, and I.V. fluids should be administered until the patient's vital signs are stable. After MAST is applied, the leg segments are inflated, followed by the abdominal segment, if needed. The end point of pressurization is determined in all instances by the stabilization of the patient's blood pressure, which must be continuously monitored. When desired blood pressure is achieved and maintained, inflation stops. During inflation, the patient's feet may turn bluish. The suit's maximum pressure, 104 mm Hg, usually is not sufficient to totally occlude perfusion; however, routine palpation of the dorsalis pedis pulses is mandatory. When deflation of the garment is indicated, the abdominal segment is depressurized first, followed by the leg segments.

34 Correct answer — C

Anaphylaxis is most commonly precipitated by antibiotics, although a variety of agents have been reported to precipitate this severe reaction. Essentially, any compound capable of acting as an allergen may cause an anaphylactic reaction. The most common examples of such compounds include antibiotics, especially penicillin (300 fatal anaphylactic reactions to penicillin occur each year in the United States), followed by medicines derived from animal sources, insect bites and stings, and iodinated radioactive contrast media.

35 Correct answer — A

After exposure to an allergen, a patient typically develops symptoms of anaphylaxis within 2 to 20 minutes. The immediate reaction is usually life-threatening and displays the symptoms characteristic of anaphylaxis. The classic manifestations of anaphylaxis include the triad of urticaria, laryngeal edema with bronchospasm, and hypotension. The intitial signs typically are cutaneous, consisting of diffuse erythema, pruritus, urticaria, or angioneurotic edema. These are frequently followed by pulmonary insufficiency from bronchospasm, laryngeal edema, or both. The patient typically demonstrates stridor and wheezing. Airway obstruction may progress rapidly and lead to severe respiratory distress. Cardiovascular collapse may occur either before or after the cutaneous and pulmonary manifestations.

An accelerated reaction, which occurs 20 minutes to 48 hours after exposure, is rarely life-threatening; typically, this type of reaction manifests as urticaria and occasionally laryngeal edema. A delayed reaction may develop 3 or more days after drug administration is initiated and typically consists of a rash.

36 Correct answer — D

Angioneurotic edema, a cutaneous manifestation seen initially in anaphylaxis, would be the nurse's lowest priority when treating a patient with altered gas exchange. Stridor, hoarseness, and inspiratory wheezing indicate respiratory compromise; treating these symptoms is the nurse's highest priority because airway obstruction and severe respiratory distress may follow quickly.

37 Correct answer — A

Corticosteroids are not used in the initial management of anaphylaxis. These drugs are used only in protracted cases and then only after I.V. fluids, epinephrine, and antihistamines have been administered. Epinephrine is regarded as the drug of choice; it can reverse all signs and symptoms of anaphylaxis. Its beta-adrenergic properties decrease

Shock Answers

histamine and bradykinin release and cause bronchodilation. Its alpha-adrenergic activity affects vasoconstriction, reversing hypotension.

38 Correct answer — B

Dobutamine hydrochloride is least likely to be used to treat anaphylaxis. During anaphylaxis, vasodilation, rather than a primary loss of myocardial contractility, is thought to be responsible for the hypotension. Thus, an agent with principally vasoconstrictive effects would be desirable. Dobutamine does not have enough vasoconstrictive effect to be useful in this situation, whereas norepinephrine does. I.V. aminophylline is indicated in instances of bronchospasm. Antihistamines are useful as adjunctive measures in relieving urticaria. Hydrocortisone, a steroid, decreases inflammation.

39 Correct answer — D

The most important principle that should be considered when caring for a patient with a history of allergies is to obtain an accurate and thorough drug history, which includes identifying and describing previous drug reactions. All of the other choices are important, but the drug history has the highest priority.

CHAPTER 15

Substance & Toxicologic Emergencies

1 A 23-year-old man who had been hiking is brought to the emergency department (ED) after having sustained a snakebite to his lower left leg 20 minutes ago. The most appropriate nursing intervention for this patient would be to:

A. Accurately identify the snake type
B. Immobilize and elevate the affected leg
C. Immobilize the affected extremity below heart level and apply a lightly constrictive tourniquet
D. Apply ice to the skin over the snake bite wound

2 Which incident is the most common cause of death from acute alcohol intoxication?

A. Respiratory depression or arrest
B. Aspiration of vomitus
C. GI bleeding
D. Accidental injury

3 Which condition commonly mimics the signs and symptoms of alcohol intoxication?

A. Diabetic reactions
B. Head injury
C. Drug overdose
D. All of the above

4 The nurse would expect the management of a patient with acute alcohol intoxication to include administration of all of the following *except:*

A. Thiamine 100 mg I.M.
B. Chlordiazepoxide (Librium) 100 mg I.M. every 2 to 4 hours as needed
C. Diazepam (Valium) 5 to 10 mg I.V. bolus for seizure management
D. Normal saline solution I.V.

5 When planning the care of a patient with alcohol intoxication, the nurse should keep in mind that alcohol withdrawal syndrome:

A. Does not cause death
B. Typically starts 6 to 72 hours after the last alcohol ingestion
C. Lasts up to 12 hours after withdrawal
D. Is best managed by restricting fluid intake

Substance & Toxicologic
Emergencies Questions

6 Many patients undergoing therapy for alcohol abuse use disulfiram (Antabuse). The nurse would anticipate the emergency management of a disulfiram-alcohol reaction to include:

A. Initiation of an infusion of normal saline solution
B. Administration of diphenhydramine hydrochloride (Benadryl) 50 mg
C. Administration of chlorpheniramine maleate (Chlor-Trimeton) or a similar drug
D. All of the above

7 A 19-year-old man arrives at the ED exhibiting signs of confusion, lethargy, dysarthria, and emotional instability. Which drug is most likely to produce these symptoms?

A. Phencyclidine (PCP)
B. Barbiturates
C. Amphetamines
D. Cocaine

8 A 22-year-old man arrives at the ED for treatment of PCP ingestion. Which of the following would be an important concern when planning the care of this patient?

A. Offering the patient constant verbal reassurance
B. Administering phenothiazines
C. Providing tactile stimulation
D. Placing the patient in a dimly lit room

9 The nurse who is assessing a patient with a methadone addiction knows that withdrawal symptoms typically appear within:

A. 8 to 10 hours
B. 12 to 24 hours
C. 24 to 36 hours
D. 36 to 48 hours

10 The correct procedure for gastric lavage in the initial management of the unconscious patient who has a substance overdose includes:

A. Instillation of 200 ml of warmed saline solution via a nasogastric tube drained by gravity
B. Instillation of iced normal saline solution
C. Performing the lavage before endotracheal intubation
D. Performing the lavage using 50% normal saline solution and 50% magnesium sulfate solution

SITUATION

A 75-year-old woman with a long history of rheumatoid arthritis is brought to the ED in a convulsive state. About 4 hours earlier, she complained to her primary physician that her arthritis was very painful. Her physician ordered methyl salicylate (wintergreen oil) to be applied topically. The patient's son tells the nurse that his mother may have taken the drug orally (1 tsp = 21 adult aspirin tablets).

Questions 11 to 15 refer to the above situation.

11 The nurse would anticipate the absorption of methyl salicylate to continue how long after ingestion?

A. 2 hours
B. 3 hours
C. 6 hours
D. 10 hours

12 The nurse would expect to note signs of acute salicylate intoxication in a patient who has taken a single dose greater than:

A. 50 mg/kg
B. 100 mg/kg
C. 150 mg/kg
D. 200 mg/kg

13 Which sign of salicylate poisoning (salicylism) should the nurse assess for in this patient?

A. Tetany
B. Coma
C. Hypernatremia
D. Hypothermia

14 The nurse would anticipate emergency treatment for this patient to include all of the following *except:*

A. Gastric lavage with activated charcoal
B. Administration of ipecac syrup
C. Administration of sodium bicarbonate
D. Hemodialysis

15 Which statement about salicylate intoxication after ingestion of enteric-coated aspirins is *true?*

A. Because of the drug's enteric coating, symptoms will not be as severe
B. Hospitalization probably will not be required
C. Toxic effects will be delayed because of delayed absorption
D. Early blood levels are a reliable guide to prognosis

SITUATION

A 3-year-old girl weighing 35 lb (15.9 kg) is brought to the ED. She is alert but has been nauseated, vomiting, and diaphoretic since this morning. Last night an open bottle of pediatric acetaminophen (Children's Tylenol) was found in a bathroom at the patient's home.

Questions 16 to 20 refer to the above situation.

16 How long after ingestion of acetaminophen would the nurse expect to note signs and symptoms of overdose in a patient?

A. 1 to 3 hours
B. 4 to 6 hours
C. 12 to 24 hours
D. 24 to 48 hours

17 The nurse knows that, if treatment is unsuccessful for this patient, all of the following complications may occur *except:*

A. Liver necrosis
B. Liver failure
C. Impaired renal function
D. Arrhythmias

18 Which laboratory value is characteristically abnormal in acetaminophen toxicity?

A. Creatinine phosphokinase level
B. Alkaline phosphatase level
C. Prothrombin time
D. Direct Coombs' test

19 The nurse is aware that the antidote for acetaminophen overdose consists of administering:

A. Activated charcoal
B. Physostigmine (Antilirium)
C. Acetylcysteine (Mucomyst)
D. Naloxone (Narcan)

20 Which nursing diagnosis is most appropriate for this patient?

A. Decreased cardiac output related to bleeding from impaired coagulation
B. Decreased cardiac output related to bleeding from irritated GI mucosa
C. Potential for injury related to seizures
D. Impaired gas exchange related to respiratory depression

SITUATION

A woman arrives at the pediatric clinic with her 5-year-old son, whom she thinks has swallowed 5 to 10 iron supplement tablets. The child is vomiting and complaining of severe abdominal pain.

Questions 21 to 25 refer to the above situation.

21 Which statement regarding iron poisoning is *true?*

A. Toxicity depends on the amount of iron salt ingested
B. Ingestion of 50 to 100 ferrous sulfate tablets is not considered fatal
C. Acute iron poisoning occurs primarily in elderly people
D. Shock is the most common cause of death in iron poisoning

22 The nurse knows that iron ingestion may be confirmed by:

A. Gastric fluid analysis
B. Serum triiodothyronine (T_3) and thyroxine (T_4) levels
C. Serum hemoglobin levels
D. Abdominal X-rays 72 hours after ingestion

23 If toxicity is suspected, the nurse would expect the physician to order which procedure first?

A. Administration of a saline cathartic
B. Administration of ipecac syrup or gastric lavage
C. Abdominal X-rays
D. Serum iron level analysis

24 Which assessment finding may indicate iron toxicity?

A. Metabolic alkalosis
B. Abdominal pain and hemorrhagic gastroenteritis
C. Seizures
D. Renal failure

25 The nurse would expect supportive care for this patient to consist of:

A. Maintaining the patient's body temperature
B. Administering antihypertensives
C. Administering diuretics
D. Dialysis

SITUATION

A 12-year-old boy arrives by ambulance at the ED. According to the boy's father, the patient drank 2 oz (57 ml) of liquid bleach (an alkaline substance) on a friend's dare.

Questions 26 to 30 refer to the above situation.

26 Which statement concerning caustic substances is *true?*

A. Acidic substances have the same effect as alkaline substances
B. The severity of an alkaline burn depends on the pH of the substance and the duration of contact with the mucosa
C. Oropharyngeal and esophageal damage is more common with liquids than with solids
D. The absence of oral burns excludes the possibility of esophageal burns

27 Which symptom of caustic ingestion should the nurse assess for in this patient?

A. Tinnitus
B. Hyperthermia
C. Drooling
D. Dyspnea

28 The nurse would anticipate treatment for caustic ingestion to include:

A. Dilution with 8 oz (240 ml) of milk or water
B. Administration of activated charcoal
C. Administration of a cathartic
D. Induction of emesis or gastric lavage

29 Which dose of a concentrated acid or alkali is considered lethal to an adult?

A. 5 ml
B. 10 ml
C. 15 ml
D. 30 ml

30 Which statement about the nursing management of a patient who has ingested or been exposed to a caustic substance is *true?*

A. Dermal and ocular decontamination should be carried out
B. Antibiotics may be administered prophylactically
C. Steroids should never be administered
D. Barium swallow is contraindicated

SITUATION

A 21-year-old woman arrives at the ED, complaining of blurred vision, sore throat, dizziness, and nausea. She reports to the nurse that her sister has similar symptoms. Both women ordered the same meal at a restaurant yesterday. The physician suspects that the patient has botulism.

Questions 31 to 34 refer to the above situation.

---

31 Which statement about botulism is *true?*

A. Ingestion of improperly home-processed vegetables, fruits, and meats is responsible for most cases of botulism
B. Botulism is not caused by fresh vegetables that have been grown in the ground
C. Danger arises when cooked foods remain at room temperature for more than 2 hours
D. The spores of *Clostridium botulinum* cannot withstand boiling for more than 30 minutes

32 Botulism is caused by a neurotoxin that blocks release of acetylcholine at peripheral nerve endings. The nurse is aware that botulism produces signs and symptoms similar to those of:

A. Guillain-Barré syndrome
B. Brown-Séquard syndrome
C. Salmonella poisoning
D. Acetaminophen overdose

Substance & Toxicologic
Emergencies Questions

33 The nurse is aware that eight serologically different toxins of *C. botulinum* exist, but Types A, B, and E most commonly affect humans. Which statement about toxin types is *true?*

A. Identification of the type of toxin requires serum or stool analysis
B. The incubation period for Type A is longer than that for Types B and E
C. Patient care is the same, regardless of toxin type
D. Respiratory insufficiency occurs with the same frequency, regardless of toxin type

34 The nurse would anticipate treatment of botulism to include:

A. Administration of magnesium salts (Milk of Magnesia)
B. Administration of acetylcysteine
C. Exchange transfusion
D. Hemofiltration

SITUATION

A 51-year-old woman was admitted to the ED about 2 hours ago. She has a history of asthma, and her admitting diagnosis is pneumonia. She is now complaining of breathing difficulty. The nurse notes an audible wheeze and an erythematous rash over the patient's entire body; the rash was not noted on admission. The patient received an initial dose of penicillin by I.V. piggyback 1 hour ago but has no history of allergies to antibiotics.

Questions 35 to 38 refer to the above situation.

35 Which sign of anaphylaxis would the nurse expect to find while assessing this patient?

A. Bradyarrhythmias
B. Cheyne-Stokes respiration
C. Laryngeal edema
D. Hypertension

36 Which statement concerning allergic drug reactions is *true?*

A. A drug reaction typically begins as a macular eruption on the head and proximal extremities that spreads in a symmetrical pattern
B. Initial episodes of an exanthematous-type hypersensitivity drug reaction always occur within 1 week after the drug is started
C. If a patient has received a drug many times without a reaction, the nurse can safely presume that a reaction will never develop
D. The morphology of the erupted rash provides clues to the causative agent

37 The nurse would expect immediate treatment of a severe allergic drug reaction to include administration of:

A. Oxygen
B. Norepinephrine (Levophed)
C. Furosemide (Lasix)
D. Prednisone (Deltasone)

38 Which nursing intervention is appropriate for a patient in anaphylactic shock?

A. Place a tourniquet on the patient's arm above the I.V. site
B. Place the patient in high-Fowler's position
C. Administer atropine sulfate to reverse bradycardia
D. Place the patient in Trendelenburg's position

SITUATION

A 15-year-old boy is brought to the ED by his father for evaluation of a painful, erythemic lesion on his right leg. The patient, who had been walking through a wooded area earlier in the day, thinks that he may have been stung or bitten.

Questions 39 to 43 refer to the above situation.

39 Which nursing intervention is appropriate when treating a patient with an insect bite or sting?

A. Carefully place a tourniquet proximal to the sting or bite
B. Ensure that emergency equipment is available in the event of respiratory failure
C. Ensure that antivenom is available for I.V. administration
D. No intervention is necessary because serious complications typically do not result

40 Which therapy would the nurse expect the physician to order for a patient who incurred any bite, regardless of the type?

A. Antibiotic
B. Antipruritic
C. Calcium gluconate
D. Tetanus toxoid

Substance & Toxicologic
Emergencies Questions

41 When advising the patient about how to reduce the risk of future bites or stings, the nurse instructs him to:

A. Wear protective clothing when hiking or working outdoors near sheds or woodpiles, and check the protective clothing before each use

B. Spray insect repellent in the yard, on himself, and on his clothing

C. Take no special precautions, as nothing can prevent bites

D. None of the above

42 The nurse's discharge instructions for a patient who suffered an insect-related allergic reaction should include information on all of the following *except:*

A. The necessity of wearing a medical alert bracelet or necklace to indicate an allergy

B. If the patient is allergic to bee stings, the importance of carrying an anaphylaxis kit and knowing its proper use

C. Avoiding the use of perfumes, sprays, and brightly colored clothing because these attract insects

D. The possibility of serum sickness, which may occur 2 to 3 days after being stung

43 The nurse knows that, unlike other bites, the bite of the brown recluse spider:

A. Can occur any time of the year, but usually between September and March

B. Can occur any time of the year, but usually between April and October

C. Can be the most disfiguring, sometimes requiring skin grafting to close the wound

D. Has no particular differentiating characteristics

SITUATION

A 24-year-old man is brought to the ED by family members, who found him slumped over in a chair at home. An empty prescription bottle for 30 100-mg amitriptyline (Elavil) tablets, with an issue date of 5 days ago, was found near the patient. He is unresponsive except to deep pain, which elicits purposeful movements. The patient has clear lung sounds; his vital signs are blood pressure, 160/96 mm Hg; pulse rate, 140 beats/minute; and respiratory rate, 14 breaths/minute.

Questions 44 to 49 refer to the above situation.

Substance & Toxicologic
Emergencies Questions

44 Considering the patient's prescription for amitriptyline, the nurse should elicit from the family whether the patient has a history of:

A. Psychotic disorders
B. Anxiety-related neurosis
C. Chronic paranoia
D. Depression

45 Which action is the nurse's highest priority during the initial management of a patient with a tricyclic antidepressant overdose?

A. Instituting cardiac monitoring
B. Performing a neurologic assessment
C. Instituting measures to prevent aspiration
D. Beginning an infusion of normal saline solution

46 During this initial phase, the nurse should anticipate the need for:

A. Evacuation of gastric contents
B. Insertion of an indwelling urinary catheter
C. Parenteral infusion of physostigmine salicylate
D. Administration of quinidine sulfate (Quinidine) for arrhythmia control

47 Which assessment finding is not typically seen in the early manifestation of tricyclic antidepressnt overdose?

A. Agitation
B. Diaphoresis
C. Dilated pupils
D. Exaggerated reflexes

48 The nurse would expect the most effective and conservative treatment for the patient who has overdosed on a tricyclic antidepressant and develops severe tachycardia to include the administration of:

A. Sodium bicarbonate
B. Magnesium sulfate
C. Diazepam
D. Phenytoin (Dilantin)

49 Upon evaluation of the effectiveness of therapy, which assessment finding indicates the need for further treatment in this patient?

A. Cardiac arrhythmias
B. Miosis
C. Urinary incontinence
D. Hypothermia

A 22-year-old man is brought to the ED by his friends, who tell inform the nurse that they think he has overdosed on cocaine.

Questions 50 to 54 refer to the above situation.

50 Which symptoms of cocaine abuse would the nurse expect to detect during a patient assessment?

A. Lethargy and obtundation
B. Constricted pupils
C. Hypothermia and tiredness
D. Euphoria and restlessness

51 Further assessment of this patient is likely to reveal which cardiovascular effect?

A. Hypotension
B. Myocardial ischemia
C. Atrioventricular block
D. Sinus bradycardia

52 Which treatment would the nurse expect the physician to order for a patient with a suspected cocaine overdose?

A. Oxygen
B. Naloxone
C. Physostigmine
D. Activated charcoal

53 When documenting suspected cocaine use, the nurse must keep in mind that cocaine can be detected in the urine for up to:

A. 12 hours
B. 36 hours
C. 5 days
D. 10 to 14 days

54 After the patient has been in the ED for some time, the nurse begins to evaluate him for signs of withdrawal. Which symptom is characteristic of cocaine withdrawal?

A. Euphoria
B. Hunger
C. Suicidal ideation
D. Lengthy sleep periods

Answer Sheet

	A B C D		A B C D
1	○ ○ ○ ○	31	○ ○ ○ ○
2	○ ○ ○ ○	32	○ ○ ○ ○
3	○ ○ ○ ○	33	○ ○ ○ ○
4	○ ○ ○ ○	34	○ ○ ○ ○
5	○ ○ ○ ○	35	○ ○ ○ ○
6	○ ○ ○ ○	36	○ ○ ○ ○
7	○ ○ ○ ○	37	○ ○ ○ ○
8	○ ○ ○ ○	38	○ ○ ○ ○
9	○ ○ ○ ○	39	○ ○ ○ ○
10	○ ○ ○ ○	40	○ ○ ○ ○
11	○ ○ ○ ○	41	○ ○ ○ ○
12	○ ○ ○ ○	42	○ ○ ○ ○
13	○ ○ ○ ○	43	○ ○ ○ ○
14	○ ○ ○ ○	44	○ ○ ○ ○
15	○ ○ ○ ○	45	○ ○ ○ ○
16	○ ○ ○ ○	46	○ ○ ○ ○
17	○ ○ ○ ○	47	○ ○ ○ ○
18	○ ○ ○ ○	48	○ ○ ○ ○
19	○ ○ ○ ○	49	○ ○ ○ ○
20	○ ○ ○ ○	50	○ ○ ○ ○
21	○ ○ ○ ○	51	○ ○ ○ ○
22	○ ○ ○ ○	52	○ ○ ○ ○
23	○ ○ ○ ○	53	○ ○ ○ ○
24	○ ○ ○ ○	54	○ ○ ○ ○
25	○ ○ ○ ○		
26	○ ○ ○ ○		
27	○ ○ ○ ○		
28	○ ○ ○ ○		
29	○ ○ ○ ○		
30	○ ○ ○ ○		

Substance & Toxicologic
Emergencies Answer Sheet

1 Correct answer — **C**

If less than 30 minutes has elapsed since the snakebite, the nurse should promptly initiate treatment, beginning with immobilization of the affected extremity below heart level and the immediate application of a lightly constrictive tourniquet. The skin should be washed, but ice should not be applied to the bite. Snake bites involving the head or trunk are the most dangerous; however, most snake bites occur below the elbow or knee. The nurse must remember to avoid elevating the affected extremity because this action increases envenomation. In the United States, rattlesnakes, water moccasins, copperheads, and coral snakes are the most common poisonous snakes. Identifying the type of snake that inflicted the bite is helpful, although valuable treatment time must not be wasted in doing so.

2 Correct answer — **A**

The most common cause of death from acute alcohol intoxication is respiratory depression. Such depression begins to occur at alcohol blood levels of 0.20%; death occurs at approximately 0.40% to 0.50%. Death also commonly results from aspiration of vomitus and accidental injury, especially from automobile accidents. GI bleeding occurs most commonly in patients who chronically abuse alcohol.

3 Correct answer — **D**

Head injury, drug overdose, and diabetic reactions can all mimic acute alcohol intoxication. Other disorders also should be considered, such as acute brain syndrome, meningitis, and psychiatric disorders. An accurate history and physical examination and appropriate diagnostic studies are necessary to arrive at the correct diagnosis.

4 Correct answer — **D**

Normal saline solution would not be included in the management of a patient with acute alcohol intoxication. The appropriate I.V. solution for treating an intoxicated patient contains dextrose (dextrose 5% in water or dextrose 10% in water) to facilitate the metabolism of the alcohol. Diazepam and chlordiazepoxide are tranquilizers that may be helpful in controlling behavior. Strong sedatives should not be used because they increase the risk of respiratory depression. Diazepam also is indicated for seizure control. Thiamine maintains or restores neurologic function that may be impaired from malnutrition and vitamin deficiency.

Substance & Toxicologic
Emergencies Answers

5 Correct answer—B

Alcohol withdrawal syndrome typically begins 72 hours after alcohol is last ingested and may continue for several days. However, its onset is unpredictable; it may begin as early as 6 hours after alcohol is withdrawn. The cause of a significant number of deaths, alcohol withdrawal syndrome has a mortality rate of 10% to 15%. Adequate hydration and proper electrolyte balance are critical to maintaining multisystem functioning.

6 Correct answer—D

Disulfiram-alcohol reactions mimic anaphylactic shock and should be managed in basically the same manner. This includes initiating an infusion of normal saline solution and administering diphenhydramine hydrochloride and chlorpheniramine maleate. Reactions may last up to several hours or as long as alcohol is in the bloodstream. Reaction also may occur from up to 14 days after discontinuation of disulfiram because of the drug's slow elimination from the body.

7 Correct answer—B

Barbiturates are noted for creating confusion along with lethargy, dysarthria, and emotional instability. Phencyclidine (PCP), amphetamines, and cocaine usually produce euphoria and increased activity.

8 Correct answer—D

A patient under the influence of PCP typically responds better to the least amount of stimulation. Therefore, the patient should be placed in a dimly lit, quiet room and should be cared for by only one nurse. Phenothiazines are clinically similar to PCP; their administration may produce an anticholinergic crisis or potentiate the effects of PCP.

9 Correct answer—C

Methadone typically remains in a patient's system for approximately 48 hours. Depending on the patient's metabolism and drug history, withdrawal symptoms may become evident in 24 to 36 hours.

10 Correct answer—A

The correct procedure for gastric lavage for a patient with a substance overdose involves the instillation of 200-ml increments of warmed normal saline solution, which is drained by gravity intermittently. Instillation of iced normal saline solution, which causes local venous constriction, is effective for a patient with a GI hemorrhage. The

Substance & Toxicologic
Emergencies Answers

airway of an unconscious patient must be protected before gastric lavage; therefore, endotracheal intubation must be performed first. Magnesium sulfate or citrate is administered after the lavage is completed to enhance excretion. Activated charcoal may also be given at this time to increase adsorption of the toxin.

11 Correct answer—C

The nurse would anticipate the absorption of methyl salicylate to continue for 4 to 6 hours after ingestion, with peak levels occurring in about 6 hours. The nurse should keep in mind that absorption may be delayed if the patient has ingested food. The absorption of regular aspirin tablets is nearly complete within 2 hours.

12 Correct answer—C

Signs of salicylate intoxication occur when more than 150 mg/kg is ingested at one time.

13 Correct answer—B

Salicylate poisoning may result in a variable degree of central nervous system depression, producing such signs as lethargy, coma, and seizures. Dehydration, hyponatremia, and hypokalemia are signs of acute salicylism, along with the hallmark signs and symptoms of tinnitus, vomiting, hyperthermia, and hyperpnea.

14 Correct answer—B

Emergency treatment for this patient would not include administration of ipecac syrup, as emesis should not be induced in a patient experiencing convulsions or an altered level of consciousness. Activated charcoal binds salicylates and prevents further absorption; it may be given via a nasogastric tube, if necessary. Sodium bicarbonate corrects metabolic acidosis and shifts salicylates from the tissues into the plasma. Indications for hemodialysis include a potentially lethal salicylate blood level (greater than 100 mg/dl), a deteriorating condition despite conservative therapy, or an inability to affect alkaline diuresis.

15 Correct answer—C

If the aspirin or salicylate product ingested had an enteric coating, the toxic effects could be delayed because absorption of these products occurs more slowly. The patient must be kept under observation for at least 24 hours because enteric-coated salicylates may not reach their highest concentration until 24 hours or more after the overdose. Since absorption occurs more slowly, early levels may be an unreliable guide to prognosis.

16 Correct answer—**C**

Initial signs and symptoms of acetaminophen overdose—nausea, vomiting, lethargy, and diaphoresis—usually occur within 12 to 24 hours after ingestion. Elevated serum aspartate aminotransferase (AST), serum alanine aminotransferase (ALT), and serum bilirubin levels, as well as a prolonged prothrombin time (PT) and tenderness in the right upper abdominal quadrant over the liver, usually occur after 24 to 48 hours. About 3 to 5 days after ingestion, the patient may experience jaundice, hepatic coma, hypoglycemia, oliguria, or a severely prolonged PT.

17 Correct answer—**D**

Acetaminophen overdose does not produce arrhythmias. The hepatotoxicity of acetaminophen is related to depleted glutathione stores and the accumulation of a toxic metabolite of acetaminophen. Liver necrosis, liver failure, and impaired renal function may occur. Renal failure, a less common occurrence, is typically mild, although severe tubular necrosis may ensue.

18 Correct answer—**C**

The PT is characteristically abnormal in acetaminophen overdose, with a prolonged bleeding time. Other hepatotoxic effects of acetaminophen include elevated AST, ALT, and bilirubin levels.

19 Correct answer—**C**

The antidote for acetaminophen overdose consists of administering acetylcysteine. Within the first 12 hours, initial treatment begins with clearing residual acetaminophen from the patient's GI tract, using emesis or lavage and saline cathartics. However, if the patient is at high risk for developing hepatic damage, the currently recommended treatment is to administer acetylcysteine within 12 to 16 hours of ingestion. Activated charcoal binds acetylcysteine and should not be given. Oxygen is not indicated as an emergency treatment. Peritoneal dialysis or hemodialysis is indicated in severe cases when early treatment is not administered.

20 Correct answer—**A**

The most appropriate nursing diagnosis for this patient is *Decreased cardiac output related to bleeding from impaired coagulation,* as the patient may have altered hepatic function and impaired coagulation

442

from decreased production of clotting factors by the liver. This may predispose the patient to decreased cardiac output from hypovolemia and hemorrhage.

21 Correct answer—D

Shock is the most common cause of death in iron poisoning. Toxicity is based on the amount of elemental iron ingested, not on the amount of iron salt ingested. Ferrous fumarate (Ferranol) has 33% elemental iron; ferrous sulfate (Irospan), 20%; and ferrous gluconate (Ferralet), 11.5%. The ingestion of fewer than 10 tablets of ferrous sulfate can be fatal. Acute iron poisoning is most common in young children and usually results from accidental ingestion.

22 Correct answer—A

Iron ingestion may be confirmed in several ways. Gastric fluid may be analyzed qualitatively by the deferoxamine color test. Plain X-rays of the abdomen may demonstrate radiopaque particles; however, iron tablets may dissolve after 4 hours and iron solutions are not radiopaque. The provocative chelation test, which uses 50 mg/kg of I.M. deferoxamine mesylate (Desferal), requires significant iron absorption before the urine appears pinkish red. Serum iron levels and iron-binding capacity should be determined in any patient who has ingested an unknown or potentially toxic amount of iron.

23 Correct answer—B

In cases of suspected iron toxicity, the nurse would expect the physician to order administration of ipecac syrup or gastric lavage, as the patient's stomach should be emptied as soon as possible. Ipecac syrup is the method of choice. However, if the patient has an altered sensorium or if hematemesis has occurred, gastric lavage is indicated.

24 Correct answer—B

Abdominal pain and hemorrhagic gastroenteritis are common assessment findings in iron toxicity. GI symptoms resulting from direct irritation of the GI mucosa occur within 1 to 6 hours of ingestion. Severity ranges from mild epigastric distress and vomiting to marked abdominal pain and hemorrhagic gastroenteritis. In patients who have taken a severe overdose, the serum iron level exceeds the iron-binding capacity and results in free-circulating iron. Free iron causes systemic symptoms to develop over 24 to 48 hours. Metabolic acidosis and shock are common early features of severe overdose. Coagulation defects and hepatic damage are variable and inconsistent.

Substance & Toxicologic Emergencies Answers

25 Correct answer — A

Supportive care for this patient would consist of maintaining body temperature, administering parenteral fluids to maintain hydration, and correcting hypotension with vascular expanders and vasopressors, if necessary. Hypoxia may be treated with oxygen therapy; metabolic acidosis may be treated with sodium bicarbonate.

26 Correct answer — B

The severity of an alkaline burn depends on the pH of the substance and the duration of contact with the mucosa. Strong alkaline products produce a liquefactive necrosis, penetrate deeply and rapidly, and result in esophageal stricture. Acidic substances cause a coagulation necrosis and thus do not penetrate as deeply as alkalis. Oropharyngeal and esophageal damage is more common with solids than with liquids. In 10% to 15% of cases, esophageal burns are present despite the absence of oral burns.

27 Correct answer — C

Drooling occurs as a result of dysphagia combined with an outpouring of saliva. Although local pain or burning is almost always present, severe burns may damage nerve endings, resulting in anesthesia. Dysphagia is common. A physical examination may reveal mucosal burns, appearing as whitish gray or red patches.

28 Correct answer — A

Dilution of the ingested acid or alkaline substance with 6 to 8 oz (180 to 240 ml) of milk or water is the preferred treatment, providing the patient can tolerate oral fluid. After that, the patient should take nothing by mouth. Induced emesis, gastric lavage, and administration of activated charcoal and cathartics are inappropriate. Airway management, adequate fluid replacement, and careful monitoring for perforation and hemorrhage are essential.

29 Correct answer — A

In adults, 5 ml of a concentrated strong acid or alkali is considered lethal.

30 Correct answer — A

Dermal and ocular decontamination should be carried out, when appropriate, for any patient who has ingested or been exposed to a caustic substance. Antibiotics are not useful prophylactically. A barium swallow 10 days to 3 weeks after the incident may help

Substance & Toxicologic Emergencies Answers

determine the severity of damage. Steroids, although controversial, may be recommended if burns are found or esophagoscopy is not performed.

31 Correct answer—A

Most cases of botulism result from improperly home-processed vegetables, fruits, and meats. The spores of *Clostridium botulinum* can withstand boiling temperatures for several hours; after cooling to room temperature, they can germinate and begin to produce toxin. Danger arises when cooked food remains at room temperature for more than 16 hours. Fresh vegetables grown in the ground also can produce botulism.

32 Correct answer—A

Botulism produces signs and symptoms similar to those of Guillain-Barré syndrome, such as muscle weakness and sudden onset of paralysis. Other differential diagnoses for botulism include basilar artery stroke, chemical intoxication, tick-borne paralysis, trichinosis, and various neuropsychiatric syndromes.

33 Correct answer—A

Identification of the specific type of *C. botulinum* toxin requires serum or stool analysis. Type A toxin is more dangerous than Types B and E because of its prolonged morbidity and increased mortality. The incubation period is shorter in Type A, with the onset of symptoms ranging from 12 hours to 8 days after ingestion of the toxin. Acute onset of respiratory insufficiency, requiring prolonged mechanical ventilation, occurs more commonly with Type A.

34 Correct answer—A

Medical therapy for botulism can include administration of magnesium salts, saline solution enemas, equine antitoxin, and plasmapheresis. Medical therapy is aimed at preventing progression of toxic effects and complications by eliminating any unabsorbed toxin and neutralizing unfixed toxin. Subsequent supportive care is directed toward maintaining body functions to allow for metabolism of the fixed toxin.

35 Correct answer—C

The nurse would expect a patient with anaphylaxis to have signs of airway obstruction, laryngeal edema, urticaria, or vascular collapse.

36 Correct answer—A

An allergic drug reaction typically begins as a macular eruption on the head and proximal extremities, then spreads in a symmetrical pattern. Initial episodes of an exanthematous-type reaction usually occur within 1 week after the patient has started taking the drug; however, occasionally, the rash appears as long as 14 days after the drug has been discontinued. A patient may be treated with a drug many times before developing a reaction. The morphology of the eruption gives no clue to the specific causative agent; therefore, a careful history of all medications and other substances that have entered any body orifice is essential to making the proper diagnosis.

37 Correct answer—A

Immediate treatment of a severe allergic drug reaction includes the administration of oxygen. The patient in this situation has signs of systemic anaphylaxis. Because she is a known asthmatic, she has a greater risk of bronchoconstriction than a nonasthmatic person. Anaphylaxis is a life-threatening condition that requires immediate treatment. Treatment is directed toward impairing absorption of the antigen, enhancing oxygenation, and treating or preventing hypotension. Besides oxygen therapy, other emergency measures include the administration of epinephrine (Adrenalin), aminophylline (Phyllocontin), and hydrocortisone (Cortef). Prednisone may take 4 to 6 hours to start working.

38 Correct answer—B

The most appropriate measure in this situation would be to place the patient in high-Fowler's position to optimize ventilation. The Trendelenburg position may be dangerous because it impairs ventilation, especially in a hypotensive patient or a patient with dyspnea and bronchospasm. Since the antibiotic was given an hour ago, it has already been distributed to the bloodstream and tissues; therefore, applying a tourniquet above the I.V. site would be of little value. Tachycardia is seen in anaphylactic shock, so atropine sulfate is not indicated.

39 Correct answer—B

Respiratory failure is always a possibility after insect stings and bites; therefore, emergency equipment must be readily available in the event of a severe allergic reaction or anaphylaxis resulting in respiratory failure. Antivenom I.V. is recommended for scorpion and black widow spider bites, not insect bites. Tourniquet application is used for scorpion bites and snakebites.

Substance & Toxicologic Emergencies Answers

40 Correct answer — D

Tetanus toxoid should be administered to any patient who has incurred a bite, regardless of the type of bite, unless the patient has received a tetanus toxoid booster within the past 5 years. Prophylactic antibiotics may be prescribed. Calcium gluconate controls muscle spasms associated with black widow spider and scorpion bites. Antipruritics reduce itching associated with tick bites.

41 Correct answer — A

Wearing protective clothing when hiking or working outdoors or near sheds or woodpiles and checking the condition of protective clothing before each use are recommended to reduce the risk of infestation and to prevent bites. Insect repellents are useful only against bees.

42 Correct answer — D

Before the patient is discharged, the nurse should inform the patient who was treated for an insect-related allergic reaction that he may experience serum sickness 10 to 14 days after the sting. The nurse also should stress the necessity of wearing a medical alert bracelet or necklace indicating the patient's allergy. Other important discharge instructions include information on the importance of carrying an anaphylaxis kit and knowing its proper use and on the need to avoid using perfumes, sprays, and brightly colored clothing, which attract insects.

43 Correct answer — C

The bite from a brown recluse spider can be quite disfiguring; sometimes, skin grafting is required to close the wound. Ulcers form and, with a graft, can take 6 to 8 weeks to heal. Brown recluse spiders are found in the South, Southwest, and Pacific Northwest. Like other spiders' bites, these bites occur throughout the year but most commonly in summer or fall.

44 Correct answer — D

Tricyclic antidepressants, such as amitriptyline, are primarily used to treat depression, which typically manifests as mixed clinical signs of lethargy, insomnia, anorexia, and agitation. Although tricyclic antidepressants are highly effective in treating nonorganic depression, these drugs should be used cautiously; patients with nonorganic depression are prone to self-destructive behavior, such as life-threatening overdoses.

Substance & Toxicologic Emergencies Answers

45 Correct answer — C

Instituting measures to prevent aspiration is the nurse's highest priority because it deals with airway maintenance. Definitive treatment for any overdose always begins with the ABCs of emergency care: airway, breathing, and circulation. All supportive care is based on the assessment and maintenance of these factors.

46 Correct answer — A

The nurse should anticipate the need for evacuation of gastric contents. Tricyclic antidepressants slow peristalsis; significant amounts of ingested drugs can be found in the stomach several hours after intake. Gastric aspiration ensures removal of stomach contents; repeated lavage removes tricyclic antidepressant metabolites that are periodically released from the liver and gallbladder. Repeated charcoal administration has been recommended in cases involving tricyclic antidepressant overdosage. Such administration allows for the continued absorption of any ingested drug that may remain in the stomach. Administering quinidine sulfate would worsen the already toxic effects, which result in prolonged QRS complexes and QT intervals. Physostigmine administration may be required if anticholinergic symptoms develop. An indwelling urinary catheter may then be warranted to measure urine output.

47 Correct answer — B

The clinical manifestations of tricyclic antidepressant overdose do not include diaphoresis. These drugs mimic anticholinergic drugs and produce fever, agitation, dilated pupils, tachycardia, and dry mucous membranes. Many patients who overdose experience twitching that progresses to tonic-clonic seizures.

48 Correct answer — A

The most effective and conservative treatment is to administer sodium bicarbonate to alkalize the blood to a pH of 7.5. Studies indicate that tachycardia usually disappears at this pH; breaking the tricyclic antidepressant bonding with body protein is the proposed mechanism by which this occurs. Magnesium sulfate speeds the slowed peristalsis and hastens the elimination of drugs absorbed by charcoal. Diazepam and phenytoin are used to treat seizure activity associated with overdosage.

49 Correct answer — A

Tricyclic antidepressant overdose causes arrhythmias, fever, mydriasis, and urine retention from the anticholinergic effects of the drug. Assessment of such symptoms indicates that further treatment is necessary.

50 Correct answer – D

Symptoms of cocaine abuse include euphoria, restlessness, excitedness, hyperthermia, and pupil dilation.

51 Correct answer – B

Further assessment would likely reveal myocardial ischemia in this situation. Cocaine produces vasoconstrictive effects on the cardiovascular system similar to sympathetic nervous stimulation. Tachycardia and hypertension are the most common effects. Myocardial ischemia, infarction, and ventricular arrhythmias are also common.

52 Correct answer – A

Because no antidote for cocaine overdose exists, the nurse would expect the physician to order oxygen administration to prevent some of the cardiovascular effects caused by vasoconstriction.

53 Correct answer – B

Cocaine can be detected in the urine for up to 36 hours after ingestion.

54 Correct answer – C

Suicidal ideation and depression are signs of cocaine withdrawal, along with sleep disturbances, lethargy, and fatigue.

CHAPTER 16

Surface Trauma Emergencies

1 After a traumatic injury, the nurse should continue to assess for signs and symptoms of compartment syndrome for up to:

A. 3 days
B. 6 days
C. 10 days
D. 14 days

2 The nurse knows that reliable signs and symptoms of increased compartment pressure include pain, weakness, hypoesthesia, and:

A. Prolonged capillary refill time
B. Cold extremity
C. Tenseness of the compartment on palpation
D. Pallor

3 A patient with a leg injury and developing compartment syndrome asks the nurse why his pain is so bad. The nurse correctly responds that the pain is most likely caused by:

A. Pressure on the nerves in the leg
B. Lack of blood flow to the muscles
C. Pressure on deep tendons
D. Bleeding into the leg

4 The nurse is aware that, in compartment syndrome, irreversible damage to nerves and muscles in the affected compartment typically occurs within how many hours after the onset of impaired perfusion?

A. 1 to 4
B. 4 to 12
C. 16 to 24
D. 24 to 48

5 Which assessment finding may be a late sign of compartment syndrome?

A. Pain upon flexion of the extremity
B. Paresthesia over the affected area
C. Loss of distal pulses
D. Edema formation

6 Surgical fasciotomy for decompression of compartment pressure is indicated when compartment pressure exceeds:

A. 5 mm Hg
B. 15 mm Hg
C. 25 mm Hg
D. 40 mm Hg

7 All of the following factors would contribute to compartment syndrome *except:*

A. Direct soft-tissue trauma, causing increased interstitial space pressure and edema
B. Tissue pressure within a fascial compartment that falls below the capillary hydrostatic pressure, preventing arterial inflow
C. Venous outflow obstruction
D. Superficial pressure sore formation

8 During triage, all of the following interventions are indicated for a severe soft-tissue injury *except:*

A. Wound culture
B. Traction
C. Sterile dressing
D. X-rays

SITUATION

A 43-year-old woman arrives at the emergency department (ED) accompanied by her husband, who states that she lost the first three fingers of her left hand while using a food processor. The husband has carried the amputated fingers in a plastic bag to the ED.

Questions 9 to 13 refer to the above situation.

9 The nurse is aware that, after amputation of body parts, the prognosis for successful reattachment is poor when warm muscle ischemia time has exceeded:

A. 1 hour
B. 2 hours
C. 4 hours
D. 6 hours

10 Which injury typically holds the best prognosis for successful reattachment of an amputated body part?

A. Guillotine injury
B. Localized crush injury
C. Diffuse crush or explosion injury
D. Avulsion injury

11 Which early nursing intervention is least desirable when caring for an amputation site?

A. Applying a dry sterile dressing to the wound
B. Applying a povidone-iodine (Betadine) dressing to the wound
C. Irrigating the wound with lactated Ringer's solution
D. Irrigating the wound with normal saline solution

12 All of the following principles of caring for an amputated part are correct *except:*

A. Debris should be washed away with irrigation using cool sterile water, normal saline solution, or lactated Ringer's solution
B. The part should be handled with sterile technique
C. The part should be wrapped in sterile gauze and placed directly on ice
D. An X-ray of the part should be obtained

13 A patient with a serious or contaminated amputation and who has no known or previous tetanus vaccination should undergo tetanus immunization. To complete the full series of tetanus immunization, how long after the first dose should the patient return to receive the second dose of tetanus toxoid?

A. 2 to 4 weeks
B. 4 to 6 weeks
C. 6 to 8 weeks
D. 8 to 10 weeks

SITUATION

A 45-year-old woman sustained an injury to her left thigh when she was run over by a bus after slipping off an icy curb. Paramedics who arrive at the scene describe the patient's condition as stable, then transport her to the ED. Though the patient has no open wounds, her thigh is markedly swollen and tense. A tire tread mark is evident on the patient's thigh, and a hematoma has formed. Distal pulses are strong, and distal sensory and motor examination is normal. No pain is noted with passive stretch of her foot. X-rays reveal no fractures.

Questions 14 and 15 refer to the above situation.

14 The nurse determines that the patient's findings are consistent with:

A. An arterial injury
B. A degloving injury
C. An occult fracture
D. A compartment syndrome

15 Which nursing diagnosis holds the highest priority for this patient?

A. Altered peripheral tissue perfusion related to edema formation in the fascia
B. Potential for infection related to altered skin integrity
C. Altered patterns of urine elimination related to associated genitourinary trauma
D. Potential for injury related to possible spinal cord injury

SITUATION

A 31-year-old man had been cutting logs when the chain saw he was using struck a knot, then kicked back and struck him on the right side of his face and right upper arm.

Questions 16 and 17 refer to the above situation.

16 The nurse knows that facial damage sustained from this type of injury would least likely involve the:

A. Lacrimal duct
B. Facial nerve
C. Trigeminal nerve
D. Acoustic nerve

17 The patient complains of loss of sensation in his right index, second, and third fingers. Based on these findings, the nurse would suspect that the patient sustained damage to his:

A. Median nerve
B. Ulnar nerve
C. Radial nerve
D. Axillary nerve

SITUATION

The ED nurse is assessing a machinist who sustained an injury to his left hand when his ring finger became caught in a baling machine. The patient sustained multiple lacerations about the wrist and hand as well as significant loss of the skin, soft tissue, and tendons overlying the hypothenar area. The skin torn from the patient's finger was transported to the ED in a plastic bag. The patient is right-handed.

Questions 18 and 19 refer to the above situation.

18 All of the following initial nursing actions would be appropriate *except:*

A. Wrapping the injured finger in sterile gauze
B. Mechanically removing large pieces of debris from the wound
C. Soaking the injured finger in povidone-iodine solution
D. Assessing the patient's distal neurovascular status

19 The nurse would expect the likely outcome in this situation to include:

A. Replacement of avulsed skin and return of normal sensation
B. Replacement of avulsed skin, decreased sensation, and cold intolerance
C. Skin graft for coverage and limited range of motion
D. Amputation

SITUATION

A 32-year-old man is admitted to the ED with a crush injury to his lower legs after having been pinned under a bucket-loader for 4 hours. His vital signs are stable; he is alert, oriented, and complaining of extreme pain in his legs. Popliteal pulses are strong; pedal and posterior tibial pulses are weak. The ankles and feet appear dusky; the skin is tense, but the skin envelope is unbroken. X-rays reveal no broken bones.

Questions 20 to 25 refer to the above situation.

20 During assessment, the patient becomes semiconscious and continues to moan with pain. His blood pressure drops and his pulse rate increases. Which of the following is the most immediate life-threatening problem for this patient?

A. Arrhythmias
B. Hypovolemia
C. Respiratory depression from pain medication
D. Fat embolus to the lung

21 Based on the above findings, the nurse would anticipate the patient's arterial blood gas measurements to reveal which acid-base imbalance?

A. Metabolic acidosis
B. Respiratory acidosis
C. Metabolic alkalosis
D. Respiratory alkalosis

22 Which symptom is considered the classic sign of a developing compartment syndrome?

A. Tenseness of the compartment envelope
B. Weakness of the leg muscles
C. Pain that is out of proportion to the injury
D. Pain on passive stretch of the compartment muscles

23 The nurse knows that, if the patient's perfusion is compromised by compartment syndrome, the expected treatment involves:

A. Elevation of the affected leg
B. Application of cold packs
C. Application of warm packs
D. Fasciotomy

24 Which early major complication of a crush injury should the nurse assess for in this patient?

A. Adult respiratory distress syndrome
B. Acute renal failure
C. Hepatic failure
D. Paralytic ileus

25 The nurse should assess any patient admitted to the ED with a crush injury for possible:

A. Substance abuse
B. Gunshot wound
C. Stab injury
D. Infection

Answer Sheet

	A	B	C	D
1	○	○	○	○
2	○	○	○	○
3	○	○	○	○
4	○	○	○	○
5	○	○	○	○
6	○	○	○	○
7	○	○	○	○
8	○	○	○	○
9	○	○	○	○
10	○	○	○	○
11	○	○	○	○
12	○	○	○	○
13	○	○	○	○
14	○	○	○	○
15	○	○	○	○
16	○	○	○	○
17	○	○	○	○
18	○	○	○	○
19	○	○	○	○
20	○	○	○	○
21	○	○	○	○
22	○	○	○	○
23	○	○	○	○
24	○	○	○	○
25	○	○	○	○

Surface Trauma Emergencies Answers

1 Correct answer—**B**

Although compartment syndrome most commonly occurs within 12 to 72 hours after an injury, it may occur up to 6 days after the initial trauma. Compartment syndrome refers to the progressive vascular compromise of a portion of an extremity that, if left untreated, results in permanent death of muscle groups and nerves.

2 Correct answer—**C**

Tenseness of the compartment upon palpation is a reliable sign of compartment syndrome. Pallor, a cold extremity, and prolonged capillary refill time are nonspecific signs seen in many states of underperfusion.

3 Correct answer—**B**

The severe pain characteristic of compartment syndrome is caused by ischemia resulting from lack of blood flow to the patient's muscles.

4 Correct answer—**B**

If compartment syndrome remains undetected, irreversible damage to nerves and muscles can occur within 4 to 12 hours of impaired perfusion.

5 Correct answer—**C**

Loss of distal pulses is a relatively late sign of compartment syndrome, indicating complete disruption of arterial perfusion in the affected extremity.

6 Correct answer—**D**

When pressure within the compartment exceeds 40 mm Hg, surgical fasciotomy is indicated to relieve the pressure before irreversible necrosis develops in muscles and nerves.

7 Correct answer—**B**

Tissue pressure within the fascial compartment that falls below the capillary hydrostatic pressure would not contribute to compartment syndrome. However, direct soft-tissue injury, causing increased interstitial pressure, may contribute to this condition. When tissue pressure in a fascial compartment rises above the capillary hydrostatic pressure or mean arterial pressure, arterial inflow and venous outflow are obstructed. The prolonged inflow occlusion produces cellular ischemia, muscle necrosis, and pressure sore formation. These allow for bacterial invasion, infection, and rapid deterioration.

8 Correct answer—**B**

Traction would not be indicated for a severe soft-tissue injury. Appropriate nursing interventions include collecting information about the mechanism of injury, contamination at the scene, and the patient's tetanus immunization status; thoroughly examining the wound area, particularly noting the underlying neurovascular structures; taking a culture specimen; bandaging the wound with sterile dressings; and obtaining appropriate X-rays. All patients should receive I.V. antibiotics. Surgical consultation may be necessary if the patient requires surgical debridement and possible reconstruction of associated nerves, blood vessels, or bones.

9 Correct answer—**D**

A poor prognosis for successful reattachment is likely when warm muscle ischemia time has exceeded 6 hours. Because muscle tissue is most sensitive to anoxia, amputated parts that have not been cooled to decrease metabolism sustain damage. Connective tissue, bone, tendons, nerves, and skin can survive for up to 12 hours. Amputated parts that contain minimal muscle, such as fingers and thumbs, have reportedly remained viable for up to 30 hours at cold temperatures. Thus, immediate cooling of the amputated part and distal extremity is necessary to improve the prognosis for successful reattachment.

10 Correct answer—**A**

A sharp guillotine injury, especially of the area beyond the proximal phalanx, holds the best prognosis for successful reattachment because minimal debridement is necessary. Such amputations typically result from accidents involving an object with a sharp cutting edge, such as a knife, glass, meat cleaver, or band saw. Crush and avulsion injuries have poorer prognoses because extensive debridement and vein grafting usually are required.

11 Correct answer—**B**

The least desirable nursing intervention in this situation would be applying a povidone-iodine dressing to the wound. Appropriate immediate care of the amputation site includes the removal of visible foreign bodies and irrigation with 2 liters of lactated Ringer's solution, cool water, or normal saline solution. The area should be covered with sterile gauze, and the extremity should be supported and elevated on a board. Applying a desiccant, such as povidone-iodine solution, to the site can dry out subcutaneous tissue.

12 Correct answer — C

Care of an amputated part does not include wrapping the part in sterile gauze and placing it directly on ice. The emergency department (ED) nurse should always use sterile technique when handling an amputated part. The part should be irrigated with lactated Ringer's solution, cool sterile water, or normal saline solution to remove debris; prolonged irrigation should be avoided. X-rays of the injured extremity and the amputated part should be done. Afterward, the amputated part should be wrapped in sterile gauze, put into a sterile container, then placed on top of ice in a large container. Another acceptable method would involve wrapping the amputated part in a sterile sponge that has been moistened in a physiologic solution, placing it in a plastic bag or cup, and inserting it into an ice bath at 35° to 39° F (2° to 4° C). Placing the part directly on ice does not provide the homogeneous cooling that occurs with insertion in an ice bath. The specimen container must also be labeled with the patient's name.

13 Correct answer — B

A full tetanus immunization series includes three doses of adult tetanus toxoid I.M. The second dose is given 4 to 6 weeks after the first dose; the final dose, 6 months to 1 year later. Obtaining the patient's tetanus immunization history and adhering to the established dosage schedule are important nursing considerations. Usually, the ED nurse administers 0.5 ml of adsorbed tetanus toxoid I.M. and 250 units of tetanus immune globulin I.M. This dosage is appropriate for any patient with a serious, old, or contaminated wound or a wound involving destroyed tissue. It is also appropriate for a patient with an uncertain or no vaccination history and for a patient with major wounds who has received fewer than three doses of tetanus toxoid.

14 Correct answer — B

The patient's findings are consistent with a degloving injury. Typically, such extremity avulsion injuries are caused by large vehicles, such as trucks and buses. The large, broad double tires produce a tremendous shearing force over a large area, resulting in partial or circumferential avulsion of the skin and subcutaneous tissue. Characteristically, the patient sustaining such an injury also has an open wound. The avulsed area typically is severely crushed; damage to the underlying structures (muscles, nerves, blood vessels, and bone) is variable, possibly resulting in extensive disruption of the skin and subcutaneous tissue from the underlying structures. Fractures occur in about 80% of these injuries.

In this case, the patient has an atypical degloving injury, which consists of a small traction-type wound on the skin and subcutaneous tissue. Most of the leg in this type of injury will appear normal, except for possible tire tread marks and a region of ecchymosis. A significant hematoma will probably occur in this area. The extent of avulsion at the fascial level is deceptive and can extend the entire length and circumference of the leg. The sequelae of such an injury are insidious because the extent is grossly underestimated. Major skin loss or sepsis from extensive tissue necrosis may occur beneath the intact skin.

Because X-rays confirm that the patient has no fracture and the patient has strong distal pulses, an arterial injury can be ruled out. Compartment syndrome, which typically occurs 12 to 72 hours after the initial injury, most commonly involves the lower leg beneath the knee.

15 Correct answer—A

The priority nursing diagnosis for this patient would be *Altered peripheral tissue perfusion related to edema formation in the fascia*, which could lead to compartment syndrome. Because the patient's skin is still intact, *Potential for infection related to altered skin integrity* is inappropriate at this time. However, as necrosis and tissue destruction set in, the patient may succumb to infection. The situation reveals nothing about the patient's genitourinary status or the possibility of spinal cord injury.

16 Correct answer—D

This type of injury is least likely to involve the acoustic nerve. A kickback injury, such as the one sustained by this patient, that results in facial damage usually involves the eye, nose, or mouth; therefore, the lacrimal duct and branches of the facial or trigeminal nerves are at risk. The acoustic nerve exits from the cranial vault through the internal acoustic meatus and is not located in a particularly hazardous position.

Over the past several years, chain saw use has increased dramatically, along with a corresponding rise of associated injuries. Treatment of these devastating injuries should include neurovascular assessment based on anatomic location, as well as debridement, antibiotics, and tetanus prophylaxis.

17 Correct answer—A

Loss of sensation in the index, second, and third fingers indicates damage to the median nerve. To test motor ability of the median nerve, the nurse should ask the patient to oppose his thumb by trying to touch his little finger (pinky).

18 Correct answer — C

Soaking the injured finger in povidone-iodine solution would be inappropriate, as use of this agent can dry out subcutaneous tissue. Appropriate nursing actions during the initial management of this patient would include wrapping the injured finger in sterile gauze after removing pieces of debris and assessing distal neurovascular status.

19 Correct answer — D

Amputation is the most likely outcome when the skin is completely detached and the finger is completely denuded. Skin replacement or grafting usually do not result in acceptable hand function in these situations.

Industrial accidents commonly involve injuries to hands or fingers that become caught in moving machinery. Such injuries can range from crushing to degloving and even result in amputation. Parts of the hand may be torn or ground off and may not be suitable for salvage. A degloving injury, which is characterized by avulsion of skin, commonly leaves underlying tendons and bones intact. The primary problem in this injury is the viability of the skin. When skin is still attached distally, vascularity is difficult to assess; however, skin replacement may be possible.

20 Correct answer — B

Hypovolemia caused by extravasation of fluid into the patient's ischemic, crushed limbs is the most immediate, life-threatening problem in this situation. As much as 8 liters of fluid may extravasate into each limb. Arrhythmias may result from hypovolvemia; therefore, the patient should be placed on a cardiac monitor. Since the patient has not yet received pain medication, respiratory depression would not be a problem. Development of a fat embolus, although a possibility, is inconsistent with the patient's signs and symptoms.

21 Correct answer — A

The nurse would expect the patient's arterial blood gas measurements to reveal metabolic acidosis. Such an imbalance would occur when decreased tissue perfusion releases metabolic ischemic by-products from crushed tissues, resulting in increased lactic acid production.

22 Correct answer — C

Pain that is disproportional to the injury is a classic symptom of compartment syndrome. The patient in this situation is complaining of extreme pain and continues moaning while in a semiconscious state.

Tenseness, muscle weakness, and pain on passive stretching are other symptoms of developing compartment syndrome.

23 Correct answer—D

If the patient's perfusion is compromised by compartment syndrome, the expected treatment would involve a fasciotomy (a surgical incision made to release pressure) to minimize neurologic deficits and promptly restore local blood flow. If direct manometry of intramuscular pressures is available, fasciotomy is indicated when pressures exceed 45 cmH$_2$O. Elevating the affected leg would not produce quick enough results in this urgent situation. Applying cold packs is an early measure and of little help at this time. Applying warm packs would intensify the problem.

24 Correct answer—B

The nurse should assess for acute renal failure. The initial hypovolemic insult causes peripheral and renal vasoconstriction. Compensatory mechanisms involving the circulation of catecholamines, aldosterone, antidiuretic hormone, and renin further decrease renal blood flow and glomerular filtration rate. Also, circulating myoglobins from rhabdomyolysis produce rapid rises of serum potassium, phosphate, and uric acid levels. Paralytic ileus may develop 3 to 5 days after the injury as a result of hypokalemia, which typically follows a crush injury.

25 Correct answer—A

The nurse should assess any patient admitted with a crush injury involving trauma to the soft tissues for potential substance abuse. Alcohol, heroin, analgesic, tranquilizer, sedative, or antidepressant drug abuse circumvents the protective effect of pain. During a period of excessive sedation, an addicted patient can sleep deeply with one or more limbs compressed by his full body weight for a prolonged period; this may cause tissue necrosis in the compromised limbs.

CHAPTER 17

Professional Issues

1 In which circumstance may a nurse use force against a patient?

A. Under no circumstances
B. To help an emotionally distraught patient regain his senses
C. To assess an unconscious patient's level of reaction to physical stimuli
D. In self-defense, but only if the nurse has reasonable grounds to believe that she is being, or is about to be, attacked

2 Which statement about oral physician's orders is *true*?

A. Oral orders should be followed with written orders to ensure the nurse's legal protection
B. Oral orders are illegal in most states
C. Oral orders are valid only when witnessed by another person
D. Oral orders should be carried out only when verified and countersigned by another physician

3 If a patient does not understand the information just given by the physician during an informed consent, the nurse should:

A. Answer the patient's questions
B. Notify the supervisor
C. Notify the physician
D. Do nothing, as the consent is already signed

4 Administering a medication to a patient against his will is an example of:

A. False imprisonment
B. Negligence
C. Battery
D. Invasion of privacy

5 When witnessing an informed consent, the nurse is attesting that the:

A. Patient is informed about the procedure
B. Patient consents to the procedure
C. Patient is sufficiently alert and oriented to consent
D. Signature is that of the patient

6 In some hospitals, the nurse legally may obtain:

A. The informed consent
B. The patient's signature for an informed consent
C. Telephone consents from the next of kin
D. Administrative consent

Professional Issues
Questions

7 If a patient has questions regarding the correctness of treatment, the nurse should:

A. Inform the physician
B. Discuss the possibility of other therapies
C. Refer the patient to other qualified physicians
D. Reinforce the appropriateness of the treatment

8 The nurse disagrees with the physician's judgment in ordering furosemide (Lasix) for a patient, feeling that, although furosemide is safe to give in this situation, dopamine (Intropin) would be more effective. If, after questioning the order, the nurse is told to administer furosemide, she should:

A. Refuse to administer the medication
B. Administer the medication, as ordered
C. Administer dopamine instead
D. Consult another physician

9 Which criterion is necessary for negligence to occur?

A. The wrong therapy must be given
B. Injury must be incurred
C. A change in the patient's condition must be overlooked
D. An error in judgment must be made

10 Which of the following is the most appropriate way to legally document patient teaching?

A. Referring to it in the nurses' notes
B. Providing the patient with written instructions
C. Conducting the patient-teaching session in the presence of a witness
D. Giving the patient a written examination

11 Which triage goal is considered the most important?

A. Giving priority care to the most critically ill patients
B. Performing a comprehensive patient assessment for each patient
C. Performing an immediate patient interview
D. Placing patients in appropriate treatment areas

12 Which nursing action would be inappropriate for the triage nurse to implement?

A. Initiating cardiopulmonary resuscitation
B. Intervening immediately in arterial bleeding
C. Splinting suspected or obvious fractures
D. Placing an adhesive closure over a minor laceration

13 All of the following are responsibilities of the triage nurse *except:*

A. Preventing cross-contamination of suspected infectious patients
B. Performing a complete and comprehensive patient assessment
C. Initiating patient or family education
D. Fostering good public relations

14 The objectives of quality assurance are to:

A. Monitor the quality of patient care
B. Identify actual or perceived patient problems
C. Identify educational or remedial needs
D. All of the above

15 Resources by which to identify patient care issues include:

A. Minutes of staff meetings and patient complaints
B. Staff suggestions and state regulations
C. Joint Commission on Accreditation of Healthcare Organizations (JCAHO) guidelines
D. All of the above

16 Components of quality assurance monitoring include:

A. Problem identification, study or survey, results reporting, and recommendations
B. Problem identification, study or survey, results reporting, recommendations, and noncompliance consequences
C. Retrospective problems, study or survey, recommendations, and noncompliance consequences
D. Concurrent problems, results reporting, and recommendations

Professional Issues
Questions

17 The emergency department (ED) nurse receives a phone call from a hysterical, nearly incoherent woman who relays that she has just been sexually assaulted. She asks the nurse what she should do. The nurse correctly responds by:

A. Telling the woman to contact the police immediately
B. Telling the woman to contact the police and to come to the hospital immediately with a change of clothes
C. Referring the woman to a rape crisis center
D. Obtaining the woman's name, address, and phone number and telling her to call the police and come to the hospital immediately with a change of clothes

18 The ED nurse is speaking on the phone with a woman who states that she has just moved into the area and would like the name of a pediatrician. The nurse should:

A. Give her the name of a pediatrician on staff
B. Give her the name of a new pediatrician who is just starting a practice
C. Give her the number of the local medical society
D. Tell her to bring the child to the ED for evaluation and follow-up

19 Following hospital policy, the ED nurse places a follow-up phone call to a patient who has recently been discharged with a prescription for an antibiotic. The patient tells the nurse that he thinks he is having a drug reaction. The nurse should advise him to:

A. Decrease the dose and see if the reaction subsides
B. Continue taking the drug along with over-the-counter diphenhydramine (Benadryl)
C. Stop taking the drug
D. Stop taking the drug and return to the ED

20 The nurse knows that, in a police investigation, law enforcement agents are entitled to:

A. The patient's name, address, and age and the extent of injury
B. All patient information
C. A copy of the patient's medical record
D. No information without a court order

21 The ED nurse should know that the sequence of obtaining and securing evidence is known as:

A. The chain of evidence
B. Evidence integrity
C. Writ of evidence
D. Habeas corpus

22 Which term best describes an emergency consent?

A. Informed consent
B. Administrative consent
C. Implied consent
D. All of the above

23 The nurse knows that the parent or legal guardian of a minor who is a suspected victim of child abuse or neglect can:

A. Withdraw consent for treatment
B. Discharge the minor against medical advice
C. Be restrained by hospital personnel from taking the minor out of the hospital
D. Be restrained by police from taking the minor out of the hospital

24 The policy of an ED where most of the patient population is non-English speaking is to provide all discharge and patient instructions in English. For a patient who does not speak English but is accompanied by a friend who does, the nurse should:

A. Have the friend interpret the instructions for the patient
B. Determine the friend's ability to understand the instructions; then have the friend interpret them for the patient, and document this in the patient report
C. Delay the patient's discharge until a hospital interpreter can be found
D. Advise the patient to take the instructions to his private physician, who will interpret them for him

25 One of the nurse's responsibilities is to determine whether the patient understands his discharge instructions. The best way to accomplish this is to:

A. Have the patient repeat the instructions verbatim
B. Have the patient sign the ED record, indicating that he received the instructions
C. Have the patient explain the instructions to the nurse
D. All of the above

26 The nurse is aware that patient education is necessary for:

A. Medical and legal reasons
B. JCAHO requirements
C. Professional responsibility
D. All of the above

27 When should the nurse begin discharge planning for a patient admitted to the ED?

A. As soon as a definitive diagnosis is made
B. When discharge is imminent
C. As soon as the patient arrives at the ED
D. When the patient shows signs of improvement and can participate in the planning

28 The goals of discharge planning are to:

A. Conform to JCAHO requirements, prevent readmission for the same problem, and provide patient or family education
B. Conform to JCAHO requirements, provide patient or family education, and enhance facility revenues
C. Prevent readmission and foster good public relations
D. Prevent the patient or family from using the ED as a primary care facility

29 Which statement regarding giving telephone advice is incorrect?

A. The nurse cannot be sued for advice given over the telephone
B. Before giving any advice, the nurse should determine whether professional liability insurance covers such activities
C. Any advice given must reflect current nursing practice
D. No fee should be charged for such advice

30 Which situation does not constitute the establishment of a nurse-patient relationship?

A. A guest at a party discovers that he is speaking with a nurse and begins asking several health-related questions
B. The day after a neighbor inquires about her child's recent behavior, the nurse pays a visit to check on the child's condition
C. A patient who had been treated recently in the ED meets the nurse in a supermarket and asks about the adverse effects of a prescribed medication
D. A patient who had been treated recently in the ED phones for a re-explanation of discharge instructions

31 Which statement reflects the legally correct action a nurse should take when a person solicits medical advice?

A. The nurse must always refer the person to a physician
B. The nurse does not need to refer the person to a physician if she is convinced it is unnecessary
C. A nurse in private practice who operates without written physicians' protocols may diagnose and treat the person without a physician's referral
D. The nurse must always follow-up on the person's status 1 or 2 days later

32 A woman telephones the ED, stating that she is pregnant and bleeding vaginally. Which response by the nurse would be inappropriate?

A. Asking the woman how many months pregnant she is because the advice will vary, depending on the trimester
B. Asking the woman if she has had any prenatal care; if not, recommending that she come to the ED immediately to rule out placenta previa
C. Advising the woman to go to the nearest ED without soliciting any further information
D. Asking the woman to describe the amount of bleeding, in terms of the number of pads used in the last hour, to determine the bleeding's severity

33 A man recently discharged from the ED telephones for advice about the adverse effects of a prescribed medication. Which nursing action is most appropriate?

A. Checking the potential adverse effects in a valid drug resource and reporting the effects to the patient
B. Referring the patient to his physician
C. Referring the patient to a pharmacist
D. Asking the patient why he is concerned, then relating the adverse effects and referring the patient, if necessary, to a physician

SITUATION

The ED is notified by emergency medical services (EMS) about a multiple-casualty accident involving a school bus and a truck carrying radioactive waste. Because of the proximity of the accident to the ED, the ED personnel prepare to receive the bulk of casualties.

Questions 34 and 35 refer to the above situation.

34 The nurse's first priority in this situation would be to:

A. Designate a decontamination area
B. Notify the admitting office to clear five intensive care unit (ICU) beds
C. Clear the ED of all nonserious patients and move those awaiting admission to a holding area
D. Notify EMS about the number of casualties that the ED can accommodate

35 Which support services would the nurse expect to be most useful in this situation?

A. Laboratory and blood bank
B. Operating room
C. Pharmacy
D. Radiology

SITUATION

A prominent member of the community is brought to the ED after an attempted suicide. The nurse receives a phone call from a newspaper reporter, who asks about the incident.

Questions 36 and 37 refer to the above situation.

36 Which nursing action is appropriate in this situation?

A. Give the reporter the information requested as stipulated by the Freedom of Information Act
B. Give the reporter the general patient information as dictated by hospital policy
C. Allow the reporter to interview the patient when his condition permits
D. Notify the hospital administrator or nursing supervisor

37 A nurse who allows a reporter to gain unauthorized access to a patient's chart is guilty of:

A. Breach of patient confidentiality
B. Malpractice
C. Professional misconduct
D. None of the above

SITUATION

An 18-year-old man is brought to the ED unresponsive, with shallow breathing and a rapid, weak pulse; blood pressure is palpable at 80 mm Hg systolic. The patient's friends state that he just slumped over. After ensuring that the patient is stabilized, the nurse searches the patient's pockets to confirm identification and discovers an envelope containing a white powdery substance.

Questions 38 and 39 refer to the above situation.

38 Which nursing action is appropriate in this situation?

A. Replace the envelope and say nothing
B. Inform the physician
C. Inform the physician and secure the envelope
D. Inform the physician and notify the police

39 The nurse may be civilly liable in this situation for:

A. Illegal search and seizure
B. Invasion of privacy
C. Violation of constitutional rights
D. Nothing, as no civil liability exists

Answer Sheet

	A	B	C	D
1	○	○	○	○
2	○	○	○	○
3	○	○	○	○
4	○	○	○	○
5	○	○	○	○
6	○	○	○	○
7	○	○	○	○
8	○	○	○	○
9	○	○	○	○
10	○	○	○	○
11	○	○	○	○
12	○	○	○	○
13	○	○	○	○
14	○	○	○	○
15	○	○	○	○
16	○	○	○	○
17	○	○	○	○
18	○	○	○	○
19	○	○	○	○
20	○	○	○	○
21	○	○	○	○
22	○	○	○	○
23	○	○	○	○
24	○	○	○	○
25	○	○	○	○
26	○	○	○	○
27	○	○	○	○
28	○	○	○	○
29	○	○	○	○
30	○	○	○	○

	A	B	C	D
31	○	○	○	○
32	○	○	○	○
33	○	○	○	○
34	○	○	○	○
35	○	○	○	○
36	○	○	○	○
37	○	○	○	○
38	○	○	○	○
39	○	○	○	○

1 Correct answer — **D**

A nurse may legally use force against a patient in self-defense but only if the nurse has reasonable grounds to believe that she is being, or is about to be, attacked. Everyone, including the nurse, has the legal right to self-protection as well as the right to work in a safe environment. When attempting to manage a combative patient and the risk of danger is imminent, the nurse has the right to defend herself as long as the defense is justified and she uses a reasonable amount of force. This self-defense must cease, however, when the apparent danger has passed and the patient is no longer combative.

2 Correct answer — **A**

An oral order given by a physician to a nurse is legally valid but should be covered with a written order to prevent any legal implications. Because a physician may deny issuing an oral order, the nurse should always strive to obtain an oral order in the presence of a witness and secure a written order as soon as possible. Being aware of hospital policy regarding oral orders is also important. Some hospitals prohibit nurses from following oral orders; negligence could be charged if injury to a patient resulted from a nurse following a prohibited oral order, because hospital policy was not followed.

3 Correct answer — **C**

If a patient does not understand the information just given by the physician during an informed consent, the nurse should notify the physician, who should return and answer the patient's questions. If the physician does not do so, the supervisor may need to be called and the procedure delayed until further explanations are rendered. The nurse should not answer the patient's questions because this would constitute assuming the role and expertise of a physician. If the patient has questions that the nurse is not at liberty to answer, an informed consent probably was not obtained.

4 Correct answer — **C**

Administering a medication to a patient against his will is a form of battery, the harmful or offensive touching of one person by another. Assault, or threatened battery, refers to any act that creates a conscious, unreasonable apprehension in an individual of immediate, harmful, or offensive touching by another person. Giving a person medication or even a back rub against his will is battery. Assault and battery are examples of legal wrongs, or torts. The nurse who commits a legal wrong may be liable for damages in a lawsuit brought by the wronged person. Preventing a patient from leaving the emergency department (ED) against medical advice is considered false imprisonment. Failing to secure the bed side rails of a confused patient who subsequently falls out of bed and fractures his leg is a form of negligence. Failing to maintain the confidentiality of a patient's record is invasion of privacy.

5 Correct answer — D

When witnessing an informed consent, the nurse is attesting that the signature is that of the patient. Such witnessing does not signify that the nurse has observed any exchange of information between the physician and patient. The responsibility for obtaining consent lies with the physician and is part of the physician-patient relationship.

6 Correct answer — B

Although only the physician can obtain an informed consent, in some hospitals the nurse may legally obtain the patient's signature after the patient has been informed about a procedure. If the patient has any questions about the procedure, the nurse should refrain from seeking the signature and notify the physician. The nurse must be aware of individual hospital policy regarding the nurse's role in obtaining the patient's signature, as such policies vary from institution to institution. A nurse may witness a telephone consent from next of kin. Two physicians' statements are required to obtain administrative consent when the patient and family cannot consent.

7 Correct answer — A

If a patient has questions regarding the correctness of a particular treatment, the nurse should inform the physician, who should answer the questions. Because the nurse's role as patient advocate in such situations is not clearly defined by state laws, the most appropriate action would be to seek out the physician. Discussing other therapies and referring the patient to other qualified physicians may interfere with the physician-patient relationship; depending on the hospital, this may be grounds for dismissal. Reinforcing the appropriateness of the treatment has no bearing on the patient's right to adequate information.

8 Correct answer — B

If the nurse disagrees with the physician's judgment in ordering a particular drug for a patient and thinks that another drug would be more effective, and if, after questioning the order, she is told to give the first drug, she should do so. A disagreement in judgment does not constitute grounds for allowing the nurse to assume the role of a physician — that is, one who prescribes one medication over another. In this situation, the nurse disagreed in theory with the physician's choice of furosemide but did not specifically question the safety of giving the medication, only the medication's appropriateness. Because the physician reaffirmed the order, the nurse should comply with the physician's wishes. If the nurse still feels uncomfortable giving the medication, she may ask the physician to administer it. Legally, however, the nurse cannot refuse to administer medication unless it is blatantly erroneous to do so.

9 Correct answer—B

For negligence to occur, injury must be incurred. The breach of duty that occurs in the negligent act must be the proximate cause of the injury; that is, the negligent act must have occurred before and resulted in the patient's injury. An error in judgment that results in an injury does not necessarily constitute negligence. If the judgment was made after careful assessment of the patient's condition and would have been made by any reasonable, prudent nurse in a similar situation, the resulting error and injury is unfortunate but not negligent. Giving the wrong therapy and overlooking a change in condition do not necessarily lead to injury.

10 Correct answer—B

The most appropriate way to legally document patient teaching is by providing the patient with written instructions. The patient may dispute receiving oral instructions even if the incident is documented in the nurses' notes. Nurses' notes are highly important, however, in legal actions. Written instructions should always accompany oral instructions; they should be detailed enough for the patient and family to refer to at home, if necessary. Conducting patient-teaching sessions in the presence of a witness and giving the patient a written examination are impractical.

11 Correct answer—A

The most important goal of triage is giving priority care to the most critically ill patients. Triage, a means of sorting patients, involves categorizing patients according to their urgency of care and placing them in appropriate, designated treatment areas. Performing a comprehensive patient assessment is the responsibility of the care providers in the designated treatment areas.

12 Correct answer—D

Placing an adhesive closure over a minor laceration is an inappropriate action for the triage nurse. All of the other choices are appropriate functions of the triage nurse, who is responsible for providing immediate care or intervention for life-threatening or potentially life-threatening injuries or illnesses.

13 Correct answer — B

The triage nurse is not accountable for complete and comprehensive patient assessment. She is the first health care provider to identify potentially infectious patients and must take appropriate precautions in preventing contamination of other patients and personnel. The triage nurse also acts as a resource for patient or family education. Lastly, because the triage nurse is typically the first contact the patient or family has with hospital personnel, she is a significant representative of the hospital and thus plays an important role in fostering good public relations for the facility.

14 Correct answer — D

The objectives of quality assurance are to monitor the quality of patient care, identify actual or perceived patient problems, and, as a result of monitoring activities, identify educational and remedial activities necessary to correct identified problems.

15 Correct answer — D

All are potential resources by which to identify patient care issues. Additional resources include specific illnesses or injuries, the condition of patients upon arrival at the facility, and the response of support services to the ED. In short, anything having to do with the processing and care of patients in the ED can be developed into a quality assurance activity.

16 Correct answer — A

Problem identification, study or survey, results reporting, and recommendations are the specific components of quality assurance monitoring as recommended by the Joint Commission on Accreditation of Healthcare Organizations (JCAHO). The absence of any one or more of these factors results in an incomplete quality assurance activity.

17 Correct answer — D

The correct response would be to obtain the woman's name, address, and phone number and tell her to call the police and then come to the hospital immediately with a change of clothes. The nurse should request the patient's demographic information (name, address, and phone number) in case the phone line becomes disconnected or the patient never arrives in the ED; the nurse would then have enough information to follow-up on the case. Besides telling the patient to bring a change of clothes, the nurse should instruct her not to change her physical appearance or clothing or to shower, bathe, douche, or urinate. Depending on the patient's emotional status, the nurse also may briefly explain the need for strict compliance with these requests to ensure that all evidence remains intact.

18 Correct answer—C

The appropriate action would be to give the woman the number of the local medical society, which will provide the names, addresses, and phone numbers of pediatricians in her geographic area. This method is the most objective way of referring patients to physicians.

19 Correct answer—D

The nurse should advise the patient to stop taking the drug and return to the ED. This is the only appropriate nursing action in this situation, as any other action could be construed as the prescribing of a medication, which is the physician's domain.

20 Correct answer—A

A patient's name, address, and age and the extent of injury are considered public information. Law enforcement agents are entitled to this information only, unless they can provide a valid court order, search warrant, or subpoena for additional information.

21 Correct answer—A

The sequence of obtaining and securing evidence—the chain of evidence—is most important in a court of law. Maintaining the integrity of evidence is best assured by limiting the number of people who have access to it and by documenting how the evidence was obtained, where it was sent, and by whom it was received.

22 Correct answer—C

Implied consent best describes an emergency consent. When a patient's condition requires immediate evaluation and intervention and the patient cannot give consent for treatment and a legal guardian or next of kin is unavailable, the implication that the patient would agree to treatment if he could give consent constitutes an implied consent. Consent also is implied whenever a patient presents to the ED; in this case, the implication that the patient came to the ED expressly for evaluation and treatment constitutes consent. Although an implied consent is valid, an informed consent should always be obtained, whenever possible, before treatment is rendered. Administrative consents involve an agreement between two physicians that a

Professional Issues
Answers

particular procedure is required for a patient who cannot consent because of his mental state.

23 Correct answer—D

The parents or guardians of a minor who is a suspected victim of child abuse or neglect can be restrained by police from taking the minor out of the hospital. All states have laws mandating the reporting of suspected or known cases of child abuse or neglect. Such laws identify who must report cases of child abuse; responsible parties include registered nurses, licensed practical nurses, and other health care providers. Law enforcement agencies must investigate and, when necessary, place the minor in protective custody. Since hospital staff are not law enforcement agents, they do not have the power to restrain a parent or guardian. However, when a minor has been placed in protective custody, the hospital may not release the child to anyone other than a court-appointed guardian.

24 Correct answer—B

In this situation, the nurse should determine the friend's ability to understand the instructions; then have the friend interpret them for the patient, and document this in the patient report. The nurse also should document the name of the person who provided the interpretation. If this situation occurs frequently, the discharge instructions should be translated into the most commonly encountered languages. Delaying a patient's discharge until a hospital interpreter can be found is impractical since an interpreter is already available.

25 Correct answer—C

The best way to determine whether a patient understands his discharge instructions is to have the patient explain the instructions to the nurse. The nurse should then document the patient's understanding of the instructions in the patient report. Having the patient repeat the instructions verbatim or sign a form indicating that he understands the instructions does not demonstrate actual understanding.

26 Correct answer—D

Patient education is a nurse's professional and legal responsibility. According to JCAHO standards, it is a primary concern of all nursing and medical staffs. The goals of patient education are to improve patient well-being, promote and foster good public relations, and reinforce the prescribed medical regimen.

27 Correct answer — C

The nurse should begin discharge planning as soon as the patient arrives at the ED to facilitate the processing and actual discharge of the patient. When possible, the nurse should include the patient in the discharge planning; doing so helps to enhance the patient's disposition and care while in the ED.

28 Correct answer — A

The goals of discharge planning are to conform to JCAHO requirements, prevent readmission for the same problem, and provide patient or family education. Discharge planning also aims to identify individual patient needs and to incorporate a multidisciplinary approach to patient care. Discharge planning does not affect the use of the ED as a primary care facility.

29 Correct answer — A

The nurse can be sued for giving advice over the phone. Although this rarely occurs, a nurse can be sued for giving incorrect information, especially when the information can be directly related to patient harm. The best way to prevent such lawsuits is to ensure that malpractice insurance covers advice (given both on and off the job), make sure that any advice given reflects current nursing practice, and avoid charging a fee for advice.

30 Correct answer — A

The guest at a party who discovers that he is speaking with a nurse and begins asking several health-related questions shows no indication that he wishes to establish an ongoing nurse-patient relationship. In an established nurse-patient relationship, the nurse is obligated to give the best nursing advice possible, which may include referral to a physician. Any misinformation could be considered, in a court of law, a breach of contract. The issue of breach of contract may be a deciding factor in a malpractice lawsuit.

31 Correct answer — B

A nurse does not need to refer a person soliciting medical advice to a physician if she is convinced that it is unnecessary. Nor does she need to follow-up on such advice, unless a nurse-patient relationship has been established. Even in private practice, a nurse can diagnose and treat only nursing, not medical, problems unless she is following standard orders.

32 Correct answer — C

Advising the woman to go to the nearest ED without soliciting further information is inappropriate. Although recommending that the patient go to the hospital regardless of her prevailing condition is safe advice legally, soliciting further information about the patient's condition may prevent an unnecessary trip to the ED as well as unnecessary patient anxiety. By finding out how many months pregnant the woman is, whether the woman has had prenatal care, and how heavy her bleeding is (in terms of the number of pads used in the last hour), the nurse can determine the appropriate advice to give this patient. For example, if the patient is 9 months' pregnant with her first child, has had prenatal care, is spotting blood, and is having mild contractions every ½ hour, the nurse would advise her to go to the hospital when the contractions are 5 minutes apart and 45 to 60 seconds long, unless heavy bleeding begins. However, if the patient has not had prenatal care, the nurse would recommend that she go to the ED immediately to rule out placenta previa.

33 Correct answer — D

The most appropriate nursing action would be to ask the patient why he is concerned; then relate the adverse effects and refer him, if necessary, to a physician. Merely supplying facts about the adverse effects of a medication may cause the patient to discontinue the medication needlessly. Investigating his concerns may prevent this.

34 Correct answer — C

The nurse's priority in this situation would be to clear the ED of all nonserious patients and move those awaiting admission to a holding area. Upon receipt of such news, the ED is responsible for preparing to receive casualties. A decontamination area should be established as soon as patient care areas become available. Requesting the admitting office to clear intensive care unit beds is inappropriate because the extent and number of casualties is unknown at this time. Notifying the emergency medical systems (EMS) about available accommodations would be appropriate only after preparing the ED.

35 Correct answer — D

The radiology department and the hospital's radiation disaster planning coordinator would be most useful in this type of accident. Even if the hospital does not receive the driver of the truck carrying radioactive waste, the school bus victims and EMS personnel may be contaminated. The help of the radiology and radiation coordinating staff is especially important in planning the management of casualties and preventing further contamination. The laboratory, blood bank, operating room, and pharmacy would be helpful in providing supportive care.

36 Correct answer — D

Notifying the hospital administrator or nursing supervisor would be the most appropriate action in this situation. Under normal circumstances, the media are entitled to public information; however, because of the sensitivity of the diagnosis and the patient's prominence in the community, the nurse's primary concern is to protect the patient's right to privacy.

37 Correct answer — A

A nurse who allows a reporter to gain unauthorized access to a patient's chart is guilty of breach of confidentiality. The nurse is responsible for maintaining the confidentiality of a patient's chart and information. Failure to do so is a breach of patient confidentiality, regardless of how that breach occurred.

38 Correct answer — C

The most appropriate action for the ED nurse to take would be to inform the physician and secure the envelope. The nurse must inform the physician of her discovery because it may directly affect the care rendered to the patient. Securing the substance is within the nurse's purview because analysis of the contents may be necessary at a future time. An appropriate action for a staff nurse would be to inform the nursing supervisor or administrator at the hospital about the discovery.

39 Correct answer — D

The nurse would not be held civilly liable because no civil liability has occurred. The nurse in this situation acted in good faith in attempting to secure a positive identification and obtain medical information necessary for patient care.

Professional Issues
Answers

CHAPTER 18

Medical Dosage Calculations

SITUATION

A 50-year-old woman, weighing 144 lb (65 kg), arrives at the emergency department (ED) complaining of a severe headache. Her vital signs are blood pressure, 220/130 mm Hg; pulse rate, 130 beats/minute; and respiratory rate, 26 breaths/minute. The physician diagnoses hypertensive crisis and orders a continuous infusion of sodium nitroprusside (Nipride). The order reads: 250 ml of dextrose 5% in water (D₅W) with 50 mg of sodium nitroprusside at 0.8 mcg/kg/minute.

Questions 1 to 4 refer to the above situation.

1 Preparation of the above solution would yield a sodium nitroprusside concentration of:

A. 50 mcg/ml
B. 150 mcg/ml
C. 200 mcg/ml
D. 250 mcg/ml

2 Which flow rate is needed to infuse the sodium nitroprusside solution at 0.8 mcg/kg/minute via an infusion system with a drip factor of 60 microdrops/ml?

A. 2 microdrops/minute
B. 8 microdrops/minute
C. 16 microdrops/minute
D. 52 microdrops/minute

3 If the dosage is increased to 0.9 mcg/kg/minute, the flow rate should be regulated at how many microdrops per minute?

A. 9 microdrops/minute
B. 18 microdrops/minute
C. 27 microdrops/minute
D. 58 microdrops/minute

4 Additional treatment for this hypertensive patient includes the administration of trimethaphan camsylate (Arfonad). A 500-mg ampule of trimethaphan is diluted in 500 ml of D₅W. The physician orders 3 mg/minute of trimethaphan. Which of the following is the appropriate flow rate?

A. 90 ml/hour
B. 150 ml/hour
C. 180 ml/hour
D. 250 ml/hour

SITUATION

A 19-year-old man with insulin-dependent diabetes mellitus is admitted to the ED with diabetic ketoacidosis. His blood glucose level is 800 mg/dl; pH, 7.10; PCO_2, 28 mm Hg; and HCO_3^-, 15 mEq/liter. He appears severely dehydrated.

Questions 5 to 8 refer to the above situation.

---

5 An insulin drip at 8 units/hour is ordered. If 200 units of regular insulin are added to 250 ml of normal saline solution, the patient will receive how many milliliters per hour?

A. 8 ml/hour
B. 10 ml/hour
C. 18 ml/hour
D. 20 ml/hour

---

6 The physician orders 30 units of NPH insulin subcutaneously. The label reads 1 ml = 100 units. How many milliliters will be administered to this patient?

A. 0.03 ml
B. 0.3 ml
C. 0.35 ml
D. 0.75 ml

---

7 Normal saline solution is to be infused at a rate of 40 drops/minute. Using an infusion system with a drip factor of 15 drops/ml, how much time will be required to deliver 1 liter of the saline solution?

A. 2 hours and 50 minutes
B. 3 hours and 30 minutes
C. 4 hours and 20 minutes
D. 6 hours and 15 minutes

---

8 The physician changes the order to an infusion of 1 liter of a 0.45% saline solution beginning at 1 p.m. The flow rate is 42 drops/minute, and the drip factor is 10 drops/ml. At what time will the infusion be completed?

A. 4:05 a.m.
B. 4:58 p.m.
C. 5:30 p.m.
D. 5:42 p.m.

SITUATION

A woman is admitted to the ED with a pulmonary embolism. She is tachypneic. The physician plans to begin therapy with aminophylline and heparin.

Questions 9 to 13 refer to the above situation.

---

9 Infusion of 1 liter of normal saline solution is started at 2 p.m. The flow rate is 40 drops/minute. The drip factor is 10 drops/ml. At what time will the infusion be completed?

A. 4:10 p.m.
B. 6:10 p.m.
C. 6:40 p.m.
D. 8:10 p.m.

---

10 The physician orders 0.3 g of aminophylline to be administered by I.V. piggyback over 30 minutes. The label on the vial reads aminophylline 250 mg in 10 ml. How many milliliters should be administered?

A. 12 ml
B. 14 ml
C. 25 ml
D. 30 ml

---

11 If 100 ml of normal saline solution with 0.3 g of aminophylline is to be infused over 30 minutes and the drip factor is 10 drops/ml, the patient will receive how many drops per minute?

A. 30 drops/minute
B. 31 drops/minute
C. 33 drops/minute
D. 42 drops/minute

---

12 The physician writes an order that reads: Add 25,000 units of heparin to 500 ml D$_5$W. Infuse 1,200 units/hour. What will the flow rate be in milliliters per hour?

A. 24 ml/hour
B. 60 ml/hour
C. 240 ml/hour
D. 600 ml/hour

13 Later, the physician changes the order to a continuous infusion of 50 mg of aminophylline per hour. One gram of the drug is to be added to 500 ml D₅W. If the drip factor is 10 drops/ml, the patient will receive how many drops per minute?

A. 4 drops/minute
B. 8 drops/minute
C. 12 drops/minute
D. 14 drops/minute

SITUATION

A 54-year-old man is admitted to the ED with a massive anterior wall myocardial infarction. Cardiogenic shock is developing. The patient weighs 154 lb (70 kg). All medications will be administered via an infusion system with a drip factor of 60 microdrops/ml.

Questions 14 to 19 refer to the above situation.

14 The physician orders 500 mg of dobutamine hydrochloride (Dobutrex) in 250 ml D₅W, infused at 10 mcg/kg/minute. What will be the flow rate in drops per minute?

A. 11 drops/minute
B. 14 drops/minute
C. 21 drops/minute
D. 42 drops/minute

15 If the order reads 250 mg dobutamine in 250 ml of D₅W, infused at 4 mcg/kg/minute, the patient will receive how many milliliters per hour?

A. 16.8 ml/hour
B. 42 ml/hour
C. 168 ml/hour
D. 420 ml/hour

16 Nitroglycerin therapy is instituted with 50 mg diluted in 250 ml D₅W, infused at 10 mcg/minute. The patient will receive how many milliliters per hour?

A. 1 ml/hour
B. 3 ml/hour
C. 10 ml/hour
D. 90 ml/hour

17 If the dosage is increased to 30 mcg/minute, the flow rate will be:

A. 9 ml/hour
B. 15 ml/hour
C. 50 ml/hour
D. 90 ml/hour

18 Sodium nitroprusside is then ordered at 0.5 mcg/kg/minute. If 50 mg of nitroprusside is added to 250 ml of D_5W, the patient will receive:

A. 5 ml/hour
B. 11 ml/hour
C. 45 ml/hour
D. 110 ml/hour

19 If the dosage is increased to 0.8 mcg/kg/minute, the flow rate will be:

A. 17 ml/hour
B. 20 ml/hour
C. 50 ml/hour
D. 140 ml/hour

SITUATION

A woman is admitted to the ED with bleeding esophageal varices. Fluid replacement and administration of vasopressin (Pitressin) is initiated, and insertion of a three-lumen, double-balloon esophageal tube is planned.

Questions 20 and 21 refer to the above situation.

20 The physician orders 200 ml of normal saline solution with 50 units vasopressin infused at 0.5 unit/minute. If the drip factor is 15 drops/ml, the patient will receive how many drops per minute?

A. 3 drops/minute
B. 5 drops/minute
C. 15 drops/minute
D. 30 drops/minute

21 If the physician orders 1,000 ml of normal saline solution to be given I.V. over 4 hours and the drip factor is 15 drops/ml, how many drops per minute will the patient receive?

A. 35 drops/minute
B. 63 drops/minute
C. 65 drops/minute
D. 240 drops/minute

Medical Dosage Calculations
Questions

Answer Sheet

	A	B	C	D
1	○	○	○	○
2	○	○	○	○
3	○	○	○	○
4	○	○	○	○
5	○	○	○	○
6	○	○	○	○
7	○	○	○	○
8	○	○	○	○
9	○	○	○	○
10	○	○	○	○
11	○	○	○	○
12	○	○	○	○
13	○	○	○	○
14	○	○	○	○
15	○	○	○	○
16	○	○	○	○
17	○	○	○	○
18	○	○	○	○
19	○	○	○	○
20	○	○	○	○
21	○	○	○	○

1 Correct answer—**C**

The correct concentration is 200 mcg/ml. To arrive at this concentration, first change the units into like equivalents (milligrams should be converted to micrograms):

1 mg = 1,000 mcg

Therefore, 50 mg = 50,000 mcg.

Then to determine the concentration of solution in 1 milliliter, divide the total solution (250 ml) into the total concentration (50,000 mcg):

$$\frac{50,000 \text{ mcg}}{250 \text{ ml}} = \frac{X \text{ mcg}}{1 \text{ ml}}$$

$$200 \text{ mcg} = X$$

Therefore, the solution would yield a concentration of 200 mcg/ml.

2 Correct answer—**C**

The flow rate needed is 16 microdrops/minute. To arrive at this rate, first multiply the dose desired (0.8 mcg) by the patient's weight in kilograms (65 kg) to yield the dose that will be delivered in 1 minute:

0.8 mcg/kg/min × 65 kg = 52 mcg/minute

Next, using the concentration calculated in question 1, find the volume per minute needed to deliver the dose:

$$\frac{1 \text{ ml}}{200 \text{ mcg}} \times \frac{52 \text{ mcg}}{1 \text{ min}} \times \frac{60 \text{ microdrops}}{1 \text{ ml}} = \frac{3,120}{200} = 15.6, \text{ or 16 microdrops/minute}$$

Remember: The concentration of 200 mcg is the denominator in the first part of the equation, so the micrograms will cancel out.

3 Correct answer—**B**

The flow rate would be increased to 18 microdrops/minute.

0.9 mcg × 65 kg = 58.5 mcg/minute

$$\frac{1 \text{ ml}}{200 \text{ mcg}} \times \frac{58.5 \text{ mcg}}{1 \text{ min}} \times \frac{60 \text{ microdrops}}{1 \text{ ml}} = \frac{3,510}{200} = 17.55, \text{ or 18 microdrops/minute}$$

4 Correct answer—**C**

The flow rate to deliver 3 mg/minute of trimethaphan is 180 ml/hour. Multiply the concentration of the solution by the dose desired, then by 60 minutes to determine the flow rate per hour:

$$\frac{500 \text{ ml}}{500 \text{ mg}} \times \frac{3 \text{ mg}}{1 \text{ min}} \times \frac{60 \text{ min}}{1 \text{ hr}} = 180 \text{ ml/hour}$$

5 Correct answer — **B**

The flow rate is 10 ml/hour.

$$\frac{250 \text{ ml}}{200 \text{ units}} \times \frac{8 \text{ units}}{1 \text{ hr}} = \frac{40}{4} = 10 \text{ ml/hour}$$

In this equation, you do not need to multiply by 60 minutes/hour because the order specified the amount to deliver per hour (8 units).

6 Correct answer — **B**

0.3 ml will deliver 30 units of insulin to the patient.

$$30 \text{ units} \times \frac{1 \text{ ml}}{100 \text{ units}} = 0.3 \text{ ml}$$

7 Correct answer — **D**

You will need 6 hours and 15 minutes to infuse a liter at 40 drops/minute using a drip factor of 15 drops/ml. Multiply the total amount of solution by the flow rate, then by the drip factor, and then by 60 minutes.

$$1,000 \text{ ml} \times \frac{1 \text{ min}}{40 \text{ drops}} \times \frac{15 \text{ drops}}{1 \text{ ml}} \times \frac{1 \text{ hr}}{60 \text{ min}} = \frac{250}{40} = 6.25, \text{ or 6 hours and 15 minutes}$$

Remember to invert the flow rate in order to cancel out the drops.

8 Correct answer — **B**

You will need 3 hours and 58 minutes to infuse the solution. If started at 1 p.m., the infusion will end at 4:58 p.m.

$$1,000 \text{ ml} \times \frac{1 \text{ min}}{42 \text{ drops}} \times \frac{10 \text{ drops}}{1 \text{ ml}} \times \frac{1 \text{ hr}}{60 \text{ min}} = \frac{1,000}{252} = 3.97 \text{ or 3 hours and 58 minutes}$$

9 Correct answer — **B**

One liter of fluid administered at a flow rate of 40 drops/minute with a drip factor of 10 drops/ml will require 4 hours and 10 minutes for infusion. If started at 2 p.m., the infusion will end at 6:10 p.m.

$$1,000 \text{ ml} \times \frac{1 \text{ min}}{40 \text{ drops}} \times \frac{10 \text{ drops}}{1 \text{ ml}} \times \frac{1 \text{ hr}}{60 \text{ min}} = \frac{25}{6} \text{ or 4 hours and 10 minutes}$$

10 Correct answer—A

12 ml is needed. 12 ml = 0.3 g of aminophylline. Remember to convert to equivalent units: 0.3 g = 300 mg.

$$\frac{10 \text{ ml}}{250 \text{ mg}} \times 300 \text{ mg} = \frac{300}{25} = 12 \text{ ml}$$

11 Correct answer—C

To infuse 100 ml of fluid over 30 minutes with a drip factor of 10 drops/ml, the flow rate should be 33 drops/minute.

$$\frac{100 \text{ ml}}{30 \text{ min}} \times \frac{10 \text{ drops}}{1 \text{ ml}} = 33.3, \text{ or } 33 \text{ drops/minute}$$

12 Correct answer—A

At a flow rate of 24 ml/hour, the patient will receive 1,200 units of heparin per hour.

$$\frac{500 \text{ ml}}{25,000 \text{ units}} \times \frac{1,200 \text{ units}}{1 \text{ hr}} = \frac{1,200}{50} \text{ or } 24 \text{ ml/hour}$$

13 Correct answer—A

For the patient to receive 50 mg/hour of aminophylline at this concentration, the flow rate should be 4 drops/minute.

$$\frac{500 \text{ ml}}{1,000 \text{ mg}} \times \frac{50 \text{ mg}}{1 \text{ hr}} \times \frac{1 \text{ hr}}{60 \text{ min}} \times \frac{10 \text{ drops}}{1 \text{ ml}} = \frac{50}{12} = 4.17, \text{ or } 4 \text{ drops/minute}$$

14 Correct answer—C

For this 70-kg patient, 21 drops/minute is the flow rate at which to administer 10 mcg/kg/minute of dobutamine. To arrive at this amount, first determine the concentration of dobutamine in micrograms per milliliter:

500 mg = 500,000 mcg

$$\frac{500,000 \text{ mcg}}{250 \text{ ml}} = 2,000 \text{ mcg/ml}$$

The concentration of dobutamine is 2,000 mcg/ml.
10 mcg × 70 kg = 700 mcg/minute

The desired dose is 700 mcg/minute.

$$\frac{1 \text{ ml}}{2,000 \text{ mcg}} \times \frac{700 \text{ mcg}}{1 \text{ min}} \times \frac{60 \text{ drops}}{1 \text{ ml}} = 21 \text{ drops/minute}$$

15 Correct answer — **A**

At this concentration, 16.8 ml/hour will deliver 4 mcg/kg/minute to this patient.
   250 mg = 250,000 mcg

$$\frac{250,000 \text{ mcg}}{250 \text{ ml}} = 1,000 \text{ mcg/ml}$$

The concentration of dobutamine is 1,000 mcg/ml.

4 mcg × 70 kg = 280 mcg/min
The desired dose is 280 mcg/minute.

$$\frac{1 \text{ ml}}{1,000 \text{ mcg}} \times \frac{280 \text{ mcg}}{1 \text{ min}} \times \frac{60 \text{ min}}{1 \text{ hr}} = \frac{840}{50} = 16.8 \text{ ml/hour}$$

16 Correct answer — **B**

At this concentration, 3 ml/hour will deliver 10 mcg/minute.
   50 mg = 50,000 mcg

$$\frac{50,000 \text{ mcg}}{250 \text{ ml}} = 200 \text{ mcg/ml}$$

The concentration of nitroglycerin is 200 mcg/ml.

$$\frac{1 \text{ ml}}{200 \text{ mcg}} \times \frac{10 \text{ mcg}}{1 \text{ min}} \times \frac{60 \text{ min}}{1 \text{ hr}} = \frac{600}{200} \text{ or } 3 \text{ ml/hr}$$

17 Correct answer — **A**

To deliver 30 mcg/minute, the flow rate must be increased to 9 ml/hour.

$$\frac{1 \text{ ml}}{200 \text{ mcg}} \times \frac{30 \text{ mcg}}{1 \text{ min}} \times \frac{60 \text{ min}}{1 \text{ hr}} = \frac{900}{100} \text{ or } 9 \text{ ml/hr}$$

18 Correct answer — **B**

A flow rate of 11 ml/hour will deliver 0.5 mcg/kg/minute of sodium nitroprusside to this patient.
   50 mg = 50,000 mcg

$$\frac{50,000 \text{ mcg}}{250 \text{ ml}} = 200 \text{ mcg/ml}$$

The concentration of sodium nitroprusside is 200 mcg/ml.
0.5 mcg/kg/min × 70 kg = 35 mcg/minute

The desired dose is 35 mcg/minute.

$$\frac{1 \text{ ml}}{200 \text{ mcg}} \times \frac{35 \text{ mcg}}{1 \text{ min}} \times \frac{60 \text{ min}}{1 \text{ hr}} = \frac{105}{10} = 10.5 \text{ or } 11 \text{ ml/hour}$$

19 Correct answer — A

A flow rate of 17 ml/hour will deliver 0.8 mcg/kg/minute of sodium nitroprusside.

0.8 mcg × 70 kg = 56 mcg/minute

The desired dose is 56 mcg/minute.

$$\frac{1 \text{ ml}}{200 \text{ mcg}} \times \frac{56 \text{ mcg}}{1 \text{ min}} \times \frac{60 \text{ min}}{1 \text{ hr}} = \frac{168}{10} = 16.8 \text{ or } 17 \text{ ml/hour}$$

20 Correct answer — D

A flow rate of 30 drops/minute will deliver 0.5 unit of vasopressin per minute.

$$\frac{200 \text{ ml}}{50 \text{ units}} \times \frac{0.5 \text{ unit}}{1 \text{ min}} \times \frac{15 \text{ drops}}{1 \text{ ml}} = 30 \text{ drops/minute}$$

21 Correct answer — B

To infuse 1 liter of fluid over 4 hours with a drip factor of 15 drops/ml, a flow rate of 63 drops/minute is required. First, convert hours into like equivalents of minutes:

4 hours = 240 minutes

$$\frac{1,000 \text{ ml}}{240 \text{ min}} \times \frac{15 \text{ drops}}{1 \text{ ml}} = \frac{375}{6} \text{ or } 63 \text{ drops/minute}$$

Medical Dosage Calculations Answers

Selected References

CHAPTER 1 — Abdominal Emergencies

Brunner, L.S., and Suddarth, D.S. *Textbook of Medical-Surgical Nursing*, 6th ed. Philadelphia: J.B. Lippincott Co., 1988.

Buschiazzo, L., and Naab, G.A., Jr. "Careful Assessment of Abdominal Pain," *Journal of Emergency Nursing* 12(2):72-75, March/April 1986.

Cardona, V., et al. *Trauma Nursing: From Resuscitation Through Rehabilitation*. Philadelphia: W.B. Saunders Co., 1988.

Chalfin, L.M. "Tricks of the Trade," *Emergency Medicine* 18(8):97, April 30, 1986.

Dunham, C.M., and Cowley, R.A. *Shock-Trauma Critical Care Handbook*. Rockville, Md.: Aspen Pub., 1986.

Fain J.A., and Amato-Vealey, E. "Acute Pancreatitis: A Gastrointestinal Emergency." *Critical Care Nurse* 8(5):47-63, July/August 1988.

Jeffres, C. "Complications of Acute Pancreatitis," *Critical Care Nurse* 9(4):38-48, April 1989.

Lanros, N.E. *Assessment and Interventions in Emergency Nursing*, 3rd ed. East Norwalk, Conn.: Appleton & Lange, 1988.

Luckmann, J., and Sorensen, K. *Medical Surgical Nursing: A Psychophysiologic Approach*, 3rd ed. Philadelphia: W.B. Saunders Co., 1987.

Semonin-Holleran, R. "Critical Nursing Care for Abdominal Trauma," *Critical Care Nurse* 8(3):48-58, May 1988.

Shires, G.T. *Principles of Trauma Care*, 3rd ed. New York: McGraw-Hill Book Co., 1985.

Trunkey, D.T., and Lewis, F.R. *Current Therapy of Trauma*, vol. 2. Philadelphia: B.C. Decker, 1986.

CHAPTER 2 — Cardiovascular Emergencies

Cardona, V., et al. *Trauma Nursing: From Resuscitation Through Rehabilitation*. Philadelphia: W.B. Saunders Co., 1988.

Goldberger, E. *Treatment of Cardiac Emergencies*, 5th ed. St. Louis: C.V. Mosby Co., 1989.

Grauer, K., and Cavallaro, D. *ACLS: Certification Preparation and Comprehensive Review*, 2nd ed. St. Louis: C.V. Mosby Co., 1987.

Henderson, E. "Thrombolytic Therapy in Acute Myocardial Infarction, Part 2," *Journal of Emergency Nursing* 15(2):145-49, March/April 1989.

Holloway, N. *Nursing the Critically Ill Adult*, 3rd ed. Menlo Park, Calif.: Addison-Wesley Publishing Co., 1988.

O'Rourke, M., et al. "Limitation of Myocardial Infarction by Early Infusion of Recombinant Tissue-Type Plasminogen Activator," *Circulation* 77(6):1311-15, June 1988.

Pasternak, R.C., et al. "Acute Myocardial Infarction," in *Heart Disease*, 3rd ed. Edited by Braunwald, E. Philadelphia: W.B. Saunders Co., 1988.

Rea, R., et al. *Emergency Nursing Core Curriculum*, 3rd ed. Philadelphia: W.B. Saunders Co., 1987.

Sheehy, S.B., and Barber, J.M. *Emergency Nursing: Principles and Practice*, 2nd ed. St. Louis: C.V. Mosby Co., 1985.

Sommers, M.S., "Cardiac Tamponade after Nonpenetrating Cardiac Trauma," *Dimensions of Critical Care Nursing* 5(4):206-15, July/August 1986.

Yee, B., and Zorb, S. *Cardiac Critical Care Nursing.* Glenview, Ill.: Scott, Foresman & Co., 1987.

CHAPTER 3 – Eye, Ear, Nose, and Throat Emergencies

Cardona, V., et al. *Trauma Nursing: From Resuscitation Through Rehabilitation.* Philadelphia: W.B. Saunders Co., 1988.

Deutsch, T.A., and Feller, D.B. *Paton and Goldberg's Management of Ocular Injuries,* 2nd ed. Philadelphia: W.B. Saunders Co., 1985.

Lawlor, M.C. "Common Ocular Injuries and Disorders: Acute Loss of Vision, Part I," *Journal of Emergency Nursing* 15(1):32-43, January/February 1989.

Rea, R., et al. *Emergency Nursing Core Curriculum,* 3rd ed. Philadelphia: W.B. Saunders Co., 1987.

Sheehy, S.B., and Barber, J.M. *Emergency Nursing: Principles and Practice,* 2nd ed. St. Louis: C.V. Mosby Co., 1985.

CHAPTER 4 – Environmental Emergencies

Bayley, E.W., and Smith, G.A. "The Three Degrees of Burn Care," *Nursing87* 17(3):34-42, March 1987.

Biddle, C. "Hypothermia: Implications for the the Critical Care Nurse," *Critical Care Nurse* 5(2):34-38, March/April 1985.

Braunohler, W.M. "Frostbite: The Critical Process of Rewarming Frozen Tissue," *Consultant* 25(2):50-54, January 30, 1985.

Brodeur, V.B., et al. "Exertional Hyperthermia, Ice Baths, and Emergency Care at the Falmouth Road Race," *Journal of Emergency Nursing* 15(4):304-12, July/August 1989.

Cooke, S.S. "Major Thermal Injury – The First 48 Hours," *Critical Care Nurse* 6(1):55-63, January/February 1986.

Lanros, N.E. *Assessment and Interventions in Emergency Nursing,* 3rd ed. East Norwalk, Conn.: Appleton & Lange, 1988.

Sheehy, S.B., and Barber, J.M. *Emergency Nursing: Principles and Practice,* 2nd ed. St. Louis: C.V. Mosby Co., 1985.

CHAPTER 5 – Facial Emergencies

Cardona, V., et al. *Trauma Nursing: From Resuscitation Through Rehabilitation.* Philadelphia: W.B. Saunders Co., 1988.

Rea, R., et al. *Emergency Nursing Core Curriculum,* 3rd ed. Philadelphia: W.B. Saunders Co., 1987.

Sheehy, S.B. *Manual of Clinical Trauma: The First Hour.* St. Louis: C.V. Mosby Co., 1989.

Sheehy, S.B., and Barber, J.M. *Emergency Nursing: Principles and Practice,* 2nd ed. St. Louis: C.V. Mosby Co., 1985.

CHAPTER 6 – General Medical Emergencies

Alspach, J.G., and Williams, S.M. *Core Curriculum for Critical Care Nursing,* 3rd ed. Philadelphia: W.B. Saunders Co., 1985.

Cardona, V., et al. *Trauma Nursing: From Resuscitation Through Rehabilitation.* Philadelphia: W.B. Saunders Co., 1988.

Chameides, L., ed. *Textbook of Pediatric Advanced Life Support.* Dallas: American Heart Association and the American Academy of Pediatrics, 1988.

Committee on Transfusion Practices. "The Latest Protocols for Blood Transfusions," *Nursing86* 16(10):34-41, October 1986.

Danis, D.M. "Reyes Syndrome—1986," *Journal of Emergency Nursing* 14(2):110-11, March/April 1988.

Goldberger, E.A. *A Primer of Water, Electrolyte, and Acid-Base Syndromes,* 7th ed. Philadelphia: Lea & Febiger, 1986.

Holloway, N. *Nursing the Critically Ill Adult,* 3rd ed. Menlo Park, Calif.: Addison-Wesley Publishing Co., 1988.

Jacobson, E. "New Hospital Hazards: How to Protect Yourself," *American Journal of Nursing* 90(2):36-41, February 1990.

Lamb, C. "Managing Sickle Cell Emergencies," *Patient Care* 19:92-105, January 15, 1985.

Lipman, T.H. "Assessment of the Child with Diabetic Ketoacidosis," *Dimensions of Critical Care Nursing* 6(2):82-93, March/April 1987.

Lumley, W. "Recognizing and Reversing Insulin Shock," *Nursing89* 19(9):34-43, September 1989.

Maxwell, M.H., and Kleeman, C.R. *Clinical Disorders of Fluid and Electrolyte Metabolism,* 4th ed. New York: McGraw-Hill Book Co., 1987.

Metheny, N. *Fluid and Electrolyte Balance: Nursing Considerations,* 3rd ed. Philadelphia: J.B. Lippincott Co., 1987.

Pauley, S.Y. "Transfusion Therapy for Nurses: Part 2," *NITA* 8(1):51-60, January/February 1985.

Payne, N. "Emergency Care of the Patient with Myxedema Coma," *Journal of Emergency Nursing* 12(6):343-47, November/December 1987.

Rea, R., et al. *Emergency Nursing Core Curriculum,* 3rd ed. Philadelphia: W.B. Saunders Co., 1987.

Reeves, K. "Management of Pediatric Diabetic Ketoacidosis," *Journal of Emergency Nursing* 14(2):115-19, March/April 1988.

Sheehy, S.B., and Barber, J.M. *Emergency Nursing: Principles and Practice,* 2nd ed. St. Louis: C.V. Mosby Co., 1985.

Swearingen, P., et al. *Manual of Critical Care: Applying Nursing Diagnoses to Adult Critical Illness.* St. Louis: C.V. Mosby Co., 1988.

Tucker, S.M., et al. "Hyperthyroidism: Thyroid Crisis," *Journal of Emergency Nursing* 15(4):352-55, July/August 1989.

CHAPTER 7—Genitourinary and Gynecologic Emergencies

Andrist, L.C. "Taking a Sexual History and Educating Clients About Safe Sex," *Nursing Clinics of North America* 23(4):959-73, December 1988.

Bates, B. *A Guide to Physical Examination and History Taking,* 4th ed. Philadelphia: J.B. Lippincott Co., 1987.

Cass, A.S., et al. "Clinical Indications for Radiographic Evaluation of Blunt Renal Trauma," *Journal of Urology* 136(2):370-71, August 1986.

Flood, S. "Pericardial Effusion in the Uremic Patient: Nursing Considerations and Management," *American Nephrology Nurses Association Journal* 12(5):294-99, October 1985.

Fogel, C.I. "Gonorrhea: Not a New Problem but a Serious One," *Nursing Clinics of North America* 23(4):885-97, December 1988.

Frauman, A. "An Introduction to Physical Assessment for the Nephrology Nurse," *American Nephrology Nurses Association Journal* 12(2):112-17, April 1985.

Freeman, S., and Chapman J. "Urologic Procedures," *Emergency Medical Clinics of North America* 4(3):543-60, August 1986.

Green, J., et al. "Extreme Unilateral Hydronephrosis with Normal Glomerular Filtration Rate: Physiological Studies in a Case of Obstructive Uropathy," *Journal of Urology* 136(2):361-65, August 1986.

Johnson, D. "Pathophysiology of Renal Failure," *Critical Care Nurse* 5(4):18-20, July/ August 1985.

Sheehy, S.B., and Barber, J.M. *Emergency Nursing: Principles and Practice,* 2nd ed. St. Louis: C.V. Mosby Co., 1985.

Whittaker, A.A. "Acute Renal Dysfunction: Assessment of Patients at Risk," *Focus on Critical Care* 12(3):12-17, June 1985.

CHAPTER 8 – Neurologic Emergencies

Bourg, P., et al. *Standardized Nursing Care Plans for the Emergency Department.* St. Louis: C.V. Mosby Co., 1986.

Cardona, V., et al. *Trauma Nursing: From Resuscitation Through Rehabilitation.* Philadelphia: W.B. Saunders Co., 1988.

Hickey, J. *The Clinical Practice of Neurological and Neurosurgical Nursing,* 2nd ed. Philadelphia: J.B. Lippincott Co., 1986.

Kinney, M., et al. *AACN's Clinical Reference for Critical-Care Nursing,* 2nd ed. St. Louis: C.V. Mosby Co., 1988.

Mainfold, S.L. "Craniocerebral Trauma: A Review of Primary and Secondary Injury and Therapeutic Modalities," *Focus on Critical Care* 13(2):22-35, April 1986.

Mitchell, P., et al. *AANN'S Neuroscience Nursing: Phenomena and Practice – Human Responses to Neurologic Health Problems.* East Norwalk, Conn.: Appleton & Lange, 1988.

Rea, R., et al. *Emergency Nursing Core Curriculum,* 3rd ed. Philadelphia: W.B. Saunders Co., 1987.

Sheehy, S.B., and Barber, J.M. *Emergency Nursing: Principles and Practice,* 2nd ed. St. Louis: C.V. Mosby Co., 1985.

Walleck, C.A. "Controversies in the Management of the Head-Injured Patient," *Critical Care Nursing Clinics of North America* 1(1):67-74, March 1989.

CHAPTER 9 – Obstetric Emergencies

Beischer, N., and MacKay, E. *Obstetrics and the Newborn,* 2nd ed. Philadelphia: W.B. Saunders Co., 1986.

Bobak, I.M., and Jensen, M. *Essentials of Maternity Nursing: The Nurse and the Childbearing Family,* 2nd ed. St. Louis: C.V. Mosby Co., 1987.

Emergencies. Nurse's Reference Library. Springhouse, Pa.: Springhouse Corp., 1985.

Hahn, A., et al. *Mosby's Pharmacology in Nursing,* 16th ed. St. Louis: C.V. Mosby Co., 1986.

Howe, C.L. "Emergency: Dealing with Third-Trimester Bleeding," *RN* 48(2):29-31, February 1985.

Lee, G. "Eclampsia: Toxemia of Pregnancy," *Journal of Emergency Nursing* 11(5):225-26, September/October 1985.

Neeson, J.L., and May, K.A. *Comprehensive Maternity Nursing: Nursing Process and the Childbearing Family.* Philadelphia: J.B. Lippincott Co., 1986.

Reeder, S., and Martin, L. *Maternity Nursing: Family, Newborn, and Women's Health Care,* 16th ed. Philadelphia: J.B. Lippincott Co., 1987.

Roberts, J., and McGowan, N. "Emergency Birth," *Journal of Emergency Nursing* 11(3):125-31, May/June 1985.

CHAPTER 10 — Organ Donation

Lewis, J.C., and Minkosky, P.D. "Organ Procurement," *JEMS* 10(4):32-33, April 1985.

Simpson, H.H. "Organ Donation: Understanding the Law — Uniform Anatomical Gift Act," *Nursing Life* 5(1):24, January/February 1985.

Sladex, L. *Organ Donor Handbook.* Louisville: University of Louisville, Independent Organ Procurement Agency, 1986.

Task Force on Organ Transplantation. *Organ Transplantation: Issues and Recommendations.* U.S Department of Health and Human Services, 1986.

CHAPTER 11 — Orthopedic Emergencies

Halpern, J.S. "Upper Extremity Peripheral Nerve Assessment," *Journal of Emergency Nursing* 15(3):261-65, May/June 1989.

Iversen, L.D., and Clawson, D.K. *Manual of Acute Orthopaedic Therapeutics,* 3rd ed. Boston: Little, Brown & Co., 1986.

Lanros, N.E. *Assessment and Interventions in Emergency Nursing,* 3rd ed. East Norwalk, Conn.: Appleton & Lange, 1988.

Lindsey, B. "Cold and Heat Application in Musculoskeletal Injury," *Journal of Emergency Nursing* 16(1):54-57, January/February 1990.

Peter, N.K. "Care of Patients with Traumatic Pelvic Fracture," *Critical Care Nurse* 8(3):62-81, May 1988.

Sheehy, S.B., and Barber, J.M. *Emergency Nursing: Principles and Practice,* 2nd ed. St. Louis: C.V. Mosby Co., 1985.

CHAPTER 12 — Psychiatric and Psychological Emergencies

Antai-Otong, D. "When Your Patient is Angry," *Nursing88* 18(2):44-45, February 1988.

Brooking, J., ed. *Psychiatric Nursing Research.* New York: John Wiley & Sons, 1986.

George, J., and Quattrone, M. "Reporting Child Abuse: Duties and Dangers," *Journal of Emergency Nursing* 14(1):34-35, January/February 1988.

Haber, J., et al. *Comprehensive Psychiatric Nursing,* 3rd ed. St. Loius: C.V. Mosby Co., 1987.

Hradek, E.A. "Crisis Intervention and Suicide," *Journal of Psychosocial Nursing and Mental Health Services* 26(5):24-27, 40, May 1988.

Johnson, B.S. *Psychiatric-Mental Health Nursing: Adaptation and Growth.* Philadelphia: J.B. Lippincott Co., 1986.

Kelley, S.J. "Physical Abuse of Children: Recognition and Reporting," *Journal of Emergency Nursing* 14(2):82-90, March/April 1988.

McFarland, G.K., and Wasli, E.L. *Nursing Diagnosis and Process in Psychiatric-Mental Health Nursing.* Philadelphia: J.B. Lippincott Co., 1986.

Muchlinski, E., et al. "Planning and Implementing a Pediatric Sexual Assault Evidentiary Examination Program," *Journal of Emergency Nursing* 15(3):249-55, May/June 1989.

Osborn, M., and Bryan, S. "Evidentiary Examination in Sexual Assault," *Journal of Emergency Nursing* 15(3):284-90, May/June 1989.

Rea, R., et al. *Emergency Nursing Core Curriculum*, 3rd ed. Philadelphia: W.B. Saunders Co., 1987.

Servonsky, J., and Opas, S. *Nursing Management of Children*. Boston: Jones & Bartlett Publishing, 1986.

Shives, L.R. *Basic Concepts of Psychiatric-Mental Health Nursing*, 2nd ed. Philadelphia: J.B. Lippincott Co., 1990.

Stuart, G.W., and Sundeen, S.J. *Principles and Practice of Psychiatric Nursing*, 3rd ed. St. Louis: C.V. Mosby Co., 1987.

Van Dongen, C.J. "The Legacy of Suicide," *Journal of Psychosocial Nursing and Mental Health Services* 26(1):8-38, January 1988.

Wells, L.A. *Psychiatric Nursing Handbook*. St. Louis: Warren H. Green, 1989.

Whaley, L., and Wong, D. *Nursing Care of Infants and Children*, 3rd ed. St. Louis: C.V. Mosby Co., 1987.

Wilson, H.S., and Kneisl, C.R. *Psychiatric Nursing*, 3rd ed. Menlo Park, Calif.: Addison-Wesley Publishing Co., 1988.

CHAPTER 13 — Respiratory Emergencies

American College of Surgeons Committee on Trauma. *Advanced Trauma Life Support Instructor Manual*. Chicago: American College of Surgeons, 1985.

Brunner, L.S., and Suddarth, D.S. *Textbook of Medical-Surgical Nursing*, 6th ed. Philadelphia: J.B. Lippincott Co., 1988.

Harmon, A.R., ed. *Nursing Care of the Adult Trauma Patient*. New York: John Wiley & Sons, 1985.

Hudak, C., and Gallo, B. *Critical Care Nursing: A Holistic Approach*, 4th ed. Philadelphia: J.B. Lippincott Co., 1986.

Knezevich, B.A. *Trauma Nursing: Principles and Practice*. East Norwalk, Conn.: Appleton & Lange, 1986.

Lewis, S., and Collier, I. *Medical-Surgical Nursing: Assessment and Management of Clinical Problems*, 2nd ed. New York: McGraw-Hill Book Co., 1987.

Lundberg, G., ed. "Standards and Guidelines for Cardiopulmonary Resuscitation and Emergency Cardiac Care," *Journal of the American Medical Association* 255(21):2905-89, June 6, 1986.

McFadden, E.R., and Dusten, E.F. "Asthma" in *Harrison's Principles of Internal Medicine*, 11th ed. Edited by Braunwald, E., et al. New York: McGraw-Hill Book Co., 1987.

McGraw, J.P. "Triage of a Patient Exhibiting Hamman's Crunch after a Fall," *Journal of Emergency Nursing* 13(1):64-65, January/February 1987.

O'Boyle, C.M., et al. *Emergency Care: The First 24 Hours*. East Norwalk, Conn.: Appleton & Lange, 1985.

Shaffer, M.A., and Walraven, G., eds. "Pulmonary Trauma," *Trauma Quarterly* 2:1-79, 1986.

Sheehy, S.B., and Barber, J.M. *Emergency Nursing: Principles and Practice*, 2nd ed. St. Louis: C.V. Mosby Co., 1985.

Summer, W.R. "Status Asthmaticus," *Chest* 87(1) Supp.:87S-94S, January 1985.

West, J.B. *Respiratory Physiology: The Essentials*, 3rd ed. Baltimore: Williams & Wilkins Co., 1985.

CHAPTER 14 — Shock

Alspach, J.G., and Williams, S.M. *Core Curriculum for Critical Care Nursing*, 3rd ed. Philadelphia: W.B. Saunders Co., 1985.

Barrett, J., and Nyhus, L.M. *Treatment of Shock: Principles and Procedures*, 2nd ed. Philadelphia: Lea & Febiger, 1986.

Billings, D. "Shock Update," *Critical Care Nursing Quarterly* 11(1) June, 1988.

Cardona, V., et al. *Trauma Nursing: From Resuscitation Through Rehabilitation*. Philadelphia: W.B. Saunders Co., 1988.

Higgins, T.L., and Chernow, B. "Pharmacotherapy of Circulatory Shock" *Disease-A-Month* 33(6):309-61, June 1987.

Holloway, N. *Nursing the Critically Ill Adult*, 3rd ed. Menlo Park, Calif.: Addison-Wesley Publishing Co., 1988.

Janssen, H.F., and Barnes, C.B. *Circulatory Shock: Basic and Clinical Implications*. London: Academic Press, 1985.

Rea, R., et al. *Emergency Nursing Core Curriculum*, 3rd ed. Philadelphia: W.B. Saunders Co., 1987.

Shoemaker, W.C. "Pathophysiology and Therapy of Shock Syndromes," in *Textbook of Critical Care*. Edited by Shoemaker, W.C., et al. Philadelphia: W.B. Saunders Co., 1984.

Swearingen, P., et al. *Manual of Critical Care: Applying Nursing Diagnoses to Adult Critical Illness*. St. Louis: C.V. Mosby Co., 1988.

CHAPTER 15 — Substance and Toxicologic Emergencies

Clark, D., and Scovill, N. "Botulism: Coping with an Epidemic," *Critical Care Nurse* 7(1):49-55, January/February 1987.

Higgins, R. "Cocaine Abuse: What Every Emergency Nurse Should Know," *Journal of Emergency Nursing* 15(4):318-22, July/August 1989.

Joubert, D.W. "Use of Emetic, Adsorbent, and Cathartic Agents in Acute Drug Overdose," *Journal of Emergency Nursing* 13(1):49-51, January/February 1987.

Lanros, N.E. *Assessment and Interventions in Emergency Nursing*, 3rd ed. East Norwalk, Conn.: Appleton & Lange, 1988.

MacDonald, K., et al. "Type A Botulism from Sauteed Onions: Clinical and Epidemiological Observations," *Journal of the American Medical Association* 253(9):1275-78, March 1, 1985.

Maroncelli, R.D. "Action Stat: Accidental Poisoning," *Nursing86* 16(7):25, July 1986.

Newton, M., et al. "General Treatment of Household Poisonings," *Journal of Emergency Nursing* 13(1):12-15, January/February 1987.

Nuckols, C.C., and Greeson, J. "Cocaine Addiction: Assessment and Intervention," *Nursing Clinics of North America* 24(1):33-43, March 1989.

Ruthman, J.C., and Hendricksen, D.K. "Emergency Department Presentation of Type A Botulism," *American Journal of Emergency Medicine* 3(3):203-05, May 1985.

Sheehy, S.B., and Barber, J.M. *Emergency Nursing: Principles and Practice*, 2nd ed. St. Louis: C.V. Mosby Co., 1985.

Thurkauf, G. "Acetaminophen Overdose," *Critical Care Nurse* 7(1):20-31, January/February 1987.

CHAPTER 16 — Surface Trauma

Cardona, V., et al. *Trauma Nursing: From Resuscitation Through Rehabilitation*. Philadelphia: W.B. Saunders Co., 1988.

Dunham, C.M., and Cowley, R.A. *Shock-Trauma Critical Care Handbook.* Rockville, Md.: Aspen Pub., 1986.

Halpern, J.S. "Upper Extremity Peripheral Nerve Assessment," *Journal of Emergency Nursing* 15(3):261-65, May/June 1989.

Lanros, N.E. *Assessment and Interventions in Emergency Nursing,* 3rd ed. East Norwalk, Conn.: Appleton & Lange, 1988.

Lucas, C.E. "Answers to Questions on Crush Injury," *Hospital Medicine* 21(5):101-112, May 1985.

Sheehy, S.B., and Barber, J.M. *Emergency Nursing: Principles and Practice,* 2nd ed. St. Louis: C.V. Mosby Co., 1985.

Stroud, S.D., et al. "Chainsaw Injuries," *Journal of Emergency Nursing* 11(5):242-45, September/October 1985.

CHAPTER 17 – Professional Issues

Cardona, V., et al. *Trauma Nursing: From Resuscitation Through Rehabilitation.* Philadelphia: W.B. Saunders Co., 1988.

Creighton, H. *Law Every Nurse Should Know,* 5th ed. Philadelphia: W.B. Saunders Co., 1981.

George, J., and Quattrone, M. "The Emergency Nurse on the Witness Stand," 15(3):272-73, May/June 1989.

Rea, R., et al. *Emergency Nursing Core Curriculum,* 3rd ed. Philadelphia: W.B. Saunders Co., 1987.

Taylor, J., et al. "Emergency Nurses' Knowledge of Legal Liability," *Journal of Emergency Nursing* 14(4):225-29, July/August 1988.

CHAPTER 18 – Medical Dosage Calculations

Olsen, J.L., et al. *Medical Dosage Calculations,* 4th ed. Reading, Mass.: Addison-Wesley, 1987.

Index

A

O

Obstructive uropathy
  catheter patency in, 237
  diagnostic studies for, 238
  nephrostomy as temporary measure in, 238-239
  patient management in, 237, 238
  urinalysis findings in, 237
Oral candidiasis, 176
Oral orders, 475
Orbital floor fracture, 126
Organ donation
  candidates for, 301, 309
  consent for, 305
  contraindications for, 307-308
  discussion of, with potential donor's family, 308
Organ donor
  cause of death in, 304
  criteria for solid-organ retrieval from, 305
  extended observation of child as, 309
  goals of maintenance of, 308
  hypotension as complication in postmortem management of, 305-306
  importance of medical history of, 309
  increased urine output as indication of diabetes insipidus in, 305
  living related, 308
  methylprednisolone in, 306
  norepinephrine and epinephrine in, 307
  nursing interventions for, 308
Organ procurement agency, 308
Organ procurement coordinator, 304
Organ recipient, criteria for evaluating, 306
Organ retrieval, payment for, 307
Otitis externa, acute, 87
Otitis media, acute, 87-88
Ototoxicity, 87

P

Packed red blood cells, transfusion and, 173
Palpation, respiratory assessment and, 380-381
Pancreatitis
  causes of, 19
  as complication of perforated duodenal ulcer, 19
  dietary regimen for, 20-21
  laboratory findings in, 19
  nursing interventions for, 20
  pain relief in, 20
  pulmonary complications of, 19
  symptoms of, 20
  treatment of, 20
Paroxysmal atrial tachycardia, 59
Patient care issues, 478
Patient education
  evaluation of, 480
  as nursing responsibility, 480
Patient positioning
  in shock, 415
  in suspected lung injury, 287
Patient referral to physician, 479, 481
Patient teaching, documentation of, 477

Pelvic fracture
  catheterization in, 321
  complications of, 320
  MAST suit in, 319, 321
  patients at risk for, 320
  stabilization of, 320
  surgical management of, 319
  types of, 319
Pelvic inflammatory disease
  causative organism in, 241
  diagnosis of, 241
  discharge teaching for, 242
  potential complications of, 241
  women at risk for, 241-242
Pelvic ultrasound, preparation for, 294
Penetrating wounds
  criteria for, 17
  diagnostic procedures for, 16
  effects of blood loss in, 17
  injuries associated with, 16
  preoperative interventions for, 16-17
  removal of object from, 16
Penicillin, 72
Penile fracture, treatment of, 226-227
Pentamidine, 177
Percussion, flatness in, 380
Pericardiocentesis, 64
Pericarditis, 55
  assessment of, 71
  causes of, 72
  ECG findings in, 71
  pericardial friction rub in, 239
  signs of, 71
  treatment for, 72
Peritoneal lavage
  contraindications for, 22
  as diagnostic aid, 26
Peritonitis, chemical, 17
Phenazopyridine, 236
Phenelzine sulfate, 350
Phenytoin sodium, 58, 59, 266, 267, 268
Pink puffer, 391
Pinpoint pupils, pons lesion and, 275
Placenta previa, 288
Pneumonia
  bacterial, 395
  signs of, 364, 386
Pneumothorax
  chest tube size for, 387
  recurrence of, 376, 399
  spontaneous, 398-399
  tension, 399
Poikilothermy, 273
Postpartal hemorrhage
  assessment of, 295
  increased blood pressure and, 292
  nursing interventions for, 293
  patients at risk for, 294
  shock in, 294-295
  vaginal laceration and, 294
Postrenal acute renal failure
  diagnosis of, 229
  fluid replacement in, 230
  nursing diagnosis for, 229-230
  signs and symptoms of, 229

1990 · 2000

Nursing Magazine
In the future as in the past...

You can rely on *Nursing* magazine to keep your skills sharp and your practice current—with award-winning nursing journalism.

Each monthly issue is packed with expert advice on the legal, ethical, and personal issues in nursing, plus up-to-the-minute...

- Drug information—warnings, new uses, and approvals
- Assessment tips
- Emergency and acute care advice
- New treatments, equipment, and disease findings
- Photostories and skill sharpeners
- AIDS updates
- Career tracks and trends

SAVE 38% Enter your subscription today.

YES! Start my subscription to *Nursing* magazine. Send me 12 monthly issues for just $19.96. I save 38%.

___ Bill me ___ Payment enclosed

Name _____

Address _____ Apt. _____

City _____

State _____ Zip _____

I am an ___ RN ___ LPN ___ Other

Do you work in a hospital? ___ Yes ___No

Clip and mail to:

Springhouse Corporation
One Health Care Drive, P.O. Box 2024
Marion, OH 43305-2024

Rates outside U.S.: Canada, $27.95 (Canadian dollars); Australia, $42 (Australian dollars); New Zealand, $47 (Australian dollars); all other foreign orders, $38 (U.S. dollars). Basic rate for 12 issues in U.S. is $32.

© 1990 Springhouse Corporation   FBBB-1